Attachments: Psychiatry, Psychotherapy, Psychoanalysi

For three decades Jeremy Holmes has been a leading figure in psychodynamic psychiatry in the UK and across the world. He has played a central role in promoting the ideas of John Bowlby and in developing the clinical applications – psychiatric and psychotherapeutic – of attachment theory in working with adults. Drawing on both psychoanalytic and attachment ideas, Holmes has been able to encompass a truly biopsychosocial perspective. As a psychotherapist Holmes brings together psychodynamic, systemic and cognitive models, alert to their vital differences but also keenly sensitive to overlaps and parallels.

This volume of selected papers brings together the full range of Holmes's interests and contributions. The various sections in the book cover:

- an extended interview – covering Holmes's career and philosophy as a psychodynamic psychiatrist;
- 'juvenilia' – sibling relationships, the psychology of nuclear weapons and the psychodynamics of surgical intervention;
- psychodynamic psychiatry: integrative and attachment-informed;
- a psychotherapy section in which he develops his model of psychotherapeutic change;
- 'heroes' – biographical pieces about his major influences, including John Bowlby, Michael Balint, David Malan, Jonathan Pedder and Charles Rycroft;
- 'ephemera' – brief pieces covering such topics as frequency of psychodynamic sessions and fees.

Attachments: Psychiatry, Psychotherapy, Psychoanalysis – The selected works of Jeremy Holmes will be essential and illuminating reading for practitioners and students of psychiatry and psychotherapy in all its guises.

Jeremy Holmes worked for 35 years as a consultant psychiatrist and medical psychotherapist in the NHS. He is currently Visiting Professor at the University of Exeter, UK, and lectures nationally and internationally. Recent publications include *The Oxford Textbook of Psychotherapy*, *Storr's The Art of Psychotherapy*, *Exploring in Security: Towards an attachment-informed psychoanalytic psychotherapy* and *The Therapeutic Imagination: Using literature to deepen psychodynamic understanding*.

World Library of Mental Health series

The *World Library of Mental Health* celebrates the important contributions to mental health made by leading experts in their individual fields. Each author has compiled a career-long collection of what they consider to be their finest pieces: extracts from books, journals, articles, major theoretical and practical contributions, and salient research findings.

For the first time ever, the work of each contributor is presented in a single volume so readers can follow the themes and progress of their work and identify the contributions made to, and the development of, the fields themselves.

Each book in the series features a specially written introduction by the contributor giving an overview of his career, contextualising his selection within the development of the field and showing how his own thinking developed over time.

Rationality and Pluralism – The selected works of Windy Dryden
By Windy Dryden

The Price of Love – The selected works of Colin Murray Parkes
By Colin Murray Parkes

Attachments: Psychiatry, Psychotherapy, Psychoanalysis – The selected works of Jeremy Holmes
By Jeremy Holmes

Attachments: Psychiatry, Psychotherapy, Psychoanalysis

The selected works of Jeremy Holmes

Jeremy Holmes

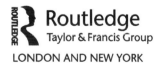

Routledge
Taylor & Francis Group

LONDON AND NEW YORK

First published 2015
by Routledge

Published 2016 by Routledge

2 Park Square, Milton Park, Abingdon, Oxon OX14 4RN

and by Routledge
711 Third Avenue, New York, NY 10017

Routledge is an imprint of the Taylor & Francis Group, an informa business

First issued in paperback 2015

British Library Cataloguing in Publication Data
A catalogue record for this book is available from the British Library

Library of Congress Cataloging in Publication Data
Catalog record for this book has been requested

ISBN: 978-0-415-64422-8 (hbk)
ISBN: 978-1-138-78286-0 (pbk)

Typeset in Sabon
by Book Now Ltd, London

To the UK National Health Service (NHS), a universal benefit, free at the point of contact, funded through general taxation, enabling sufferers – rich or poor, in sickness and health – to seek, and offer, help, expertise and succour, unencumbered by the lure and selectiveness of lucre.

CONTENTS

PREFACE

When my stalwart Routledge editor, Kate Hawes, invited me to contribute to her World Library series I was of course delighted, and gratefully accepted her offer at once – how could one not? But the experience of reviewing my work over 40 years – can it *really* be that long? – has not been entirely comfortable. For a start I seem to have been saying much the same things over and over again. My leitmotiv list runs roughly as follows: diseases, psychological and physical, arise in the context of relationships, past and current; narrative approaches must stand alongside so-called evidence-based practice if something vital in our medical culture is not to be lost; psychiatrists need to take account of unconscious as well as the more overt aspects of the mind; 'gut feelings', aka transference and countertransference, influence the doctor–patient relationship no less than its rational purposes, and need to be aired and examined; psychotherapists need Bowlby as much as Freud; psychotherapy integration is the way forward for our discipline. One might ask why it is necessary for psychodynamic psychotherapists to bang these recurring drums. Is there an inherent resistance to the uncomfortable message of the unconscious? Is the instrumentalist quick-fix zeitgeist against us? Or is it that ongoing verities need constantly to be discovered anew by each generation of practitioners? All of these possibilities, and others, are considered in the chapters which follow.

Another challenge, in trying to select pieces which show at least some traces of originality, has been to pinpoint what my specific contributions have been. Such as they are, they consist mainly of little phrases and *bons mots*: the idea of 'optional illness' as an aspect of general medicine; 'autobiographical competence' as a mark of psychological maturity; contrasting strategies for therapists depending on their patients' attachment styles as 'story-making' (ambivalent attachment) or 'story-breaking' (avoidant ditto); mentalising as the ability to 'see oneself from the outside and others from the inside'; and finding a 'vantage point' from which to view feelings and relationships as a therapy goal. Stepansky's (2009) answer to the decline of psychoanalysis is a wistful advocacy of 'optional marginalisation', a distinct if necessarily adjunct role in the medical pantheon. Discussing his book at a seminar at the Anna Freud Centre, a colleague pointed out that Holmes appears as a footnote in Stepansky's analysis. Perhaps my overall contribution could be described as a 'footnote to a footnote to footnote'!

Even that is perhaps preferable to total obscurity. But, more seriously, lest all this self-deprecation be deemed no more than inverted narcissism, these reflections have usefully served to remind me that I am not primarily a theoretician, a system-builder, a researcher even, and certainly no guru. I remain a clinician psychotherapist with minor academic leanings. My 'contribution', such as it is, flows, therefore, from the skills and purposes of psychodynamic practice. These I group under four headings, each of which goes some way to explain what I have been doing – and not doing – in the writings collected herein and elsewhere.

First, there is the therapeutic 'stance' itself, the so-called analytic attitude: a knight's move position; fluid, orthogonal to action; looking from the aforementioned vantage point (safe, yet blessed with vision) at roles and assumptions; commenting; refusing to be pinned down, pigeonholed or categorised; in search of what cannot being said, or maybe even thought. This necessary indeterminacy cascades down through the roles. Despite Freud's attempt to compare psychoanalysis with surgery, as a psychiatrist one cannot, in my view thankfully, without some sleight of hand be a 'proper doctor', a diagnoser and a curer of illness. One is always primarily a wounded healer, face to face with the sufferings of the other, trying to understand and transcend them in the context of an evolving life-story. Similarly, as a psychotherapist one does not fully embrace the mores and habits of psychiatry – always interested more in the therapeutic relationship and its meanings than, as a colleague mock-ironically used to put it, in 'stamping out mental illness'. Perhaps controversially, I believe the same stricture applies to one's role as a psychotherapist. While psychoanalytic theories are embraced by some as absolute truths, I prefer to see them as provisional heuristics, to be viewed with a degree of affirming scepticism.

Perhaps, then, I'm not a 'proper' therapist either, conceiving psychodynamic ideas as intrinsically elusive, tentative, subject to endless 'vision and revision'. But how does one decide whether an idea is true and valid or self-deceiving or irrelevant? Here I rely on two separate realms of truth-checking. A theory is plausible if it meets the normal standards of science: replicability, falsifiability, generalisability, compatibility with the wider scientific edifice. One of the great attractions of attachment theory is that, unlike some species of psychoanalysis, it fits happily into this world of mainstream scientific discourse. Alongside this there exists an entirely different approach, relying on the therapist's subjective, affective, 'counter-transferential' responses to the patient and the meanings these generate. Here an idea is true if, and only if, it 'feels right'. The negotiation is not with the verdict of reality, which is how conventional science works, but with the interpersonal field between therapist and patient, their engagement and dialogue, and whether, in the end, a 'fusion of horizons' can be arrived at (see chapter 15).

For those who need constantly to refer back to psychoanalysis' founding father, this dichotomy corresponds fairly closely with Freud's delineation of the secondary and primary processes. A valid psychodynamic epistemology requires, in my view, constant interchange between the scientific and humanistic poles. The scientific findings of psychotherapy research, neuro-psychoanalysis and, indeed, attachment theory need to be checked for their relevance to the interpersonal realities of the therapist–patient encounter. Equally, the affective ambiance of the therapeutic relationship impels scientific scrutiny via audio or video recording of sessions, qualitative studies and discourse analysis, combining physiological and meaning-focused methodologies.

A second relevant aspect is the therapist's 'maieutic' or midwife role, helping patients to give birth to self-understanding or, occasionally, to a 'new self', albeit one that will essentially be a more self-possessed, confident, mature, tolerant, open-minded, robust version of the old one. Much of my work has been in a comparable maieutic position vis-à-vis the concepts and contributions of my heroes (see Part V), mentors, friends and colleagues – Freud of course, Balint,

Bowlby, Rycroft, Ryle, Pedder, Bateman, Fonagy and Target, among others. My role model here is Huxley, Darwin's 'bulldog'. I have tried to champion attachment theory in the world of psychoanalysis and psychoanalysis among psychiatrists, and to persuade both doctors that, to use the College of Psychiatrists' slogan, there can be no health without mental health and fellow psychiatrists that there can be no mental health with psychodynamic understanding.

A third aspect is the use of language. Therapists, whether 'oracular' (Fink, 1997) or dialogic in style, need to be a good communicators, using simple, direct, context-appropriate, un-pompous, jargon-free, succinct language in which to express their questions, comments, clarifications, confrontations and interpretations. 'Moments of meeting' (Lyons-Ruth, 1999) may be silent or primarily non-verbal, but in the end it is the *logos* that emerges from reverie (Holmes, 2013) that matters, so perhaps those scraps of phrases do have an enduring value. I strive to write in a transparent, unembellished way that puts psychodynamic ideas across without hiding behind obscurantism, flag-waving or reverential psycho-scripture. To the extent that has succeeded – and of course it often doesn't – this represents perhaps my main contribution to the field.

Finally, one might point to the role of the psychodynamic clinician in bringing the past to life in the present. In Freud's much quoted remark on the value of transference: 'For when all is said and done, it is impossible to destroy anyone *in absentia* or *in effegie*' (a typical Freudian linguistic trope – from plain-man 'all is said and done', then segueing seamlessly into Latin). From this perspective, psychoanalysis is unashamedly *un*-original; there is nothing new under the (s)un-conscious. Much of my work, especially in my biography of Bowlby, has been to bring to light the contemporary relevance of past ideas and to show their continuing influence, even if recast in new language.

I end this introduction on a practical note, outlining the principles on which this volume has been compiled. I have divided the papers into six self-explanatory sections, each of which is preceded by a brief introduction. My work is made up of four main strands: attachment theory; the connections between literature and psychoanalysis; integrative approaches to psychodynamic psychiatry; plus a minor interest in psychotherapeutic philosophy and ethics (Holmes & Lindley, 1997). The first is covered in my five attachment books (Holmes, 1993/2013, 1997; 2001; 2010; Slade & Holmes, 2013). The sister volume to this one, *The therapeutic imagination: using literature to deepen psychodynamic understanding and enhance empathy* (Holmes, 2013), brings together my main papers on literature and therapy. The focus here, therefore, is on psychodynamic psychiatry, as well as tracking a quasi-biographical pathway through my professional life. I have chosen papers and chapters in journals or multi-author collections which might have escaped the notice of the average reader, previously uncollected, but which nevertheless seem apt expositions of my overall position and philosophy, in theory and in practice. I hope, at the very least, the reader will enjoy them, and that someone, somewhere, may be inspired to carry forward the sometimes guttering flame of psychodynamic psychiatry into the new era of relational neuroscience (see chapters 7 and 10) that I see as the paradigmatic future for our discipline.

ACKNOWLEDGEMENTS

Chapter 1 was originally published in *From id to intersubjectivity: talking about the talking cure with master clinicians*, by Dianna T. Kenny (published by Karnac Books in 2013), and is reprinted with kind permission of Karnac Books.

Chapter 2 was originally published in the *British Journal of Psychiatry* (2001), 179: 468–71, and is reprinted here by permission.

Chapter 5 was originally published as 'The psychology of nuclear disarmament' in the *Psychiatric Bulletin* (1982), 6: 136–8, and is reprinted here by permission.

Chapter 11 was originally published as 'Family and individual therapy: comparisons and contrasts' in the *British Journal of Psychiatry* (1985), 147: 668–77, and is reprinted here by permission.

Chapter 12 was originally published as 'Psychoanalysis and CBT' in Del Loewenthal and Richard House (eds), *Critically Engaging CBT*, © 2010. Reproduced with the kind permission of Open University Press. All rights reserved.

Chapter 14 was originally published in the *International Journal of Psychoanalysis*, Volume 92, Issue 5, October 2011 (pp. 1221–40), and is reprinted here by permission.

Chapter 16 was originally published as 'John Bowlby's "trilogy"' (2013) in the *British Journal of Psychiatry*, 202: 371, and is reprinted here by permission.

Chapter 20 was originally published as 'John Pedder' (2010) in *The Psychiatrist*, 34: 358, and is reprinted here by permission.

Chapter 21 was originally published in *Analyst of the imagination: the life and work of Charles Rycroft*, ed. Jenny Pearson (published by Karnac Books in 2004), as 'Charles Rycroft's contribution to contemporary psychoanalytic psychotherapy', and is reprinted with kind permission of Karnac Books.

PART I

AUTOBIOGRAPHICAL

Dianna Kenny and I have never met, yet, in the spirit of the age, we have had several in-depth transcontinental conversations via the internet. Professor Kenny and her publishers have kindly allowed me to include an extract from her book *From id to intersubjectivity: Talking about the talking cure with master clinicians* (London: Karnac Books, 2013), which enables me to set the scene for the rest of this volume and gives the reader some idea of my background, education, and development as a psychiatrist, attachment enthusiast and psychotherapist. 'Ten books' is a regular series in the *British Journal of Psychiatry* in which psycho-therapists of differing persuasions are invited to reflect, *Desert Island Disc*-style, on the reading that has shaped their thinking.

CHAPTER 1

INTERVIEW WITH DIANNA KENNY

DK: Let's start by your telling me about the personal and/or professional experiences that directed you into the profession of psychoanalysis and, in particular, attachment-informed psychoanalysis?

JH: I am the oldest of three, with two younger sisters. I sometimes describe myself as culturally Christian, intellectually atheist, ethically Buddhist, and ethnically Jewish – our mother was a secular Jew and Freud's *Introductory lectures* was sitting on our parents' bookshelf. Our father was an actor, newsreader and poet; we had a liberal upper-middle-class London upbringing with rural overtones – my father had grown up on a farm. There were no scientists in the family, although there was a great-aunt who was a doctor – quite something for a girl in the 1920s. The family culture was in humanities and arts, but I was fascinated with physics, cosmology and biology, and my career ambition was to become a research scientist. Once I got to Cambridge I realised that I would never make a real scientist and, more to the point, that I needed to earn my living. This, together with vague adolescent aspirations to alleviate Third World suffering, and thinking that another three years as student would not come amiss, I decided to train as a doctor.

This was the heyday of R. D. Laing. His associate David Cooper came to Cambridge and gave a lecture; we all crammed in to hear him. I can't remember a word he said. Until that moment, as an 'infantile leftist', I wanted to change the world. Cooper's message was: you can't change the world; you can only change yourself. That was the moment I decided to do medicine and then psychiatry. My clinical years were at University College London. We had some wonderful lecturers – Michael Balint and Heinz Wolf, who were very charismatic, especially for medical students. I learned from them that psychiatry can be humane and psychodynamic. For a while, however, I was diverted out of psychiatry and became a physician, with a particular interest in psychosomatics. After that I started psychiatry training and gravitated naturally to the psychodynamic end of psychiatry (the science/arts divide is ubiquitous, like left and right in politics). I also then went into analysis myself. I needed help. Charles Rycroft was my analyst. Despite retrospective reservations about Charles clinically (he was far too 'supportive' and didn't seem to understand transference), I see myself as within his tradition. I am highly sceptical of psychoanalytic fundamentalists. But John Bowlby was my intellectual father; I revere Bowlby – he is a giant. He brought a humane yet scientific approach to the mind, as opposed to dogma and doctrine. In terms of my own development, I suppose I identify to some extent with Bowlby, although he came from a much 'posher' background than I did – we both had war-torn childhoods. Bowlby was a bit avoidant, as was I. Both our fathers were absent during crucial years. Charles Rycroft's father died when Rycroft was 11 – so there's some sort of 'paternal deprivation' story there. Attachment theory felt like a natural home to me – it's a marriage of psychoanalysis and evolutionary biology and ethology. Jung said that psychological theories are a disguised form of autobiography. Unconscious forces influence our conscious thoughts – we need to understand imaginative leaps in great scientists in the light of their developmental history, as Bowlby did in his last great work, the Darwin biography.

DK: **How do you identify yourself?**

JH: As a medical doctor, a psychiatrist and a psychoanalytic psychotherapist. I am not a member of the International Psychoanalytic Association (IPA) because I have not trained as a psychoanalyst. I side-stepped this form of control and this hierarchy – but of course also missed out on the cross-fertilisation and camaraderie and evaded the necessary submission to the yoke of authority. I was, naturally, influenced by Rycroft, who eventually left the IPA, and Bowlby, who remained a member of the IPA but was *persona non grata* for many years within the British society. I am also a maverick. Maverick was a cattle rancher. Cattle ranchers branded their cattle to prove ownership, but Maverick refused to brand his – a humane move, but it meant they got muddled up with everyone else's! I am a natural integrative psychotherapist. I have been influenced by a range of therapies, including CBT, psychodrama and family therapy; I am totally anti-branding.

DK: **Could you say something more about how you define psychoanalysis and the nature of the relationship between analyst and patient?**

JH: My basic model of the analytic relationship is the parent–child relationship – securely attached children have a different developmental history compared with insecurely attached children. Maternal sensitivity correlates with security. But there is a 'transmission gap' – the term 'sensitivity' is vague: what is it that makes mothers sensitive? There is a similar issue with defining the therapist–patient relationship. We know that therapy 'works' but not what it is that produces change – is it therapist sensitivity? If so, what are its components? This is still an empirical question.

Beebe (Beebe *et al.*, 2012) is very interested in facial gestures between mothers and infants. One of her studies looked also at vocal communication. She got mums to sing along with their babies and recorded the melodic relationship between mothers' and infants' vocalisations. When the children reached one year of age, she classified their attachment using the Strange Situation. Mothers fell into three categories: one group was tone deaf; the second group sang in unison with their infants; and the third group sang in a more harmonic and jazzy way. The infants of these mothers were more likely to be secure than the infants of either of the other two groups of mothers. This was a lovely empirical demonstration of what I call partially contingent mirroring. 'Photographic mirroring' is not sufficient; partially contingent mirroring seems to be one of the things that therapists do with their patients. They mirror, and then take them a step further.

DK: **Is there a meaningful distinction between psychoanalysis and psychodynamic psychotherapy?**

JH: There is no absolute distinction between these terms; they are terms of convenience, of politics. Timing/frequency has little to do with the definition of how 'analytic' a therapy is. The discrepancy between what people say they do and what they actually do is one of my hobby-horses. Nothing extraordinary will happen just because someone is having a therapy five days a week. All frequencies of therapy will involve transference and counter-transference and defences if the therapist is working from a psychoanalytic perspective.

The main power of therapy can't be fully defined in terms of specific elements. Change comes as much from the 'non-specific' aspects, especially from the therapeutic relationship. There is an established relationship between good outcomes and length of treatment, but the theoretical position is not so important. The skill of the therapist is a better contributor to outcome than the type of therapy practised. We also know that, the longer a therapy goes on, the less theoretically driven it becomes. The quality and character of that relationship is a feature of those two individuals, so each long-term psychoanalytic dyad has its own character. As a therapy goes on, so the 'third' takes over and is a manifestation of the joint projects and personalities of analyst and patient.

DK: What aspects of classical Freudian analysis remain in attachment-informed psychotherapy?

JH: In the classical paradigm, defences are forms of affect regulation. In the attachment paradigm, the purpose of defences is also affective regulation, but, in addition, they are ways of maintaining contact with an object in suboptimal environments. It is the type and quality of interpersonal contact that creates the defence. In the classical psychoanalytic model, defence mechanisms are located within the individual. In the attachment relational model, they are essentially interpersonal. I am interested in the way in which the care-giver helps the infant cope with his overwhelming affect of fear or hunger or feeling of abandonment – and, indeed, excitement – and how this interpersonal field is translated into the consulting room, where there is a reworking of the handling of affect. That can be done 'defensively', where affect is suppressed, as in the deactivating strategy. In a secure-making relationship, the affect can be dealt with in manageable small amounts through the presence of a sensitive care-giver. I think there is a radical difference there. The role of the analyst isn't just to interpret the defence mechanisms; it is to rework the defence mechanisms while at the same time commenting on them. That, I think, is the essence and the skill and the difficulty and the excitement and the frustration of psychoanalytic work. One is simultaneously engaging with the patient and helping the patient to find a vantage point from which they can observe this relationship.

My latest idea is that there is this five-stage model that I think applies to all intimate relationships.

Stage one is what I call the *primary attachment relationship*. A lot of the attachment literature focuses on the care-seeker, on the child and the infant, and how stress and threat and illness activate the attachment dynamic and then a secure base is sought. But there is a parallel process in the care-giver. When we are presented with distress, we are biologically programmed to respond to that distress, whether it be a small animal, a stranger who is injured, or one of our loved ones – children, spouses, partners, pets, or even our plants – that needs attention. I live in a rural area; there are sheep and lambs there. When the ewes see me coming, they immediately call their infants, their baby lambs, to come them because they see a potential threat. There is this reciprocal biological relationship. In Stage one, we as therapists respond to distress; and what do you do when you respond to distress? You set your own preoccupations to one side. You immerse yourself in the vulnerability of the care-seeker. From an attachment perspective, Bowlby saw this in terms of what he calls the environment of evolutionary adaptation. Infants are not going to survive in the primitive savannah unless adults are highly protective of them. This primary attachment relationship is a little bit like Winnicott's notion of primary maternal preoccupation, which is unconscious, not in the classical psychoanalytic sense, but in the sense that it is biologically programmed.

Stage two is what I call *reverie*. Now you allow yourself to enter empathically into the inner world of the patient, so you can, to use Thomas Ogden's phrase, dream your patient. You experience your patient inside yourself. We are beginning to understand the neurobiological aspect, including mirror neurons. Something is triggered off in us by our patient's distress which enables us imaginatively to put ourselves in the patient's shoes.

Stage three I call *logos*, and this is related to interpretation. The empathic resonance of stages one and two is only part of the story because it has to be turned into a shared meaning between patient and therapist, which they can then use. You are giving this logos, this interpretation, this comment, to the patient, but you must be in empathic resonance with her also in order to help with that patient's affect regulation. The great thing about the consulting room is it doesn't matter what you say because it's a hypothetical situation; you can do things there that you wouldn't perhaps be able to do in real life.

Stage 4 is what I call *action* or decision or consequence. This flows from the therapeutic relationship in terms of change in the person's life but also from the arrangements of therapy, how long to go on, when to terminate, etc.

Finally, Stage 5 is *reflection*. You loop back and look at the whole process, finding a vantage point from which to view what happened, what went right, what didn't, and so on.

DK: Let's go back to the interpersonal, attachment models of defences.

JH: They are certainly interpersonal at the start. Let's say you are a six- or nine-month-old child and you have a stressed mother. She may be stressed socio-economically, she may be wondering where she is going to get her next meal from or how she can pay the mortgage, she may be having marital conflict, she may not have a partner. But you are an infant and you need your mother's protection because, as Winnicott says, there is no such thing as a baby. An infant without her parent or protector will die. You become distressed; if you express too much affect, your mother, rather than being able to help you with that and soothe you, may push you away. It may be too much for her. So you learn a defence mechanism – let's say deactivation. You close down your feelings. That way your mother will protect you but you pay a price: you are not so much in touch with your feelings; your affective universe is diminished, your pleasure in life may be diminished; your flexibility is compromised. There are trade-offs in all aspects of psychological life. Here the trade-off is that security takes precedence over affective expression. That's looking at a defence mechanism from an interpersonal perspective. There are continuities between defensive and interpersonal patterns in early childhood and adult life, which is quite remarkable and just what Freud predicted. The child I have just described may grow into an adult who is 'dismissive', as measured in the adult attachment literature – someone who needs relationship but, when in a relationship, is unable to express themselves fully; they are unable to respond to their partner's emotional needs or they expect their partner to be responsive to their emotional needs. They will be relationally compromised, handicapped even. If that person then comes into therapy, that relationship will be reproduced in the therapy situation. The patient will present a rather affectless account of their life. If therapy is successful, therapy provides a setting in which it gradually becomes more and more safe to express the affect which they suppress, and that enables a reworking of the defensive structures and perhaps possibly a move to more mature defensiveness. They may be able to make a joke about their feelings, which is better than not expressing feelings at all. That would be a move from repression to suppression to using a mature defence such as humour. That is an attachment perspective on the psychotherapeutic task.

One of the crucial growth points currently in this way of looking at things is the concept of disorganised attachment and the relationship between disorganised attachment and psychopathology. Disorganised attachment is relatively uncommon in non-clinical populations but very common in psychopathology. Where you have highly stressed care-givers, where children present to clinics, where there is a history of physical or sexual abuse in the family, then disorganised attachment is very prevalent. Splitting, dissociation and role reversal are the common defences, whereby you project your own vulnerability onto another person and look after it 'over there' rather than in yourself. Those are typical patterns you see in disorganised attachment, and they are highly relevant to one of the big issues for psychoanalytical psychotherapy, Borderline Personality Disorder, and the kinds of therapeutic strategies that are going to be helpful with such people.

DK: Can you say something about 'mentalising', a term that is much used in the attachment-informed therapeutic literature these days.

JH: The word 'mentalising' comes from the francophone literature and was introduced into English by Peter Fonagy in the late 1980s. That flowed directly from Mary Main's notion of 'meta-cognitive monitoring'. What goes on in the consulting room is a way of fostering the client's capacity to mentalise. I mentioned the metaphor of a vantage point. Therapy, the consulting room, provides a vantage point from which a person can begin to look at themselves, especially themselves in relationship. Therapy is a relationship that can also look at itself. Therapist and patient together look at themselves in action, and this process fosters the capacity for mentalising. Borderline Personality Disorder is a disorder of affect regulation in the sense that the borderline person very quickly becomes affectively aroused – 'I have had enough of this, I'm off' – and they storm out of the session. I heard a lovely example in a supervision session recently where the patient looked at the therapist's bookshelf and said, 'I am going to pick all those books up and throw them across the room', and the therapist, who in a previous life had been a school-teacher, said, in a very 'school-marmy' voice, 'You most certainly will *not*.'

Now, that would actually be a very good example of the kind of thing that Allen (Allen, 2013a) writes about, because one of the features of mentalising is that you can't think unless you feel safe. Arousal drives out mentalising. I usually say, if you are just about to be eaten by a lion, you don't sit there and say, 'Now, what is going on in the mind of that lion? What's going on in my own mind?' You just get the hell out! The problem that a lot of borderline patients have is that they so easily become aroused but they are unable to think about thinking. That's the essence of mentalising, being able to think about your feelings – the 'knowledge of the heart', as George Eliot calls it. When that therapist said, 'You most certainly will not', although that sounds about as unpsychoanalytic as you could get, she was actually saying, 'We are not going to be able to work together unless this is a safe space, and I am going to make sure this space *is* safe.' Without that security, there can be no mentalising. The basis of the attachment paradigm is what I say in the title of my book *Exploring in security* (Holmes, 2010). You cannot explore, you cannot think, you cannot play unless you feel safe. In therapy there is always an oscillation between dealing with arousal and stress and fear and helping that to be assuaged, and then beginning to think about what is going on. There is the constant dialectic between the affect and thinking about the affect; gradually the capacity to mentalise, to monitor oneself, to think about oneself becomes internalised. That's possibly one reason why effective therapy takes time, because that is a complex skill to learn. Malcolm Gladwell (2008) makes the point that no leading musician, no leading sportsman, no leading thinker has ever got there without putting in 10,000 hours of practice. Learning the skill of mentalising may not need 10,000 hours of analysis, but it needs quite a few hundred! That's possibly what Freud was intuitively getting at when he coined the phrase 'working through'.

DK: **It brings to mind Barbra Streisand, who forgot the words to one of her songs in a concert in Central Park in 1967, and who subsequently gave up public performances for 27 years. In her comeback concert in 1994 in Madison Square Garden she came out on stage and said, 'The only reason I am standing here before you is my $350,000 worth of psychoanalysis.'**

JH: That's really interesting … obviously very relevant to performance anxiety, which I know you are an expert on (Kenny, 2011). I have a counter-example to that story about the famous British actor Laurence Olivier. My father was an actor, so I heard this sort of in-joke. Olivier was playing Hamlet, and he was in the middle of one of the most famous speeches ever – 'O, what a rogue and peasant slave am I!' But he suddenly 'dried': he couldn't remember a single word of the speech, so he simply started reciting the London Underground Tube names, but in Shakespearean rhythm: 'Charing Cross, Waterloo, Paddington …', saying them in a very theatrical voice, and of course the audience didn't even notice, and especially with Shakespeare where you only understand about a half of it if you are lucky anyway, and then finally he got back on track. This is an example of someone who had a tremendous amount of self-confidence that would carry him through. It's put me in mind of a really important issue: rupture and repair.

One of the features of secure relationships is a good rupture/repair mechanism, because the fact is that parents are out of tune with their infants a lot of the time. The same is true of couples, of romantic relationships, where the partners are out of sync with each other quite a lot of the time. But in secure relationships that get out of sync, you cycle into repair mode. The child whose mother is thinking about something else or is worried about paying the bills or has gone off to the loo or something – the child then expresses distress and the mother immediately responds and re-establishes some contact with the child. So there is Laurence Olivier who has a major rupture but also confidence; he has the trust, he knows that his memory will be there for him when he needs it, just like he knew possibly that his care-giver would be there for him when he needed her. Maybe Barbra Streisand took $350,000 worth of psychoanalysis to acquire that sense that there would be somebody there for her when she was in distress. Psychoanalysis may have an idealised theory of what help is, so that, when you have had your psychoanalysis, you can sail through life with no problems at all, which is of course nonsense; we all face problems and some of them are of our own making. One hopes that there will be fewer of our own making after we have had psychoanalysis, but nevertheless some will be of our own making and some will be things over which we have no control whatsoever. We are all going to die; having loved ones means we are 'hostages to fortune', as Francis Bacon put it. Psychoanalysis equips us with the capacity to cope with loss and stress and difficulty rather than moving us into some idealised world in which none of that ever happens. I think it has to do with the scaffolding, the architecture, of the therapeutic relationship and the parallel between that and the parent–child relationship.

DK: **You wrote a paper in which you said that the superego is concerned as much with safety as with sex and that it is 'heir' to the attachment relationship. I wonder if you could comment.**

JH: Well, this is the heretical thing where I don't see eye to eye with my psychoanalytic colleagues. I don't believe in infantile sexuality; I think it's a myth. That's not to say, of course, that infantile *sens*uality is not hugely important. Of course, the body of an infant and the body of a mother and a father are drawn to each other like magnets, and the child seeks warmth and physical protection from her care-givers. When the child is at the breast the child is not just having some feeding experience, because we know that infants go on sucking at the breast long after their need for milk has been satisfied. The whole mouth is drawn to the breast and presumably achieves or receives sensual satisfaction. If you want to call that sexuality, fine, but I don't – in fact I think that's a projection of adult meanings onto infants and is a kind of intellectual mis-attunement, which goes back to Freud. Similarly, of course, there are sexual issues between parents and children – there is no question about that. Little boys have erections. Little girls may have sexual feelings that we can we detect and record, and similarly of course some women, when breast feeding, experience some sexual feelings. Fathers can get erections from time to time when their children are on their knee, and I don't think that's necessarily an abusive situation. So I am not denying that sex is totally absent in the parenting relationship, but I don't see it as central or primary, and I think Freud was just plain wrong, and his successors just use flimsy and convoluted arguments to try to stay true to their founder, even though the wrongness of it is staring them in the face. And I think the reason for his being wrong was because he wanted a coherent theory. Since his theory is based around libido and he sees libido as a form of sexuality, then he has to have infantile sexuality. That leads on to the Oedipus complex. I want to rewrite the Oedipus complex in attachment terms, to look at it from an evolutionary perspective – that is, a child's need for the parent is not the same as the parent's need for the child.

Here I have been influenced by the anthropologist Sarah Hrdy (1999). She has studied infanticide; parents sometimes kill their children. This happens in non-human mammals too. The child has a paramount need for its parent, but the parent's need for the child is mitigated because they may also have other children; they have a partner by whom they can generate more children. Attachment theory is essentially an evolutionary theory and, although Freud was Darwinian, it was not in the same way that Bowlby was. I see the Oedipus complex in terms of the conflict between the child's absolute need for the mother and the mother's need to balance her love for the child, her protection of that child, with a love for her other children and her love for her partner. Freud argued that the little boy had sexual feelings for his mother and saw the father as a sexual rival. I see it much more in terms of an evolutionary or genetic rivalry. A superego in classical psychoanalytic terms is an internal representation of Oedipal prohibition. It constitutes the father saying to the child, 'No, that woman, your mother, my wife, belongs to me.' So the child suppresses his sexual needs and his sexual feelings under the influence of the superego. Well, I am trying to rewrite the superego in attachment terms, and in my view this prohibition is essentially a way of protecting the child so that a mother who says to the toddler, 'No,' when the child goes towards an electric light socket is installing in the child a superego, a prohibitive superego that keeps that child safe. That's the basic idea. But there is a difference between a benign superego and a harsh punitive superego, because we all have to learn to take risks. Our primitive superego says, 'No, don't do this, don't do that', but in order to develop and progress we need to feel enough security in ourselves to say, 'Well, I know this is a risk. I know if I kiss this girl I may be rejected.' Or 'I know if I do a bungee jump off this bridge I may die. But in order to enlarge my sense of self, in order to explore the world fully, I am going to have to do things that feel a bit risky. I have got to feel sufficiently secure inside myself to be able to undertake this task.' So, on the basis of secure attachment, we can begin to take risks, whether these are sexual risks or risks in a wider sense. I don't think it is a particularly successful paper; I think it fell on deaf ears.

Another aspect is the theory of therapeutic action. A person comes into therapy with a whole set of defences. If the therapist provides sufficient safety, the patient moves to a less defended position. My metaphor for this is the kangaroo's joey: as I understand the biology, you have got this little tiny little creature that emerges from the womb and then has to climb up the mother's belly to get into the pouch for further development to take place. Now, that's a very scary thing to think about because that joey is incredibly vulnerable at that moment of climbing. In therapy the patient has to become incredibly vulnerable before the developmental process can resume. What one is doing in therapy is simultaneously giving a message to the patient that it is safe, that the therapist is going to look after them, he is not going to push them further than they can tolerate, but at the same time will not collude, but will challenge and create a different relational environment from what they expect and have had instilled in them through their developmental experience. So, therapy is all the time playing with challenge and security.

DK: You have written that the therapeutic situation is a place where the therapist creates maximum security but, at the same time, also maximum uncertainty.

JH: Yes, I really believe that. It is a very simple point, but when you go to see a therapist you absolutely need to know that that person is reliable; they are as good as their word. If they say they will see you next week at 10 o'clock, they will see you at 10 o'clock. You also need to know that this person isn't going to exploit you sexually, financially or through gossip, i.e. in terms of confidentiality. That space, that hour that you are offered, is inviolable; people aren't going to intrude on it because it is going to be quiet and comfortable. This creates conditions of security. Then the patient comes in and essentially the therapist doesn't say very much. Now, in other forms of therapy, such as CBT, the therapist directs the patient, the therapist takes control of the session, the therapist continues to be reassuring, whereas in psychoanalytic work one is really rather unreassuring. One might not even say anything when the patient comes in – I sometimes just make a gesture to indicate 'The floor is yours' or 'Where do you want to start?' or 'Tell me the story.' That's pretty scary. Silence can be very persecutory if it goes on too long. But there must be a reticence: the therapist holds back and creates a space into which, with luck, the patient will be able to express herself, feel safe enough to take a risk. It's quite risky talking about yourself, and the more you trust your therapist the more likely you are to be able to take that risk. It's really a simple point, this idea of maximum security and maximum uncertainty.

DK: **Simple, yet also paradoxical and profound.**

JH: Yes … the patient says, 'Well, what am I supposed to talk about?' or, 'Ask me some questions', and I would probably say, 'Well, what kinds of questions you would like me to ask you?', or something like that, pushing it back.

DK: **If the patient then tells you what questions to ask, what happens then?**

JH: Yeah. Well, let's imagine a patient comes in and I say, 'The floor is yours', and the patient says, 'I don't know what to talk about. Please give me some guidance here.' So I might say, 'Well, what kind of guidance are you looking for?' And the patient might say, 'Well, I don't know where to start. Should I talk about my childhood? Should I talk about what's going on now?' I really believe in a light touch in therapy, not exactly making jokes all the time, not a Woody Allen situation – but just playing. Winnicott said psychoanalysis is learning to play, so you are playing. If it's the first session I might say, 'Okay, let's hear a story which has led up to your coming to see me and sitting in this room on this particular day, and maybe that will give us a clue as to where we want to go next.' When you are up against so much anxiety, the first thing is to lower that anxiety so you can begin to do some work. If I felt the patient was so panicky that their mind had gone blank, I would definitely make some semi-helpful remark. So, again, it's all the time the balance between security and exploration. If there is a paramount need for security, if the attachment system is activated, no exploration is possible. If I feel a person is just so anxious that they are in a state of attachment panic, then that has to be dealt with. I might say, 'It sounds like you are feeling really, really panicky. Perhaps you are wishing you had never come here in the first place', so we might focus on that. I tune into the affect – that's what I call the reverie – I am feeling the patient's anxiety, and then I am giving a *logos*, I am trying to give a name to it, and then assess whether the patient picks up on that *logos*. I feel that psychoanalytic theory is so far removed from this kind of issue, and this is really where I feel we need to focus our attention and where we need theoretical models. That's where the attachment paradigm provides such a good context for that because it's a) really interested in the minutiae of relationships and b) has this experimental empirical culture, where you are saying, 'Well we don't really understand this. What kinds of exploration would help us to understand it better?'

DK: You said in your book *Exploring in security* that co-constructed meanings are the only therapeutic truths. This statement is almost an aphoristic way of summarising what you have just been saying. It seems to be that, in using the phrase 'fusion of horizons', you are talking about co-constructed meaning.

JH: Yes. It takes us back to Tom Ogden and the 'psychoanalytic third' and the fact that, in the end, you are working together with somebody to try to create something that makes sense to both of you; it's a joint project. Another metaphor that I rather like comes from Donnel Stern (1997, 2010), a relational theorist. Stern is interested in Hans-Georg Gadamer, a Heideggerian philosopher. Gadamer proposed the concept 'fusion of horizons'. He says that all truths are conversational truths. The patient comes in with his world-view, the therapist comes in with her world-view, and then they have a conversation and attempt to achieve a fusion of horizons in the sense that they are then both looking at the same thing in a way that satisfies both of them.

DK: I would like to move on to a discussion of some of the key elements in the psychoanalytic approach and get a response from you on some of the issues, for example, the use the couch.

JH: To some extent the couch is a bit like the QWERTY keyboard. We are stuck with the QWERTY keyboard because the early typewriters used to jam up if they put the letters in more logical order. From a logical point of view there is no particular reason why we should use the QWERTY keyboard, because we all use electronic keyboards now, but we are just stuck with it. It goes back to hypnosis, and Freud's pre-psychoanalytic hypnotic arrangements, and we are all heirs to Freud, so we use the couch. There is nothing wrong with the QWERTY keyboard; we are all used to it and we all use it. I personally don't feel that one necessarily needs to confine the use of the couch to the more frequent – three times or five times a week – analyses. Some of my once-weekly patients use the couch. We need to consider the benefits or otherwise of the couch. I think there are huge advantages. There is a sense in which you are held, you are lying down, you can dream more easily, daydream, you can pursue your unconscious more easily. Tom Ogden says there is something about sitting behind patients and not having to interact with them in a facial way that enables the analyst to dream their patient and more easily pursue their own counter-transference. Empathic responses perhaps follow more easily. So using the couch can foster the psychoanalytic process. But there are disadvantages too. A patient who has been dropped affectively or emotionally as a child or who has been insufficiently 'held' may need the reassurance of actually seeing a responsive analyst/therapist in front of them – to feel that they have got someone who is really attuned and responding in a minute-to-minute way via facial contact. Another downside to the use of the couch is that it may foster dependency and regression that doesn't actually lead anywhere, so one needs to be aware of that. I refuse to be pinned down by the concrete, that's why I don't think psychoanalysis can be equated at all to the use of the couch or to sessions five times a week. The essence of the psychoanalytic approach is that it is an exploratory culture as opposed to a supportive culture. There are various aspects of the couch which foster that exploration, but at times they may be inimical to it as well. In my practice I use a mixture of lying down and sitting up, as indeed I experienced myself as a patient. So that's my 'position' – sometimes 'up', sometimes 'down'!

The important thing is the meaning. I have a patient whom I thought would be suitable for the couch and she said, 'No way, I can barely get into the room, let alone lie down.' That's the state we are still at, but it's possible that in a few months, or even years, she will feel safe enough to get onto the couch. There are other patients whom I feel possibly get onto the couch a bit too readily because they are slotting into a preconceived psychoanalytic model without actually looking at what the meaning of it might be. If a patient has been on the couch and then suddenly decides to say, 'I don't want to be on the couch anymore, I want to sit up', that is neither good nor bad; it's something to be explored. Maybe they don't really trust the analyst or they are terrified of what they might find if they really regress. Or they feel they have had enough, they need to move on, they want to have a fair fight with the analyst and get into some aggressive competitiveness that is really not so easy when you are lying down and the other person is sitting up. There are 101 different issues to canvass about the couch. It's what we do, what we feel comfortable with, that's how we have been analysed, that's the culture. This is one of the paradoxes that I still struggle with, which is this idea that I am an integrative, maverick therapist but I also have a mother tongue. Esperanto and a general language do not really work. Everyone speaks his own language, whether it's English or Chinese or Italian or Dutch. In order to express yourself fully, you have to be absolutely conversant with the particular, to use Hobson's (1985) phrase (which he got from Coleridge), the 'minute particulars'; you have to be absolutely conversant with your own particular language. And for most psychoanalysts the couch is part of their language, and if you don't use the couch, well, in a way you are restricting your linguistic universe; even though in calling a table *la table* or *la tavola* we are still referring to the same object, we nevertheless all have a slightly different perspective on it.

DK: What are your thoughts on therapeutic regression?

JH: Regression. Yes, I noticed I was using that word and I don't think I have got anything terribly useful to say about it. Winnicott talked about regression in the service of progression, and I sometimes use the French proverb *reculer pour mieux sauter*. In other words, you run back in order to jump better. So, in order to progress, and I do believe you need to – as I was saying with my joey and kangaroo model – you need to be able to divest yourself of your habitual defences in order to move to a more mature and sophisticated use of defences. In that sense, I think that effective therapy is inherently somewhat regressive. The controversy arises when a patient curls up on the couch like a little a little foetus and says, 'I want to be fed by my mummy.' There was a culture in the 1950s, 1960s and 1970s of going along with that. You will find it in the literature; you will find it particularly in people like Winnicott. I, on the whole, am rather against that sort of thing. I feel maybe it's because I am a psychiatrist who sees a lot of borderline patients. We know that inappropriate psychoanalytic treatment can actually make borderline patients worse. And we are talking here about very difficult patients.

My general rule is, if you are working with a very difficult patient, you need two professionals. You need a psychoanalyst and you also need a case manager. It's the job of this case manager to deal with suicidal crises, to admit the patient to hospital when they need it, to prescribe medication when it's appropriate, to help with the practical problems of housing, and so on. It may be, and in fact I think it sometimes is the case, that a psychoanalytic treatment precipitates some kind of breakdown. I certainly don't think it's a good thing, and I don't think it's really the psychoanalyst's job to manage that break-down. I feel the case manager has to deal with that. It's the psychoanalyst's job to help the patient look at and understand whatever is going on for them, including a breakdown that might require them to go to hospital. The analyst cannot move out of his analytic role into a case-management role. For psy-chotherapy to work, the patient needs to have a sufficiently functioning ego to get him- or herself to therapy, to be able to talk to the therapist – in private practice, to pay for the therapy. The regressive aspect needs to be handled by a case manager rather than by the therapist. I am a bit suspicious – let's put it that way – I am a little bit suspicious of regression. Of course, regression does happen, but it's in the context of the therapy. The patient needs to be able to get up off the couch and walk out and continue with their basic coping, their basic living. Going back to Heinz Wolf, he used to say, 'Well, it's nearly time to stop now, and I am going to have to hand you back to yourself.' That's like saying, yeah, OK, regression happens in the session, but it's got to be reversible. If it's irreversible, it may sound heroic and wonderful, but I am a little bit sceptical and suspicious. I don't really believe in heroic psychoanalysis. One hears about it and people like to write about it, but I am sceptical.

DK: **Would you call encouraging regression heroic?**

JH: We all tell stories. Everything everyone writes about their psychoanalytic work, including myself, is a story. The fly on the consulting room wall isn't telling stories; it is actually observing what really goes on. I am not saying that those of us who write about what goes on in the consulting room are making it all up – and we have a problem with confidentiality, so it all has to be disguised in some way – but we inevitably choose particular cases that are telling a story that we want to tell.

DK: **You were saying earlier that psychoanalysis is not very good at defining its aims or what would constitute a positive outcome or what mental health is. Peter Lomas invokes a moral dimension and says that psychoanalysts are trying to help people become better people, to live a 'good life' in the sense meant by Aristotle, so I am wondering about your perspective on these issues and how attachment and sexuality figure.**

JH: I do agree about the Aristotelian idea of what it is to lead a good life, and that to be a 'good person' means being a coherent and integrated person rather than being riven by splits and repressions. Aristotelian 'virtue ethics' is different from utilitarianism, and as a huge generalisation I would say psychoanalysis is more virtue-ethics oriented as compared with CBT, which is essentially utilitarian. That said, I don't believe in psychoanalysis for its own sake as a kind of secular religion. From my (medical perhaps) point of view, the point and purpose of therapy is to alleviate suffering and help overcome psychological difficulties, including illness. Most people manage to live good(ish) lives without recourse to therapy. So that is a utilitarian aim, you might say, but it uses Aristotelian virtue-ethics means to achieve that utilitarian end.

DK: Where does sexuality fit into in your attachment perspective?

JH: My immediate response to that is to recall a colleague of mine. Morris
Eagle's (2007) view is that – and I don't actually fully agree with him –
we have two separate dynamics, the sexual behavioural system and the
attachment behavioural system, and that a long-term partnership, such as
a marital relationship, is always a bit of a compromise between those two.
One interesting point is statistics show that, when couples start dating, on
average they have sex after around seven meetings, whereas it takes two
years for a fully attachment relationship to develop – so there are separate
dynamics, with differing time-scales, and it takes a while for them to
converge – for their horizons to fuse, as it were! A marriage – this could be
a homosexual marriage, so I am not just talking about it heterosexually – a
marriage obviously contains both attachment and sex. You can get extreme
examples of those, where there is one without the other. At one end is the
unconsummated marriage, which has attachment with no sex. At the other
end, there is rape. In rape, there is no attachment at all; there is just some
kind of sex going on, at least from the male point of view. I think where I
subscribe to the Oedipal idea that everyone has to cope with rivalry, envy
and jealousy. We underestimate the role of the sexual dynamic at our peril,
and I am not in any way underplaying it. But I believe that the sexual
dynamic really kicks in only during adolescence; that's when teenagers
begin, to some extent, to undo their attachment relationships with their
primary care-givers, their parents. They then move their attachment relationship into their peer group and, as development progresses, pair off, and
sexual partnership emerges out of that. Adolescence has these three stages,
it seems to me: first, the undoing of the intense attachment relationship
with parents; then the forging of the beginnings of attachment relationships
with peers and mentors so that their secure base becomes their peer group.
You see this in extreme forms with gang formation, which often happens
when there's no father. These boys move from an attachment relationship
to their mother to a gang that then becomes their secure base. In stage three,
there is the differentiation out of a sexual relationship where sexuality and
attachment are a counterpoint one to the other.

Now, is this resolution of the Oedipus complex – and, indeed, what does
one mean by resolution of Oedipus complex? It seems to me that resolution
is the development of the capacity to tolerate a three-person relationship.
Clearly, one of the purposes or functions of marriage is reproduction. If
prospective parents are going to be effective parents, they are going to have
to tolerate the presence of a third person in their relationship. It is well
known that the sexual relationship becomes relatively sidelined in the early
days following the birth of a child. The father needs to develop the capacity to allow his partner to have this intimate, physical, sensual relationship
with their baby. His capacity to do that must relate to some extent to his
own developmental experience of having been able to tolerate his parents
having a life apart from him while at the same time knowing that, if he is in
distress, they would respond to him. I think one way of looking at it takes
us back to exploring insecurity. In other words, resolution of the Oedipus
complex in attachment terms, I think, would be to say sex is all about
exploration. You can only explore your sexuality or your bodily feelings,
and your partner's, if you both feel safe. People normally have sex in safe
places – that's why it takes place in bedrooms, in dark places, in secluded

places, where you know that you are safe, where you are not going to be attacked by a predator. Only when you are safe can you reach heights of excitement – another paradox, perhaps, or more of a dialectic. From the attachment point of view, there needs to be a degree of security; you need to be able to trust in order to have a sexual relationship. Equally there needs to be, I suppose, a sense that if there is a security need it will be met. In that classic situation where the parents are having sex or want to have sex and the baby cries in the night, how does that couple and that family cope? Is the – this may be a rather sexist way of looking at it – but is the father able to switch off and say, 'Okay, baby's distress takes precedence over my sexual needs. My partner has got to be available for our baby's security, and that is more important than my sexual need.' Children need developmental experiences in which they don't feel so driven by envy and rivalry and exclusion and fear that they have to intrude on the parents' sexual relationship, while at the same time knowing that if there was a crisis the parents would respond to them.

DK: **How well does attachment theory deal with negative emotions?**

JH: The main negative emotion that attachment theory writes about, and Bowlby was interested in, was anger. Whether or not that is a negative emotion may be open to debate, but obviously envy and rivalry can manifest themselves as anger. If you discover your partner is having an affair, you respond to that with anger, but underneath the anger may lie Oedipal insecurity, envy and rivalry. I would say that attachment theory does have something to say about negative emotions, but it sees them in terms of attachment – the primary function of anger is to activate attachment behaviour. It works both ways: if the child feels angry, he will activate the care-giver to attend to him. The first thing that happens if you feel threatened and the parent isn't there is you get angry.

I sometimes give an example from adult life: if you arrange to meet your partner at such and such a place and time for coffee and they don't turn up, or they turn up half an hour late, and you say, 'Where the hell were you?', you are expressing anger, but that anger is actually fuelled by an attachment dynamic – their non-appearance activates your attachment needs, and in order to re-establish contact with your secure base you express anger. It's about rupture and repair. I'll give another example from the developmental origins of attachment. I remember as a child when I was probably aged about eight. I grew up in London and there was a big main road near where we lived and my mother was very keen on walks so we used to go to the park a lot. On the way back, we had to cross this main road. I was with my mother and she would have been pushing a pram with my younger sister. Anyway, I ran ahead across the main road, and when she caught up with me she hit me and said, 'Don't you ever do that again.' I thought, 'I don't get this, why is she hitting me? She should be pleased that I am here and I am still alive and we are reunited.' But, of course, by hitting me she was ensuring that it didn't happen again, because I would think twice about running across the road if I thought I was going to get a slap for doing so. Maybe this is why I became a psychotherapist!

So, going back to the question as to whether attachment theory theorises negative emotion, I would say, yes. Now, how does this relate to envy and jealousy or the Oedipal situation? Well, let's go back to a pathological scenario – a couple with a new baby and the baby cries while the parents are in the middle of having sex. One or other of the parents might get very angry with that child, and I think that can be understood in terms of attachment rivalry. The father is saying to or about his wife, 'You belong to me. What the hell are you doing disrupting our sex life by going off to look after your crying baby?' Because the parents don't come, the baby is saying, 'Look, I am going to die in here if you don't come soon.' In both cases, the negative emotion is attachment related. I am very interested in the neo-Kleinian model of the Oedipus complex, which is quite relevant to mentalising. Ron Britton is the probably the best exponent of the neo-Kleinian model. He recasts Oedipus in mentalising terms and argues that the Oedipal child, the three-year-old child, whose parents are off behind the bedroom door having sex, will feel excluded and has to experience loss and loneliness. But, in that process, that child also acquires a mind of his own. He thinks, 'Well, I am free, I can think my own thoughts. I am no longer so dependent on my mother; I am an independent being.' These are the beginnings of mentalising. The beginnings of thinking your own thoughts can be seen in terms of the Oedipal dynamic. Here we are moving away from a concrete infantile sexuality model to a much more metaphorical one that includes this attachment aspect and the mentalising. Another key aspect is the idea of 'affect regulation' – with the help of the care-giver, a child can 'regulate', face and cope with their negative emotions – that's a hallmark of secure attachment; insecure children either suppress or soup up their negative emotions. In avoidant attachment, affects are not available for reworking and maturation and so remain in primitive forms, which can be very disruptive to interpersonal life. A lot of therapy is about co-regulation of negative emotions, so that, in time, the patient can begin to self-regulate and use their negative feelings to enhance their sense of autonomy and build more satisfying relationships.

DK: **Your reference to the metaphorical just now leads us nicely into the next discussion – on language. Could you comment about language in psychoanalysis?**

JH: Where to start? I think at the end of my book *Exploring in security* I make a semi-joking point that I sometimes ask colleagues: 'You have had ten years of analysis. What do you remember? What stays with you?' And usually it's relatively few things, but I think it's often a metaphor; it's often a really powerful image. I'll give an example. It's just one word, and that word is 'dumped'. This was somebody who had some problem in childhood which meant that they were dumped by their parents with their grandparents, who were actually hopeless with children. This patient was somebody who subsequently abandoned ('dumped') other people – wives and girlfriends and his own children. The analyst picked this up and used the word 'dumped', and somehow that word became a talisman for everything significant in the person's psychopathology. So I do think language is very important. When I am with clients I notice something that intrigues me and I try to foster this. But what I say just 'comes out'. Now we are talking and I am trying to be quite thoughtful and to answer your points and set them in a framework. Whereas when I am with a client I just try to experience myself almost like a vessel or vehicle out of which emerges language. That's what I am calling *logos* in the model that I outlined earlier.

As a psychiatrist and therapist I have seen a lot of psychiatric interviews or seen videotapes; I believe that the effective therapist intuitively, without even realising that they are doing it, adjusts their language and their linguistic universe to that of the client and to the client's vocabulary, the client's IQ, the client's linguistic skills. I like Jonathan Lear's word 'idiolect'. Couples and families have certain key phrases that mean something to them but do not mean anything to anyone else; it may be a family joke or something like that. That's what I call idio-language – in other words, it's a unique, specific linguistic world that intimate partners share. I think the same is true in psychotherapy and psychoanalysis: one develops – one begins to develop – an idio-language with one's patient, so you don't have to explain everything because you know what they mean and they know what you mean. The capacity to pick up on the patient's metaphors and play with them is a really important part of therapeutic work. I am very intrigued by what metaphor is, and I still don't really know the purpose of it, but I think it's something to do with how the metaphor gets you inside somebody else's head. You want to create the third; the route to the third is through metaphor, and that applies to poetry because you then share the experience, the affective experience of the poet – it somehow resonates with your own. For example, a patient might say, 'I have had a really rough day today.' Now, that actually is a dead metaphor. So the therapist might say, 'Well, rough in what way? Was it like walking through a ploughed field or walking on glass?' I am just making this up now. Then the patient might say, 'Oh, yes, it was really like wading through a ploughed field, my legs felt heavy', and then the therapist might say, 'Well, how are we going to get the mud off those boots today?' I feel that that kind of communication is an integral part of good therapy. Dream analysis is really metaphor work because a dream is a kind of metaphor. Every dream analysis to me is metaphor work. I suppose the final point about language is a correlation between good outcome in therapy and the therapist's use of metaphor. We are usually taught to play with the patient's metaphors, but sometimes therapists come up with something that really strikes home to the patient and makes the patient feel that they are understood. The difference between saying to a patient, 'Well, it seems as though you suffer from anxiety' – that's the kind of thing a psychiatrist might say – versus, say, 'Well, sometimes it feels as though you are a frightened child and haven't got anyone who is there to protect you.' That metaphor of a frightened child is a cliché but it's still a metaphor. Let me give you an actual example. My father-in-law is now dead, but when the First World War was over he was five years old and he was at school, and the entire school left to go and celebrate the end of the war and he was forgotten; he was stuck in the school and he was obviously completely terrified. The patient might then come up with a memory like that. I feel this metaphorical way of working is absolutely integral to what we are trying to do as therapists, and I think it's something to do with empathy. I think that empathic resonance is communicated via metaphor. This also happens in literature and poetry.

Going back to the Oedipal issue, I think I am a rebellious adolescent who, because of the war and because of my father's injury – I had a slightly handicapped father – I never really had my Oedipal battle. I got away without the Oedipal battle. One of the things about attachment theory for me is that Bowlby became my father. I shied away from psychoanalysis because it was a bit of a matriarchy. I am not saying this is in any way consciously matriarchal, but the predominant culture in British psychoanalysis is Kleinian. So it's a kind of matriarchy even though many of the Kleinians are male, and Ron Britton is a good example. Nevertheless, I think I needed to find a good father whom I could feel was stronger than me and cleverer than me and more powerful than me and whose example I could follow. Rightly or wrongly, I tended to see psychoanalysis as a rather closed system with totalitarian tendencies. Maybe totalitarianism is non-Oedipal in the sense that a totalitarian regime is a homogeneous regime; it's not a marriage. A marriage is always a mixture, and the question is to what extent the British Psychoanalytic Society is a marriage. I would say it isn't. It's an uneasy compromise, the so-called gentlemen's agreement. But it wasn't a proper marriage; it was a semi-peaceful co-existence. It remained a series of independent, sequestered, isolated groups that haven't fully cross-fertilised with the predominant regime, which is the Kleinian model. I think that may be changing now. I think that this is probably relevant to Rycroft as well, because Rycroft was really driven away by the Kleinians. I have identified with him but I needed to get beyond him – which is why Bowlby was so important – to resolve my Oedipus complex. And of course, ironically, attachment theory is mainly about mothers!

DK: Before we conclude today, I wanted to ask you how psychoanalysis, and attachment-informed psychoanalysis in particular, helps us to manage our existential anxieties.

JH: That's a nice little question. I suppose the fundamental existential anxiety is the fear of death. It's highly relevant to someone of my age and stage of life. How do you come to terms with death? To the extent that I am able to do so, I think of neither psychoanalysis nor attachment theory but probably of a Buddhist approach. Change and transience and life and death are all part of a continuous process. But maybe the way in which people relate to the idea of death is influenced by their attachment perspective; I was having a conversation with my wife about this the other day. It is how one visualises the moment of one's death. As an avoidant, deactivating character, I see it as a completely isolated moment. In my fantasy of death I am not surrounded by loved ones who are holding me and moving me into this world of non-being. I am alone. This event that stimulated this conversation was a recent visit to one of my sons – and grandson – in a foreign country. I was saying goodbye to him at the airport and then I went through into the waiting lounge. I thought that there is now no way I can communicate with my son. Perhaps this is what death is like. You can no longer look after your loved ones. You are alone; you are cut off from your attachments. I think it would be quite an interesting study to relate a person's attachment style to their fantasy of the nature of death.

I don't believe in infantile sexuality and I don't believe in the death instinct. From the psychoanalytic point of view, existential anxiety relates to the death instinct, and it would be to do with how one deals with one's existential anxiety by coming to terms with one's rage, one's destructiveness, one's murderousness. I see rage and destructiveness and murderousness all as perversions of attachment. Rage and destructiveness are ways of trying to establish a connection with the object, with the inaccessible object. 'Rage, rage against the dying of the light' is Dylan Thomas's model. I think that's an attachment rage that is saying, 'Where are you? I need you. I need you to be with me.' From an attachment point of view, if you have come to terms with existential anxiety, you know that there is a good object inside you, so the security is there; you don't need to rage against the dying of the light. Dylan Thomas is praising this protest against the dying of the light.

That's healthy anger, healthy aggression: why have I got to die, why has my Dad got to leave me/us? I suppose the only other point that I would make about dying and about death is the question, 'If I could lead my life again, would I make the same mistakes?' From a Buddhist perspective I realise – not that I believe in any literal way in reincarnation – but the knowledge that you have acquired through learning from your mistakes isn't completely lost; it's passed on to the next generation in some way. I suppose one way of dealing with one's existential angst is the idea of the next generation and your legacy to your children, your grandchildren, your friends, all our relationships, brothers, sisters, spouses, which is a completely relational picture, it seems to me. One might say the psychoanalytic model is a much more individualistic one – each of us must come to terms with our death instinct. Anyway, I don't know, it's a really interesting issue.

CHAPTER 2

TEN BOOKS

Being asked to write this piece was for me an honour and strangely exciting. Admittedly, that pleasure was tempered by the realisation that one's career has to have become somewhat crepuscular before such an invitation is likely to arrive. Another unwanted thought was the worry that perhaps books themselves, not just this particular author, are becoming obsolete. I sometimes think that everyone I know is writing a book, while no one reads them these days – it's all blogs and tweets, TED lectures and abstracts. Academics insist that writing, and presumably reading, books is a waste of time: they do nothing for one's department's research rating. Even novels nowadays tend to be reserved mainly for holidays, although membership of a 'book group' has been for many years a pleasurable part of my non-working life.

Like many psychiatrists, I see our discipline at its best as a happy marriage of art and science; it would be nice to believe that all the psychiatry worth knowing is contained in the literary canon. Here, though, I have decided to confine myself to works that would be found on the psychiatry and psychotherapy shelves in a library or bookshop. For the record, my personal top-ten non-psychiatric books for psychiatrists (cf. Holmes 2013) are: Tolstoy's *Anna Karenina* (marital breakdown, sex and suicide, with a dash of train-spotting); Dickens's *David Copperfield* (loss, bereavement and regeneration); Eliot's *Middlemarch* (the perils of pedantry, subservient women's awakening and the sociology of medicine); Austen's *Emma* (manic omnipotence, the depressive position and the acquisition of reflexive function); Conrad's *Heart of Darkness* (madness, cross-cultural studies and the inner journey); Gosse's *Father and Son* (filial piety versus individuation); Chekhov's short stories (the doctor as impartial yet compassionate observer); Proust's *Swann's Way* (narcissism and obsessive-compulsive disorder); Heller's *Catch 22* (post-traumatic stress disorder and black humour); and the *Oxford Book of English Poetry* (emotion into words: the essence of psychotherapy); with Shakespeare and the Bible taken for granted.

The divided self

Now to serious business. My first book, which I blame entirely for my choice of career as a psychiatrist, is R. D. Laing's (1960) *The divided self*. It was impossible to have been a student in the 1960s without reading this extraordinary, powerful and utterly original-seeming work by a 28-year-old Glaswegian who, against all the odds, took the Tavistock Clinic by storm in the 1950s. I say 'original-seeming', because in fact a lot of its ideas were drawn from therapists such as Bateson (1972), Searles (1965) and Fromm-Reichman (1959) in the USA and Winnicott (1971) and Rycroft (1985) in the UK who pioneered working with patients with psychosis. Nevertheless, the synthesis was truly 'Langian', and how many psychiatrists have an adjective made from their name?

Between, roughly, 1960 and 1980 no medical student, however illiterate, would have admitted to not having read Laing. Then, as his drink- and drug-befuddled powers began to wane, he disappeared from view, and today it is only the exceptional student who has even heard of *The divided self*, let alone read it. To me it seems as good and as relevant as ever: an essential antidote to biomedical reductionism, and a celebration of psychiatry as a guardian of individual experience and life story. Without Laing I doubt if the current interest in family intervention, and even cognitive-behavioural therapy (CBT) in psychosis, or user movements such as Hearing Voices Network, would have happened. Despite a reputation for mysticism and a penchant for LSD, Laing was keen to operationalise his ideas in a scientific way. His concept of 'ontological insecurity', in which patients with Borderline Personality Disorder lack a secure base either within themselves or their environment, is close to current ideas about disorganised attachment, and may be due for a revival.

Introductory lectures on psychoanalysis

Laing was trained as a psychoanalyst. Much of my early reading in psychiatry consisted of working through the bibliographies of his books. So my next choice is, of course, Freud. Reading *Introductory lectures on psychoanalysis* (Freud, 1916) for the first time was one of those overwhelming experiences that are increasingly remote as one gets older. The lecture format, and Freud's subtle mastery of persuasiveness and rhetoric, as well as his self-made subject matter, make it as unputdownable as a detective thriller (Michael Shepherd once cleverly compared Freud and Sherlock Holmes). Freud's paradigm shift seems as relevant to psychiatry today as it was nearly a century ago. Pitting himself against conventional psychiatry, he argues:

> Now you will have a right to ask the question: if no objective evidence for psycho-analysis exists [...] how is it possible to study the process at all or convince oneself of its truth? [...] second [...] your training will have induced in you an attitude of mind very far removed from the psycho-analytical one.
>
> (Freud, 1916, p. 15)

He goes on to show, in a way that was to my psychiatrically naïve mind utterly convincing, how the phenomena of mental illness, not to mention those of everyday life, are incomprehensible without the notion of the unconscious and acknowledgement of the ubiquity of sexuality. He expounds a developmental model of human motivation and the biographical meaning of psychiatric symptoms that continues to provide a programme of research and debate for contemporary psychiatry (Fonagy, 1999).

Psychoanalysis and beyond

Psychoanalysis is more than merely a powerful scientific or literary theory – it is also an ideology. The past 50 years have seen the gradual decline and, possibly, demise of grand theories in the West, but to be a student in the 1960s meant taking a position on the dominant ideologists of the time. I embraced both Freud and Marx, no doubt using them as a container for much of my own adolescent disturbance. I remain deeply grateful to my analyst, Charles Rycroft, who managed to tread softly on my dreams and at the same time to interpret them. He showed me that it was possible to respect a patient's beliefs, while at the same time gently deconstructing them and the projections they represent. Having an analyst who is also a well-known author can be a mixed blessing, but for me it was comforting, especially in his absence. Rycroft's best-known and most useful book is the *Critical dictionary of psychoanalysis* (1972), still in print after more than half a century; his own personal favourite was *The innocence of dreams* (1979). But I have chosen as my third book *Psychoanalysis and beyond* (1985). It is a collection of essays showing the range of Rycroft's interests, psychoanalytic, literary and political, and his mastery of the essay format, with a fascinating biographical introduction by Peter Fuller (no doubt satisfying some of my Oedipal curiosity). Rycroft's skill as both exponent and critic of psychoanalysis, as well as his lucid prose style, is fully displayed. One of the most scurrilous pieces in the book is his essay 'Ablation of the parental image', in which he discusses the motivations that draw people towards psychoanalysis as a career. He argues that the attempt to find a 'new beginning' can be an omnipotent fantasy, an attempt to wipe out the reality of one's own history and graft oneself onto a new one, adopting one's analyst and supervisor as surrogate parents.

Playing and reality

One of the most charismatic psychoanalytic figures of the 1960s was Donald Winnicott, who became President of the British Psychoanalytic Society just around the time that Rycroft began his 'strategic withdrawal'. *Playing and Reality* (1971) is surely Winnicott's best, most creative and accessible book. Like much psychoanalytic writing, it is a collection of essays, and it includes Winnicott's famous paper propounding the theory of transitional objects. I was stunned by this simple idea, which builds a whole theory of cultural life out of a child's favourite rag or teddy bear. *Playing and Reality* is permeated by Winnicott's unique style: evocative and provocative, authoritative and authoritarian, profound and elusive. It also contains detailed descriptions of sessions that enable one to see a master clinician at work. He was extraordinarily sensitive to nuances of emotion, used very simple, direct, yet profound language when talking to patients, and had a huge capacity to tolerate silence and regression.

Childhood and society

Those qualities are not easy for less gifted therapists to emulate, and indeed represent pitfalls for the unwary beginner. Winnicott was not afraid to break the rules, which can be confusing for those who are trying to learn them: the best practitioners do not always make the best teachers. One outstanding teacher who influenced several generations of medical students to become psychiatrists was Heinz Wolff, a consultant at University College London (UCH, as it then was) and the Maudsley. He introduced me to Erik Erikson's work. Erikson, like Heinz, was a free spirit with an intuitive feeling for children, an integrator who used psychoanalytic ideas to study history and cultural difference. Heinz recommended *Young*

Man Luther (Erikson, 1959), with its notion of the 'moratorium', a pressure-free moment between childhood and adult responsibility where identity can be forged and new ideas germinate – dangerous ideas for students nearing their finals! But *Childhood and Society* (Erikson, 1965), my fifth choice, is Erikson's deservedly classic work. His version of the 'ages of man', and the tension between autonomy and dependency, creativity and despair, provides an essential developmental framework for thinking about the maturation or disintegration of the personality throughout the life cycle; they can even be related to cognitive therapy's attempts to substitute positive for negative thought patterns in depression.

The doctor, his patient and the illness

Another outstanding teacher at UCH was the psychoanalyst Michael Balint. His classic work *The Doctor, His [sic] Patient and the Illness* (DPI; Balint, 1957) is my sixth sine qua non. This single work, together with the Balint groups – case discussions for general practitioners (GPs) in which they are encouraged to talk about their feelings and reactions to their patients – transformed the face of general practice in the 1960s and 1970s. When we were students, DPI and Balint's groups opened our eyes to the fact that behind the cases we were being asked to see on the medical and surgical wards were people with stories to tell, whose illnesses arose as much out of their biographies as they did from the 'causes of disease' we were expected to memorise. DPI shows how talking to patients is more than 'just chatting'; a psychotherapeutic conversation can help create new meanings and overcome illness. Oddly (and here I again reveal my incipient fogyism), few now seem to read his books, but the Balint spirit informs contemporary writers on general practice and has helped to make GP training the innovative experience it is – in my view, far in advance of most psychiatric training programmes. Today it seems that GPs are being encouraged to use CBT rather than Balint's modified psychoanalytic approaches with patients suffering from 'common mental illnesses', but for difficult cases – often the rule rather than the exception – DPI is a book that reaches parts inaccessible to simple CBT and problem-solving approaches.

Individual psychotherapy and the science of psychodynamics

One of the most attractive aspects of DPI, albeit in an era where attitudes towards consent were, by today's standards, cavalier, is its use of brief pithy case histories. David Malan, one of Balint's pupils and colleagues, brought the use of the case history as a teaching device to a fine art in my seventh choice, the clumsily titled but beautifully written *Individual psychotherapy and the science of psychodynamics* (Malan, 1979). This account of brief psychodynamic psychotherapy, what it is and how to do it, is essential reading for any self-respecting psychiatrist. Malan's 'triangles' – 'anxiety', 'defence and hidden impulse' and 'other, therapist and parent' – form a heuristic framework within which much psychodynamic work can be conceptualised. Finding a pattern that runs through the patient's relationships – past, present in the outside world and current with the therapist – is the cornerstone of the psychodynamic formulation, which, I am delighted to note, is now seen as a skill candidates for psychiatric examinations are expected to be able to demonstrate. If they read Malan they should have no trouble with this task.

Malan was a pioneer in several ways. He was one of the first psychoanalysts to undertake research that does justice both to accepted methodology and to the realities of dynamic therapy. His finding that interpretations that link parent and therapist (i.e. transference interpretations) are associated with good outcomes in brief therapy has, on the whole, been confirmed by subsequent studies. *Individual psychotherapy* is also one of the relatively few books that actually tell psychiatry residents and other beginner psychodynamic psychotherapy students how actually to do dynamic therapy – when and how to say what and in which situations. Here, dynamic therapy has lagged drastically behind CBT and other more manualised models. I suspect that this is because it was always assumed that students would be in therapy themselves, and that the experiential learning of the training therapy, backed up by supervision, would be a sufficient model for their own practice. There are other useful books in this area – Storr's *The art of psychotherapy* (which I have updated; Holmes, 2012) and Casement's (1985) *On learning from the patient* are both excellent, but Malan's is still for me the richest blend of theory and practice.

The social origins of depression

I have divided my working life between general psychiatry and psychotherapy; I often wonder why I continue to sit on this potentially volcanic fault line. The tension between coal-face and contemplation is a perpetual challenge. Whatever the reason, a seminal book which has helped to bridge the divide is Brown and Harris's (1978) *The social origins of depression*, my eighth choice. For nearly 40 years George Brown, although himself not a clinician, has been Britain's most creative and original social psychiatry researcher. Starting with his early research on mental hospitals and expressed emotion in schizophrenia, his definitive studies on the role of adversity in depression have provided an indispensable evidence-based counterweight to the biomedical model in psychiatry. Without Brown, the selective serotonin reuptake inhibitors might have swept the psychiatric board entirely. Beneath the academic façade of his work, which has a statistical rigour few psychotherapists can hope to follow in its entirety, the spirit of Marx and Freud lives on. Brown and Tirril Harris (an attachment-based psychotherapist) methodically build up their case: showing beyond reasonable doubt that depression is related to loss; that loss is a function of poverty and social adversity; and that the greatest bulwark against depression is the presence of an intimate confiding relationship. One of the fundamental aims of psychotherapy is, of course, to equip its patients with the capacity to form more satisfying confiding relationships, so here social psychiatry and psychotherapy come together.

A secure base

Brown and Harris's book was strongly influenced by the work of John Bowlby, who also conceptualised separation and loss, and how they are handled, as crucial elements in the origins of psychiatric illness. I have spent the past decade or so working in the field of attachment theory, and a book by Bowlby would be an essential component of my psychiatric desert island library. The monumental 'trilogy' is an obvious choice, and *Handbook of attachment* (Shaver & Hazen, 2008) is state of the art, but my favourite is Bowlby's penultimate work, *A secure base* (1988), published just a year before his biography of Darwin. Here Bowlby's simple, logical, dogged and committed approach to stating the almost obvious, which most of us are too blind, or enamoured of our own ideas, or threatened by simplicity, to notice, shines through. His chapter 'On knowing what you are not supposed to know and feeling what you are not supposed to feel' is a classic example of this, in which he insists that the majority of people with psychological disturbances have experienced major trauma in their lives, which, because they have been prohibited from speaking about their experiences, has remained unmetabolised and a potential source of vulnerability and psychological illness. Helping clinicians to value and find ways of enabling their patients to get in touch with these forbidden stories of loss and pain is one of the central tasks of psychotherapeutic psychiatry.

Psychodynamic psychiatry in clinical practice

Finally, what about a textbook? As a callow neurology Senior House Officer destined for psychiatry, on leaving the firm I was presented with the rather daunting black-jacketed *Clinical psychiatry* (Mayer-Gross, Slater & Roth, 1969) by my consultant, Richard Pratt, a wonderfully kind and psychotherapeutic man who happened to be a neuropsychiatrist at the National Hospital, Queen Square. Bergin and Garfield's (1994) *Handbook of psychotherapy and behaviour change* is essential reading for anyone interested in psychotherapy research. The various Oxford textbooks are always worth consulting, and the most recent, the unrivalled two-volume *New Oxford textbook of psychiatry* (Gelder, López-Ibor & Andreasen, 2000), contains almost everything anyone could possibly want to know about our subject. But, weighing in at exactly a stone on my bathroom scales, it is not exactly light reading. My last choice then is Gabbard's (1994) *Psychodynamic psychiatry in clinical practice.* This is a tour de force in which the author, displaying his usual fund of erudition and humour, systematically describes how psychoanalytic and other psychodynamic approaches can help us understand, treat and survive all of the major psychiatric disorders. Gabbard, a psychodynamic psychiatrist's role model, is an integrator who pays due respect to biomedical advances while continuing to insist on the contribution a dynamic approach can make to the everyday practice of psychiatry.

And a few more

Now that I have used up my ten slots, I am embarrassed to acknowledge all that I have left out, especially those that have been influential in my practice. For family therapists, Bateson's (1972) *Steps to an ecology of mind* and Haley's (1977) *Problem solving therapy* are essential reading. Also, caught up in my anecdotage (and envy?), I have omitted many excellent books by contemporaries, such as Clare's (1976) *Psychiatry in dissent*, Fulford's (1988) *Moral theory and medical practice*, Hamilton's (1982) *Narcissus and Oedipus* and Wright's (1991) *Vision and separation.* I realise, too, that I have chosen nothing about philosophy or religion, both of which provide an essential underpinning to psychiatry and are primarily book-based. The link with philosophy is perhaps that I have chosen authors – Laing, Freud, Rycroft, Winnicott, Balint, Erikson, Malan, Brown, Bowlby and Gabbard (and not forgetting Bateson) – as much as specific works, just as one tends to think of a philosopher's world-view, as opposed to any particular book from his or her œuvre.

It is hard for someone of my generation to imagine a world without books – although my wife is constantly encouraging me to reduce the number of those that furnish our rooms. So, to conclude: what are books, and why do they matter? A book is a friend, companion, whiler away of time, transporter to another world, a bridge across geography and history, a refuge from the rigours of work, not to mention a possible bed prop and aid to deportment. To use Winnicott's term, a book is transitional: an inanimate object, a set of arbitrary marks on a piece of pulped wood, yet one that has a life of its own. Reading is a key that simultaneously opens up our own inner world and that of others. I end, then, with the thought that reading books is a kind of therapy – one that, like psychodynamic psychiatry, will continually renew itself.

PART II

JUVENILIA

Apart from student journalism, 'Varicose veins' was my first published paper. As a 'Balintian', it was my would-be psychiatrist's way of getting through the mandatory 'pre-registration' surgical internship. As an author one has no idea who, if anybody, reads one's work, so I was delighted by Herman's little piece which appeared in the *BMJ* many years later, and which is reprinted here. 'The sibling', another early paper, emerged from my placement with the maverick Kleinian analyst Henry Rey during my training at the Maudsley Hospital in the UK. Trainees would sit in with Rey as he did psychotherapy assessments, and I noticed how, in his typically warm yet confrontational style, he often explored the patients' sibling relationships. Yet, in my combing of the psychoanalytic literature, I found few attempts to theorise the sibling relationship other than as a pale reflection of Oedipus. Coles's (2003) excellent collection goes some way to redress that, but I like to think that in 1980 I was ahead of my time. The same is true of my 'Nuclear disarmament' paper (1982), also written as a trainee. It prompted the comment from one of my supervisors 'What's going on, Holmes, does this mean you're become a Kleinian?' This was the first and last occasion on which I have been so designated! The paper is a not entirely successful attempt to link the turmoil of inner world with that of geopolitics. In the post-Cold War era, it seems something of an anachronism, but I include it here as some aspects are applicable to our current global threat: anthropogenic climate change. And at least it predated Segal (1987).

CHAPTER 3

VARICOSE VEINS
An optional illness

In 1962 at least 40,000 patients in England and Wales had operations on their varicose veins. Why? These operations are quite simple, fairly safe, and a basic part of any surgical registrar's repertoire. But what are the indications for operation?

Basic questions

Some patients have complications from their veins: dermatitis, thrombophlebitis, ulcers, or haemorrhage. These are a minority. Most patients present simply with the veins themselves, visible, unsightly, and often associated with vague symptoms like aching, cramps, or a feeling of heaviness in the legs.

Most of the patients who come to their doctor must have had clinically obvious varicose veins for years, and there are many women with veins who never present at all. Why does the patient come when she does, and not last year or next? When asked, almost all patients will say that they have had some symptoms from their veins. Why do some patients develop these symptoms and others not?

There seems to be some mystery surrounding this basic question. As one textbook puts it: 'The character of the patient with varicose veins seems to be largely responsible for the severity of the symptoms.' This explains very little, although one might imagine that some patients have a lower pain threshold, or have more perivascular nerve endings, or are simply less stoical than others.

An 'optional' illness

This article looks at the problem from a different perspective. It suggests that a patient with varicose veins goes to her (or his) doctor because of a temporary *need to be ill*; vein-strip operations provide a brief *optional illness* which meets this need.

This may seem paradoxical, for in our culture illness is conceived as being in essence *obligatory*. A person has no choice but to fall ill, and this misfortune entitles him, as a victim of fate, to care, sympathy, and, if possible, repair work on our part. But illness is a social as well as a biological event: to fall ill is to be treated in a particular way, and to be expected to behave in a particular way. One could say that the ill patient is playing a sick-role, and that, as Balint (1957) has suggested, a person becomes a patient, or is cast in this role, only after negotiation and mutual agreement with his doctor.

Once the illness is 'established', however, this early phase is forgotten and the patient is then treated *as though* his illness were obligatory. Those 'optional' illnesses which are not accidental, but which may arise from a person's needs and desires, tend to be overlooked or misunderstood. Varicose veins provide a simple model of this type of problem: to have them is an affliction; it becomes an illness only when the patient (now defined) asks the doctor to do something about them.

This article looks at the reasons why patients are in need of a period of illness.

Methods

This report is based on a study of 24 consecutive patients admitted to a general surgical ward, where I was house officer, for vein strip. On this firm the waiting list for vein operations was short: about four weeks. On admission, each patient was asked why he (or she) had gone to his doctor when he did, and a brief psychiatric history, with particular emphasis on recent worries, family crises and emotional problems, was taken. No interpretations were made, and in fact most patients needed only minimal encouragement before they were prepared to talk.

Each patient was scored as having severe (+ +), mild (+), or no (0) emotional upset. Patients were also classified by the presence or absence of complications and by the length of history, either short (less than 18 months) or long (more than 18 months).

A similar study of 31 patients with inguinal and femoral hernia repair was made.

Results

The overall numerical findings are summarised in Table 3.1. Table 3.2 breaks down the indications into those with complications and those with only symptoms, whilst Table 3.3 shows how the psychological score changes with the length

Table 3.1 Severity of emotional upset in 55 patients undergoing operation for varicose veins or hernia

Operation	Score			Total
	+ +	+	0	
Veins	11	10	3	24
Hernias	2	1	28	31

Table 3.2 Severity of emotional upset according to indication for operation

Indication		Score			Total
		+ +	+	0	
Veins	Symptoms	11	7	2	20
	Complications	0	3	1	4
Hernias	Symptoms	2	1	21	24
	Complications	0	0	7	7

of history. Table 3.4 shows the sex of the patients, and Table 3.5 shows the age distribution.

Some typical case histories

Here are some examples of typical case histories.

> *Case 1*   Mrs EF, aged 51. Vein strip. This patient, who married when she was pregnant, had left her home town, husband and three small daughters and moved to a different part of the country, where she settled. There she met another man with whom she was now living. She did not want to marry him. She had missed her family, particularly her own mother and her youngest daughter, but had had scanty contact with them over the past twelve years. Just before coming into hospital she had been home for the first time to help her youngest daughter, now aged 17, and unmarried, have her baby. Her family begged her to stay, but after the baby was born she returned to her 'boyfriend'. Her family was furious and refused to answer any of her letters. This had thrown Mrs EF into despair. She hoped that when her family learned that she was in hospital they would pity her and make contact again. (They did.) Score + +.

Table 3.3 Severity of emotional upset according to length of history

Length of history		Score			Total
		+ +	+	0	
Veins	Short	1	3	0	4
	Long	10	7	3	20
Hernias	Short	0	0	28	28
	Long	2	1	0	3

Table 3.4 Sex of patients

Operation	Women	Men
Veins	20	4
Hernias	3	28

Table 3.5 Age of patients

Operation	Age	
	Median	Mean
Veins	37	44
Hernias	40	36

Case 2   Mrs PG, aged 50. Vein strip. She had been a happily married woman, with two sons aged 19 and 17, until one year before the operation. Then her eldest son had been killed on the way to work on his motor-cycle. She had been miserable for a short time, but could not cry, and then had returned to work. Now she was insomniac, plagued by cramps in her legs at night, and terrified every time her younger son and husband, both of whom rode motor-cycles, left the house. She felt that if her veins were done she would be able to sleep. Score + +.

Case 3   Mr GM, aged 55. Herniorrhaphy. This man had been unhappily married for the past ten years to his second wife. She grumbled constantly and criticised his dead wife and children. Recently his son and daughter-in-law had been evicted, and so Mr M had put them up in his house while they looked for a flat. His wife was furious and refused to speak to Mr M or his son. Mr M then went to his general practitioner about the hernia he had had for twenty-five years; he thought that being in hospital would 'bring her round'. (It did.) Score + +.

Case 4   Mrs CK, aged 45. Vein strip. Married to an alcoholic and recidivist. His first prison sentence was when the children were aged 7, 4, and 1 years. He was inside for four years; in this time they were evicted, and she worked, paid for and furnished the flat where they now live. When he came out she 'took him back' on condition he went straight. Six months' later he was in prison again. He had been released just before she came into hospital. She 'wished she could leave him', and hoped that her illness would show him what 'she had done for the children'. Score + +.

Case 5   Mrs PS, aged 49. Vein strip. This woman adored her eldest son, aged 23. She had become very unhappy recently because his fiancée (now wife) had 'turned him against her'. She felt that they did nothing but laugh at her behind, or even in front of, her back. Her son rarely visited her now; she hoped that in hospital she would be able to speak to her son away from his wife. (She couldn't.) Score +.

Discussion

The main conclusion of this study is that, when patients with a longstanding surgical condition seek operation, many do so because they have considerable emotional problems. Accepting (for the moment) that this is valid, we can ask why this might be so. There are many reasons why people may need a period of illness.

1   *Operation as a way of showing one's wounds*   A number of these patients felt hurt, misunderstood, unloved by their families. They also felt very angry about this. They seemed unable to express these feelings directly. Instead, by becoming ill, they made a covert demand for sympathy and, by inducing in others the guilt-feelings which illness evokes, expressed their secret anger and resentment, Cases 1, 3 and 5 all hoped that a relative would be more loving to them after the operation. Another example was:

Case 6   Mrs PD, aged 43. Vein strip. This patient had a near-psychotic delusion that her husband was having an affair: she would imagine this whenever she saw him talking with another woman. She saw the operation as a crucial test of his fidelity: if he was by her bedside when she came round from the anaesthetic, this would prove that he loved her. (He was.) Score + +.

These sorts of feelings are reminiscent of those in some attempted suicides, where the patient may cut her (wrist) veins to show people how much they are hurting her.

2   *Operation as a way of being babied*   In hospital, patients are expected to be passive and compliant, and in return may wish that their every need will be satisfied. In fantasy, patients are fed, washed and dressed by cool and clean and beautiful women.

> *Case 7*   Miss SB, aged 27. Vein strip. This girl was very close to her parents, who lived in Scotland, but she had recently left home for the first time, coming to England to take up nursing. She was very homesick and felt safe only when she went out with middle-aged men. She was happy as a patient, but when the time came for her discharge after her vein strip she became very agitated, and insisted that the other leg, which had minimal vein varicosity, be done as well. Score + +.

This patient was a nurse, perhaps trying to master her own need to be looked after by caring for others. As a patient, her unfulfilled dependence needs were satisfied. Case 4 is another example of a patient who saw the operation as a chance to 'have someone look after her for a change', as she put it. Another was:

> *Case 8*   Mrs PL, aged 57. Vein strip. She was married to an older man, now a bedridden chronic bronchitic. She had nursed her own parents for years, until they died, and also her grand-daughter while her daughter went out to work. She felt that everyone 'just used her', and that in hospital she could relax 'for the first time in years'. Score +.

3   *Operation as a cry for help*   It is well known that patients who are basically depressed may present with a physical illness. Case 2 is a clear example of this. Another was:

> *Case 9*   Mr JM, aged 56. Vein strip. An insurance salesman who had failed to get promotion and so was still doing door-to-door selling in which he felt he could no longer compete with younger men. He was apathetic, sleeping badly, frightened of old age, and wanted the vein strip 'in case anything worse happens'. Score + +.

4   *Operation as a penance*   The idea of purification through suffering may seem anachronistic, but several of the patients clearly hoped that they would in some way be purged by the operation. This feeling is even recognised in the surgical homily 'There's no such thing as painless surgery', delivered in a grin-and-bear-it voice. One good example was:

> *Case 10*   Mr GR, aged 33. Hernia repair. He had had the hernia since he was 6 years old. Now a married man with four children, he smoked 100 cigarettes

a day and spent all his evenings in clubs. He was rarely at home, but after leaving hospital he was going to 'give it all up and become a family man with a pipe and slippers'. He gave up smoking for two days after the operation, but could stand it no longer, hated the ward, started again, became very agitated, and took his own discharge. Score + +.

5   *Operation as a way of getting a new personality*   Some of the younger patients fall into this group. They are insecure in their self-image, cannot see themselves as sexually desirable, and focus their discontent on some often quite minor blemish, which they see as the root of all their anxieties. For example:

Case 11   Miss CW, aged 33. Vein strip. An attractive girl who thought that her slight varicose veins were 'absolutely disgusting', she felt self-conscious although superficially poised; felt she was too thin and was always trying to put on weight; had a steady boyfriend, but was sure that he didn't really like her. She had made a minor suicide attempt when she was 17 'because my parents don't really care about me'. Score +.

Conclusion

Two facts emerge from this study. One is that, when patients with varicose veins present, about half of them are in the throes of some significant emotional crisis. The other is that patients with hernias usually present within weeks of first noticing their lump, and they are rarely emotionally disturbed.

These facts can be explained in a number of ways. Taking the veins first, one could say that the typical varicose-vein patient is a middle-aged woman who is in any case facing the psychological problems of the menopause, and there is no causal connexion between her emotional disturbance and presentation for vein strip. Alternatively, I suggest that it is precisely these psychological difficulties which create in certain types of patient a need for illness as a solution or pseudo-solution to their problems.

This article does not contain the data which would enable one to distinguish these possibilities. To do this the inpatient group would have to be compared with a matched group of ambulant sufferers from varicose veins, but there are two points which tend to support the causal theory. One is that those patients who had *complications* from their varicose veins, for whom the operation was more or less obligatory, showed no severe emotional disturbance. Secondly, it is striking that the only hernia patients in whom there was any significant emotional disturbance were those with longstanding lumps, for whom, like the varicose-vein patients, the operation was now 'optional'.

Although a hernia, like varicose veins, is a minor surgical condition and patients are put on a waiting list before operation, they seem to form psychologically a quite distinct group. The patients, often men in their thirties, are in a less stressful phase of their life-history. Also, it is likely that almost any man will find a lump in his groin sufficiently threatening to show it to his doctor, who, since the complications are more serious, may put more pressure on the patient to accept an operation than he would if they had varicose veins.

These patients all presented with a commonplace surgical condition. Their doctor is faced with two problems: why did the patient present, and what is wrong with him? The organic diagnosis is simple, but it may be a way of *not* seeing that the patient is a person with a problem. Pathological processes cause organic disease for good physico-chemical reasons; people need to be sick for equally good but quite different reasons, and we should try to understand both.

Summary

Eleven out of twenty-four patients admitted for routine vein strip for varicose veins were involved in recent emotional upsets or family crises. It is suggested that they may have become troubled by their veins in response to these difficulties and have sought an operation as a way of resolving them.

I am grateful to Mr L. A. Ives, F.R.C.S., Sister Kay Donovan, Dr H. H Wolff and Dr M. Balint for help in preparing this article.

A PAPER THAT CHANGED MY PRACTICE: OPTIONAL ILLNESS

Joseph Herman

Assia Community Health Centre, Jerusalem

Certain articles have a way of following you throughout your entire career, cropping up in widely differing circumstances. In my case, one such article would be 'Varicose veins: an optional illness' … The paper is elegantly designed and its conclusions go no further than the facts at hand allow. It suggests that there can be a temporary need for falling ill, leading to negotiation with a physician and the transforming of an affliction or a blemish into an illness. For the patient, undergoing surgery can be a way of showing hurts, doing penance, being babied, crying out for help, or even getting a new personality. For the doctor, making the diagnosis of varicose veins may be a way of not seeing the patient's problem of living.

Dr Holmes's paper has had an extraordinary influence on my own practice, thinking and teaching in the quarter century that has elapsed since my first reading of it. It is as applicable today to coronary bypass and operations for degenerative disease of the knee joint as it was then to varicose veins. Time and again, I have encountered patients who, through a feeling of neglect by family or society, chose to undergo surgery for doubtful indications, even excusing suboptimal outcomes by a process of cognitive dissonance. Despite my awareness of some of the problems these people were facing and of the idea of a temporary need to be ill, I was never able to 'rescue' anyone from the fate on which he or she had decided.

My next encounter with Dr Holmes's paper took place recently. I have become interested in how descriptions of disease and mortality seem to move back and forth between medical sources, on the one hand, and the popular sphere or fiction, on the other … imagine my astonishment when I came across the following lines by Camus in his essay 'The enigma', written in 1950: 'Doctors know that certain illnesses are desirable: they provide, in their own way, a compensation for a functional disorder which, in their absence, would express itself in a more serious disturbance. Thus there are fortunate constipations and providential attacks of arthritis.' Is this not an early formulation of optional illness?

CHAPTER 4

THE SIBLING AND PSYCHOTHERAPY

Psychoanalytic and other literature relevant to the sibling relationship is reviewed. Cases are presented illustrating the role of feelings towards the sibling in psychothera-peutic practice. Three main areas are discussed: (1) the birth of a sibling as a 'fixation point'; (2) the effect of the sibling on identity formation; (3) the role of the sibling relationship in treatment, especially the importance of acknowledging sibling rivalry.

Review

The importance of the sibling relationship in the psychodynamic understanding of the person is well established. As a research topic, however, the sibling vector has been relatively neglected. This article consists of a review of some of the relevant literature, examples of the place of the sibling relationship in psychotherapeutic practice, and a short theoretical discussion.

The psychoanalytic view: the sibling as rival or parent substitute

For Freud, the central human drama, the 'kernel of the neuroses', was the Oedipal situation (Freud, 1916). He was aware of the part played by the siblings, but in his writings they are given few lines. When they do appear it is usually as understudy for one of the parental roles: as substitute for the longed-for parent, or as another rival for their love. He seemed to view the primary sibling relationship as hostile, only to be 'overlaid' later with affection. He visualised far-reaching effects of this on the personality.

> A child who has been put into second place by the birth of a brother or sister and who is for the first time now almost isolated from his mother does not easily forgive her this loss of place; feelings which in an adult would be described as greatly embittered arise in him and are often the basis of a permanent estrangement.
>
> (Freud, 1916)

> The boy may take his sister as a love object by way of substitute for his faith-less mother. When there are several brothers all of them courting a younger

sister, situations of hostile rivalry, which are so important for later life, arise already in the nursery. A little girl may find in her elder brother a substitute for her father who no longer takes an interest in her as he did in her earliest years. Or she may take a younger sister as a substitute for the baby she vainly wished for from her father.

(Freud, 1921)

Subsequent psychoanalysts have generally followed Freud's emphasis on the negative aspects of the sibling relationship and seeing in it a reflection of the child's relationship with his parents. Anna Freud (1998) cites her experience with the Bulldog Bank orphans as the exception which proves the rule. She claims these children showed little evidence of normal sibling rivalry and attributes this to the lack of intimate parental relationships about which to feel rivalrous. Bettelheim (1969) has also maintained that sibling rivalry is inconspicuous in communally raised children.

Anna Freud points out that hostile and erotic feelings towards siblings are often less repressed than those towards parents, and thus siblings may be 'used for the discharge of libidinal trends deflected from the parents'. She also sees an influence on future character development: 'Since contemporaries outside the family are treated like the siblings, these first relationships to the brothers and sisters become important factors in determining the individual's social attitudes' (Freud, 1969). Fleugel (1921) quotes mythology from Cain to Chronos revealing the unconscious significance of the sibling relationship. He saw the displacement of libido from parents to siblings not as a defensive manoeuvre but as an important part of normal maturation.

Adler: personality and birth order

Freud remained, to the last, his mother's first son – although he did have two much older half-brothers by his father. Among the early psychoanalytic writers it was Adler, a fourth-born, who emphasised the importance of sibling relationships as one of the primary determinants of personality (Ansbacher & Ansbacher, 1958). For him, the sibling relationship was an issue in its own right, not merely a screen where the elemental Oedipal triangle could be projected. Adler claimed that personality types could be derived from birth position. According to him, the eldest is the one who has been 'dethroned' by the arrival of the next child: he is the conservative, interested in the past, longing for the good old days, hoping to win parental approval by being a good organiser and protector of the weak; the second-born, never special, has always to contend with feelings of envy and slight; while the youngest, never to be dethroned, is the favoured one, the youngest son of fairy stories who, against all the odds, 'gets the fame and the money all at one sitting' (Larkin, 1955).

There have been many attempts to put Adler's ideas to the test, mostly based on studies of 'normal' US college students (Warren, 1966). The results have generally been equivocal or contradictory, or both. For example, McArthur (1956) found first-borns were more serious, sensitive and parent-oriented than their placid, easy-going, peer-oriented second-born fellow students; Greenberg *et al.* (1963), however, found no significant correlation between birth order and personality variables; and there is no correlation between MMPI neuroticism score and birth order (Altus, 1966). It is noteworthy that the majority of these studies are both male-oriented and success-oriented.

Birth order *per se* is probably not a simple determinant of personality any more than it is of psychiatric illness (Hare & Price, 1969). In studies of life events and depression, Brown *et al.* (1975) have shown that it is not necessarily the life event itself which leads to breakdown, but its 'contextual meaning' in the micro-social environment of the individual. Similarly, although sibling position is clearly a significant part of an individual's self-experience, it is the context, social, famil-ial, psychological, which will determine the effect of such position of his personality or proneness to psychiatric illness.

Child observation studies

Child observation studies are just such an attempt to study the microsocial environment: they suggest that there are indeed birth-order-related differences in parental handling and child behaviour, and that many of these differences persist over time (Sutton-Smith & Rosenberg, 1971); it is not known whether they persist into adult life. According to Waldrop (1965), differences may start even in the neonatal period when, she claims, high 'sibling density' infants (i.e. from close-spaced families) cry and suck less vigorously than others. Mothers interact about twice as much with their first-born at the toddler stage as they do with second-borns. Although at a given age they *expect* first-borns to be more independent, the first child is actually *more* distressed by a short absence of mother from the room than are his younger sibs.

Lasko (1954) showed how first-borns experience a greater *change* in parental handling than subsequent children: around the time of birth of the second sibling there is a sudden decrease in intensity of interaction, with a changeover from warm positive reinforcement to the use of punishment and prohibition. Second and subsequent children tend to get more consistently warm handling, albeit at a lower intensity. Interpreting these findings, Sutton-Smith and Rosenberg (1971) suggest the first-born is treated as a kind of 'mini-adult' by the beginner mother, who has unrealistic developmental and emotional expectations for her first child, which she then readjusts for her later offspring.

Koch (1955, 1956), in an ambitious study, set out to relate the behaviour of pre-adolescent children in home and school to their sibling position. She found that the intensity of sibling rivalry depends on the age- and sex-gap between siblings: where the age-gap is more than four years, the older child is most jeal-ous of a same-sex sibling; where the gap is less than four years, then opposite-sex siblings excite greatest rivalry.

Koch's interpretations of her complex results have been criticised (Brim, 1958); they are certainly open to a number of different explanations. A psychoanalytic view of the above might be as follows: if a same-sex baby is born when the older child is in the Oedipal phase, i.e. three to five, this will be felt by them as a threat to their relationship to the opposite-sex parent and rivalry will be intense. When the gap is narrow and the older child is still in the oral phase, they may then be most threatened by an opposite-sex sib and come to feel they are the 'wrong' sex, or that they have the 'wrong organ' to get maternal attention. As one of Koch's little interviewees said in reply to the question 'Would you like to be like your new baby brother or sister?', 'Yes, I would; then I could yell my head off and my mamma would take care of nobody but me.'

Looking at personality, Koch found definite sex/positional effects. For example, girls with older brothers tended to be more tomboyish than those with older sis-ters. Boys with older sisters tended to be more self-confident, less attention-seeking, less aggressive, than those with older brothers. This would follow if parents tend to favour their first boys, who are then able to build their identity as they like, or 'personally', to use Slater's (1961) personal/positional classification. Girls, or second-born boys, on this view, would be tempted to build their identity 'positionally' rather than 'personally', via envy of the favoured sib's position or 'identification with the aggressor' (A. Freud, 1936).

Child analysis: the sibling as a trigger for regression or maturation

The influence of the sibling relationship on identity formation and its pathology has been noted by many child analysts. Rollman-Branch (1966) suggests that, when a new sib arrives, the older child faces a developmental challenge to which he may react in one of two ways: he may identify with the parent, moving in the direction of greater autonomy and ego-development; or he may identify with the newborn child, leading to regression and loss of independence.

Since presumably all non-only children have to face such a challenge, the question remains whether, and under what circumstances, the sibling relationship becomes a significant determinant of psychopathology.

David Levy (1935), a child analyst particularly interested in the subject, maintained that sibling rivalry becomes important only when there is also disturbed relationship with the mother. He postulates a 'mother, ignorant and emotionally immature, who over-indulges her infant, creating excessive dependency on her, and when as a result the child becomes difficult, discards it.' The 'discarded' child may then become excessively rivalrous towards the new arrival who, in his turn, begins to feel guilty about this, and may himself later feel discarded if a further sibling is born. Klein (1969) said of such youngest children:

> Youngest and only children often have a strong sense of guilt because they feel their jealous and aggressive feelings have prevented their mother from giving birth to any more children. I have frequently found that fear and suspicion of schoolmates or of other children were linked with phantasies that the unborn brothers and sisters had after all come alive, and were represented by any children who appeared hostile. The longing for friendly brothers and sisters is strongly influenced by such anxieties.

The sibling relationship in clinical practice

Psychoanalytic observation and child observation studies have suggested that the sibling relationship may influence the adult personality in a number of different ways: the birth of a sibling may become a 'fixation point'; there may be effects on character formation and sexual identity; and the sibling relationship may be intricately linked with the Oedipal situation. I shall now try to exemplify these points with cases taken from once- or twice-weekly out-patient NHS psychotherapy practice.

(1) The birth of a sibling as a fixation point

Feelings aroused at the time of birth of a sibling may become a focus around which neurosis is organised in adult life. The birth of a child or an abortion may reactivate emotions from this period.

Case 1 was a young woman whose symptoms of recurrent depression, and inability to sustain relationships with men, dated from an illegal abortion some years previously, in which she had become ill with a uterine infection and had to go into hospital. At the time she thought that she was dying. She had never felt fully herself since. She was the older of two sisters: the younger was mother's favourite. The patient had turned to father but, when she was eight, he had died. She described her guilt and depression about the abortion; she then linked this to the wish that her mother had never had her sister, and her envious anger at her sister for taking her mother away from her. She made a link between her abortion and her childhood wish that her sister would die. Illness and depression were her punishment.

Comment

The pregnancy and abortion acted as a seed around which her sibling jealously crystallised out. In this were condensed her murderous feelings towards the younger sister; guilt about this; self-punishment in an attempt at expiation; the reparative implication of pregnancy; envy of her mother's capacity to have intercourse with her father and produce children; and sadness at the loss of her father. Sibling jealousy was the thread on which she could hang these many feelings.

Abraham (1924) claims that one of the precursors of adult depression is 'a severe injury to infantile narcissism brought about by disappointments in love', and cites the birth of a sibling as one such possible disappointment. The next case exemplifies this.

Case 2 was a markedly depressed young man. He felt that life had never been fair to him: he had always got the worst of things, the worst jobs, the worst girls. Everyone was better off than he. In the course of treatment he recalled that these feelings had started with the birth of his sister when he was three. After she was born everything was different. All the attention went to her, father loved her, no one put pressure on *her* to do well at school or made her life a misery, as his was.

After the session in which he had recalled these feelings, he dreamed that he stabbed his sister with a long knife pushed through a letter box, and then was arrested for killing some 'old folks'.

Comment

In the dream sexual and aggressive impulses towards the sibling are explicit, while the parents are only dimly present as 'old folks'. The sibling relationship may be accessible to consciousness while the underlying oedipal structure is still buried.

---

(2) The sibling relationship in identity formation

Patients with character disorders form an increasing proportion of psychotherapeutic practice, and the influence of the sibling relationship on the psychopathology of such patients will now be discussed.

Lewin (1951) described the 'oral triad' of mother, baby-at-the-breast, and watching older sibling. The older sibling may feel excluded and enjoys the excitement vicariously, by identifying with one or other pole of the mother–child dyad. Where the envied sibling is of the opposite sex, there may be an envious cross-sex identification. This paradigm is exemplified by the next two cases.

Case 3 was a man who became depressed when his divorced wife refused him access to their daughter on the grounds that he was homosexual. He was the oldest child, with two younger sisters, one only a year younger than he.

He described the family scenario: his mother preferred his sisters; the parents did not get on; his father rejected him; the only person he felt close to was his sister; the only way to get love in the home was to be a girl; even now, he and his sister are so close that when he feels suicidal he imagines she must too. Being homosexual was being 'like a girl' and so being liked like a girl, as his sister was.

Case 4 was a young woman who presented with depression. She was the only girl among three boys. Her parents did not get on; her father was a drunkard; her mother preferred the boys; at the age of five she said to herself, 'I don't belong to this family', imagining that she was adopted, and disowning her mother. She started to rock herself to sleep every night, thus 'becoming' her own mother. The only happy memories of childhood were when she was out in the woods with her father climbing trees, when she performed more daring exploits than her brothers. Her depression started at puberty, when she had to give up her fantasy of being a boy perforce.

Comment

In the oral triad the watcher is estranged from his true identity, identifying instead with the envied sibling, or mother, or both at different times. In case 4, the patient tried first to 'be' her brothers (climbing trees, etc.) then at puberty switched to 'being' the mother she felt angry with for preferring the brothers, i.e. a useless mother. Both patients became depressed when they could no longer maintain a fantasy identification with the opposite sex which flew too blatantly in the face of reality. In case 3 the patient was confronted at his divorce with the fact that he was not really a 'mother' to his daughter. In both cases it seemed that the father was not available as an alternative reliable source of love for the child who felt their mother was preoccupied with the other siblings. Thus the role of the father may be crucial in facilitating adjustment to sibship. Progress in therapy seemed to depend on the therapist providing a safe base from which the patient could deal with their feelings of sibling rivalry.

The Argentinian peasant mother says to the whiny displaced older child, 'Go suck your father's testicles' (Levy, 1939). If a father, or grandparent, is not available at this time, the older child may remain psychologically trapped in the oral triad long after the younger sibling has been weaned from it.

---

(3) The sibling relationship as a key to the Oedipal situation

In the next case I shall try to show how understanding the sibling relationship provided the key which unlocked some of the core psychopathology as treatment progressed.

Case 5 was a young man in his early thirties: he was severely obsessional; he had great difficulty in separating from his parents; he had never had sexual intercourse; and he had powerful sado-masochistic fantasies in which he was alternately tied up and beaten by, and tied up and beat, an older man. He had one sister, three years older than he.

He described himself as a complete 'failure': he had gone into the same profession as his father, but could never hope to rival his eminence in it; he was a failure with girls, his father had married a former beauty-queen, how could he hope ever to marry someone like that? He denied any rivalrous feelings towards his father, who, he said, was a kind man who helped him in every possible way, even though he was such a disappointment to him. In the transference he reproduced his relationship with his father, making constant efforts to please the therapist by applying for new jobs, taking girls out, but the end was always the same: failure. At this point he would turn triumphantly to the therapist and say 'What did I tell you? I'm a failure, why don't you get rid of me and take on a patient who will be a success?'

When asked his fantasies about this hypothetical patient, she turned out to be a woman, a little older than himself, rather like ... his sister.

This fantasy unlocked a flood of material about his sister: she was their father's favourite, always sat next to him at table, could do no wrong. As a child he used to get into her bed when he felt frightened, and at the start of his depression he had felt intense sexual desire for her.

In the next session he brought a dream, the first in the therapy: he was taking a girl home to meet his parents; the four of them sat round the dinner table, mother and father, he and the girl; he looked at her and suddenly saw she was so ugly she would never be acceptable to them. He said the dream showed how he wanted to be close to his father, but his 'sister' (the girl) was there sitting next to him, how envious he felt of her, and how this made her ugly in his eyes.

He suddenly saw that the girl was like every girl he had been attracted to: they all had qualities which he envied, then he revealed how he then had compulsively to find something wrong with them. At this point he started to feel angry at father for making him feel that sister was better than he, and he finally accepted the often-repeated interpretation that his self-punishing 'failure' was a reproach to his father for this, as well as a punishment for having these ungrateful angry feelings.

Comment

The movement here was from 'I am unsuccessful with girls' through 'I am only attracted to girls whom I envy' to 'I envy my sister's position *vis-à-vis* my father'. At this point the underlying father–sister–self triangle was uncovered. He was unable to make this movement until he could face his sibling rivalry. This fits with Beiber *et al.*'s (1962) finding, in a study of the psychotherapy of homosexuality, that a good prognosis was associated with an ability to acknowledge sibling rivalry.

---

(4) The sibling relationship in therapy

In the last example I want to show how sibling rivalry reached near-psychotic intensity in the treatment of a depressed patient with a severe schizoid personality disorder, and how understanding this helped in the minute-by-minute maze of her sessions.

Case 6 was a woman in her middle thirties who presented with depression. She dressed and behaved for the most part like a small child. She had lived alone for most of her adult life. The only beings she loved were her two cats. If only cats could talk, she said, she would be perfectly happy.

Her sister was two years younger; soon after she was born their mother left home and they were brought up together in institutions and with relatives. She stated that she had 'no' childhood and had been 'given away' by her mother.

I shall now describe two consecutive sessions.

In the first she started by talking about cats. How was my cat? Did it miss me while I was at work? Her cats got jealous of one another: the older one pushed the younger one off her bed where they slept.

Then she drew a picture. It showed a house, divided down the middle. In each half there was a female figure and a clock. The figure on the left was young and pretty, the clock showed 3 o'clock; the figure on the right was old and untidy, the clock showed 4 o'clock. Her comment was 'This shows how you can grow old in an hour.'

Then she became quiet and lethargic. She tried to draw again, but couldn't. 'What do other people draw?' she asked. Then she showed me her bag. It had been given to her by a friend, a fellow student from college days. This girl had invited her to her art exhibition but the patient couldn't go. 'I just couldn't bear it, it wasn't like ordinary jealousy.'

Now it was time to stop. Do the 'others' mind if she comes again next time? (She asks this often.) She rang later in the day and asked: 'Could I come and sit in your room, not to disturb you?'

Comment

This session is saturated with the feeling of sibling jealousy. The older cat is jealous of the younger one. She is worried about my cats, are they jealous of her? When her sister was born she had to 'grow old in an hour'. Her anger made her grow ugly. She felt unwanted. The only hope was to find what 'other' people drew, to imitate them; but it is impossible, her jealousy is so strong she can't bear to look at her friend's pictures. Leaving me means being replaced by 'others'; she rings later to check if a rival is with me.

The next session starts with her apologising for ringing me: she felt so alone: she had been alone all her life. 'My mother didn't like children.' She draws a picture: a large voluptuous reclining female figure; below is a smaller, frightened looking female.

Then comes an early memory. She had to have her photograph taken. She was frightened of going into the dark room; a man gave her a doll to comfort her. After the picture was taken she had to give it back. This made her cry. She commented: when her sister was born she was 'given away' like that by her mother.

She remembers how her mouth used to hurt when her teeth came in: how she used to bite the other children at school. 'You wouldn't believe it now, but I was a real terror at school.' Once she tried to kill another child.

It is near the end of the session. Do I really want to see her next week? It is such a long time to wait. Nothing happens in between.

Comment

In this session she shows her feeling that her mother betrayed her by bringing a rival into the world. She had to give her mother 'back' like the doll in the memory. She felt murderous towards the rival: she could bite and scratch – like a cat perhaps. She can get mother back by being mother to her little cats. Sometimes she can imagine me as her mother, but the illusion is shattered by the end of the session when I 'give her away'. 'Nothing' happened between sessions, just as she had 'no' childhood. She has built her life around this denial of the painful reality of being a sibling.

Discussion

At the core of the sibling relationship is an ambivalence: the paradox of rivalrous allegiance of two children to the same parents. As Hopkins (1953) put it: 'Abel is Cain's brother and breasts they have sucked the same'; or, in Freud's formulation,

> Each of us wants to be the favourite; the older child would like to eliminate his successor, to rob it of his privileges. At the same time he recognizes that his rival is equally loved by his parents; he cannot destroy him without destroying himself.
> (Freud, 1921)

This rather grim view of the sibling relationship runs through the psychoanalytic canon. But there is a positive side: if the 'belly of the mother is the universe of the infant' (Klein, 1969), then to be a sibling is to find one is not alone in the universe. Acceptance of siblings seems to be associated with health, and coming to this acceptance an important ingredient in treatment. A preliminary to this, however, may be the acknowledgement of feelings of sibling rivalry.

Thus, the arrival of a sib, whether in reality for the first-born, or psychologically, in the developing consciousness of the later-born, presents the child with a developmental challenge. The child has to accept that he or she is not the sole object of parental love, but that love has to be shared with others. The child's earliest emotions centre on the parents. When siblings arrive the situation changes: he is now for the first time faced with an equal to whom he has mixed feelings.

The child may deal with hostile impulses towards his equal in a number of different ways. There may be open hostility, with remarks such as 'Why don't they send the baby back to the shop?'; the hostility may be directed towards himself, when he becomes whiny and miserable or withdrawn; or the child may deny the reality of the newcomer altogether, ignoring him or pretending that he doesn't exist.

Other children may want to play with their new sib at once and feel furious at their unresponsiveness. The child may cope with hostile feelings by regressive identification, with temporary bedwetting for example. Finally, the child may deal with his rivalry by becoming a 'little mother' to the baby, helping with nappy-changing, feeding, etc.

These reactions are probably seen transiently in all children (Sturge, 1977). Which of them predominates, and whether or not they stick in the child's character, may depend on the family context in which they occur.

How can we characterise this context? Parsons and Bales (1955) have pointed out that entry into the Oedipal phase involves moving from a two- to a four-body system, not to a three-body system as it is usually construed. As the child becomes aware of his parents as separate entities, and of the differing roles of his father and his mother, simultaneously he becomes aware of the fact of sexual differentiation among children: his gender is his destiny, and he or she is a little boy or a little girl and cannot be both. As Freud (1916) puts it, 'When other children appear on the scene the Oedipus complex is enlarged into a family complex.'

The world at this stage can be divided 'vertically' into males and females and 'horizontally' into parents and children. This gives a four-way matrix with which the child can categorise himself and his family. This matrix contains the Oedipal triangle of mother–father–child but also two more triangles: mother–sib–child and father–sib–child. Each of these can be 'positive' or 'negative' (Freud, 1923), loving or hating, and each interlocks with the others.

The predominant mode of the sibling relationship depends on this four-way matrix and its vicissitudes. A range of environmental constellations can be imagined. A crucial factor may be the availability of the father. Thus he may be physically absent, or angry at mother's preoccupation with the new baby, or he may vent his feelings on the other child who has turned to him. Conversely he may mediate between the displaced child and his newly preoccupied mother – after all they are both in the same boat. The mother may be able to relate easily to only one child at a time, thus fostering feelings of exclusion in the others. She may sexualise her relationship with the infant, encouraging an envious cross-sex identification in the older child; she may favour older children, which may lead to self-denigratory or depressive feelings in the younger ones, especially if of the opposite sex. On the other hand, she may have the happy knack both of being able to respond to her children's individual needs and of maintaining a balance in the whole family so that those needs can be best met.

Where one child is handicapped or exceptional, there are important reverberations throughout their sibship. Their brothers and sisters frequently feel neglected and may experience intense guilt at their own hostile reactions to their disadvantaged sibs – they may imagine themselves responsible for the handicap. Excessive guilt, or even somatising reactions modelled on the sibling illness, may follow in later life.

Finally grandparents, like fathers, may play a vital role in helping families to adjust to a new member. The older children may be handed over to their grandparents and so for a while enjoy the advantages and disadvantages of the grandparental relationship. This is often a unique blend of indulgence and conflict-free love, together with a lack of the normal intensity of parent–child feelings.

The grandparent is often a focal point in the family network, and the child may feel – through contact with other family members via his grandparent – an enrichment that more than compensates for his lost sense of specialness. But if the 'handing over' is felt to be irreversible and the child feels he has lost his parent for ever, however loving the grandparent, there may be an enduring sense of loss.

Family growth links through the sibling relationship with the growth of the individual. Here the family matrix offers the growing child a chance to develop a sense of equality and ability to share; it is also at the critical point that family difficulties may be internalised as individual pathology.

CHAPTER 5

THE PSYCHOLOGY OF NUCLEAR DISARMAMENT

A case study

The psychology and psychiatry of the nuclear arms race have been discussed in three main ways. One approach has looked at the possible psychological consequences for the surviving population of a nuclear war. These studies, which have covered a wide range of catastrophies, including the Hiroshima and Nagasaki bombs and Nazi concentration camps, as well as natural disasters such as floods and cyclones, all point in the same direction. When half or more of a person's social and physical environment is destroyed, the effects on the human psyche are devastating. The phrase 'the survivor syndrome' has been used to describe the state of psychological shock and disablement which results in those that are left behind by the dead. Its effects outlive the physical sequelae of such disasters and are matched in longevity only by the slowly developing cancers which manifest themselves two or more decades after a thermonuclear explosion. These studies make the scouting-for-boys and cricketing atmosphere evoked by the British Government pamphlet *Protect and Survive* or the Civil Defence exercise 'Square Leg' in the 1970s seem remote from the likely psychological reality of a post-nuclear-attack world.

A second type of study assesses the effects of living in a nuclear age on the psychological development of the population. Mack (Sagan et al., 1986), for example, suggests that feelings of powerlessness and pessimism among the young, and even their penchant for disaster films, can be understood as a reaction to the nuclear threat. Against this must be set the fact that apocalyptic movements predicting the end of the world, espoused especially by young people, existed long before the advent of nuclear weapons.

Thirdly, the arms race itself can be considered in psychological terms, extrapolating from individual psychology to the behaviour of nations. In stepping out of its professional role to comment on wider issues or world affairs, psychiatry runs the risk of irrelevance or arrogance. However, it is this approach that I shall follow. This is justified on two grounds. The difficulties of disarmament are so great, and the dangers of the continuing arms race so worrying, that any new angle may be helpful. Also, for those who are prepared to recognise them, the fears created by the threat of nuclear war can now be seen directly affecting our professional lives. This discussion is based on a case seen in a psychiatric out-patient clinic in which fear of imminent nuclear war was a central issue in the patient's illness.

Case history

The patient was a single woman in her early thirties, middle class, professional, feminist; she had had a brief, childless marriage some years before. She came for help because over the previous weeks she had developed a state of paralysing panic. The basis of it was simple, she said: she was convinced of the imminent probability of nuclear war. Every time she heard a plane pass overhead she feared that it was a bomber carrying nuclear warheads. Every time the traffic made a loud noise it made her think of invading tanks. Worse than noise was news. She was unable to watch television, listen to the radio, or read a newspaper. She could not use public transport in case she saw the newspaper headlines of her fellow passengers. When she did encounter the media, their message all pointed in the same direction – war was inevitable. Every action of the world leaders suggested it; every local conflict might provide the spark that would ignite the final conflagration. To survive this nightmare she had built a complicated cocoon for herself in which she was protected from daily reminders of the holocaust which she was convinced was to come. Yet within her psychological bunker she was still far from safe. After feeling a little better one evening, she went to visit some new friends, and was horrified after an excellent dinner to be given a tour of inspection of the house, including the cellar which had been converted into a fall-out shelter!

By most standards she was a brave woman: she had travelled widely on her own, and had a demanding job which exposed her to much human suffering. Beneath her anxiety and phobias she was clearly depressed. The origins of her breakdown gradually unfolded. The immediate precipitant seemed to be a conflict aroused by her wish to have a child. She longed to commit herself to her lover, and to have a baby by him, but feared that she would not be good enough as a mother, that she might damage the child. Because of similar doubts she had previously had an abortion, which had left her feeling guilty and regretful, although still convinced it was the right decision.

Her worries and guilt about her aggressive feelings, and doubt in her capacity to care for a child, went further back than this. They seemed to centre on an adoring father in whose eyes she could do no wrong. Envious and angry towards her brother and sisters, and cut off from her mother by her 'special' relationship to her father, she would often behave badly, but he could find no fault in her.

She was offered a series of psychotherapeutic sessions. A turning point came when she had a dream in which she had been in the audience at a lecture where she had felt 'bludgeoned' by the male speaker, a doctor. This related in part to her presenting symptom in which she was the silent witness to the world's aggression. It also referred to her position as a patient and to her envy of doctors. However, there was a curious reversal in the dream: through most of the sessions her doctor-therapist had been a nearly silent audience to her anxious and at times demanding discourse. Eventually he suggested that the dream perhaps contained a reference to this rather 'bludgeoning' part of herself. At this point she recalled that as a small child she had been left alone with her baby cousin and had viciously hit him on the head. He appeared to pass out and she was terrified that she had killed him. She had never dared to tell anyone (including her previous therapist) of this incident. It seemed as though the discovery of this residue of apparently gratuitous aggression, and having the chance to reveal it in an accepting but not uncritical atmosphere, was a great relief to her. Her panic about the impending end of the world lessened. Her other symptoms began to recede. Another crisis arose when she became pregnant, but this time she was able to accept it, and soon afterwards she married her lover, though not without more misgivings.

Discussion

When the patient came for treatment she was locked in a fierce and incapacitating internal battle. This was her neurosis. However real the threat of nuclear war, and however healthy it may be to be anxious about it, her fear was so great that we must call it a neurosis. Healthy anxiety produces the arousal needed to act to try to remove its cause – hers made her less able to act. It should be said, however, that, if her neurosis was one of exaggerated sensitivity to nuclear threat, there is an equal and opposite and usually undiagnosed affliction of excessive indifference to the possibility of nuclear war. She had confused her own inner violence with an external threat. Later – partially disarmed – she began to trust herself. She could then co-operate with her aggression and put it to good use in her struggle to per-suade her lover that their relationship and her pregnancy were a good thing, for he had been as ambivalent as she. Her fear of disaster became a rational concern about nuclear weapons.

Can we learn any wider lessons from this case of personal disarmament? The first point is a general one. The difficulty which nations face in trying to disarm is not unlike the problem of the neurotic patient. It may be generally agreed that it would be desirable to disarm and that nuclear weapons are unacceptably danger-ous; the neurotic patient is often prepared to try any measure to rid himself of his symptoms; yet in both cases it is extraordinarily hard to make progress. Rational effort alone seems inadequate. In both, it seems likely that there are powerful unknown forces maintaining the status quo.

What are these forces? No doubt for disarmament these are economic, politi-cal and social. They may be psychological as well. The patient's fear was of attack from without. She was frightened of the bomb which would drop on her and her world. Her recovery began when she realised that she was as persecuted by her *own* aggression as she was by any external enemy. She had projected long-forgotten destructive impulses, never adequately acknowledged by her father, on to every passing aeroplane. When she faced up to, and could begin to accept, her warlike wishes, her peace of mind returned.

Projection is intrinsic to the arms race, too. *We* have defensive, deterrent, peace-keeping nuclear weapons, while *they* have aggressive, expansionist, first-strike bombs. By locating all the aggression in the enemy we avoid looking at the threat we pose to them. The remoteness of nuclear weapons and the 'unthinkability' of nuclear war provide excellent vehicles for such projections. They become beautiful machines whose impact is far removed from any direct experience we may have of hurting or being hurt. Military personnel in charge of nuclear warheads are deliberately not told where their weapons are aimed. One such soldier had no difficulty in visualising his own family and city being destroyed by a Soviet attack. When he was then asked to imagine the effects which his weapons would have on his oppo-nent in the Soviet Union he demurred, saying that this was unthinkable, that it would undermine his whole job if he were to begin to consider it. He was far more disturbed by the thought of his own destructiveness than by that of the enemy.

There are two aspects to the process of projection. First, there is the projection itself, then there is the content or nature of the projection. This is often a primitive and distorted fantasy. The patient imagined that her little cousin was dead, that she had annihilated him: in fact she had simply given him a nasty bruise. In adult life her violent inner wishes were transformed into horrifying images of nuclear attack, which paralysed and terrified her. When she took the projections back into herself and saw them for what they were – a residue of childish feelings which she had long outgrown – their spell was broken.

Similarly, each of the superpowers sees in its opponent an image of its own ambition, expansionism and desire for absolute superiority. This terrifying vision of the enemy then fuels the race for more fearsome deterrents on each side. In this atmosphere of mutual projection it is impossible for each side realistically to assess the threat which the other poses. For example, commentators seem to have great difficulty in gauging the likelihood of a Russian invasion of Great Britain. If each side were able to acknowledge its *own* wish to attack and humiliate the enemy, rather than steadfastly insisting that its armaments were merely defensive, it might then be easier to look at how great the actual threat is, and whether it is more or less dangerous than possessing nuclear weapons. Unfortunately, there is an important difference from the neurotic patient. Her childish fantasy of the damage she had done far exceeded the reality. It was reassuring for her to realise this. Nuclear weapons, on the other hand, are almost certainly *more* damaging than we imagine, despite the efforts of the military to 'normalise' our attitude towards them.

To summarise: an important impediment to disarmament lies in the fiction, fiercely held by both sides, that neither has aggressive intentions towards the other. The moral argument for disarmament turns on this point, since it questions the rightness of being prepared to destroy a civilian Soviet population – the very basis of deterrence. It is not merely 'good', but good psychological sense, to start from this point. It encompasses the paradox that the fight for peace is often proclaimed with such violence by its protagonists. It might also lead to the conclusion that defence *is* necessary, but that nuclear – as opposed to conventional – weapons are unrealistically dangerous. An aggressive approach to disarmament would be putting each side's wish to beat the enemy to good use.

There are three other psychological themes relevant to disarmament that arise from this case. The first concerns defence – a term common to both psychiatry and military strategy. So great were the patient's anxieties that as her neurosis developed she diverted more and more of her energies into defending herself, leaving correspondingly less and less drive for a productive life. A similar process may affect nations, whose economies become increasingly distorted by their defence budgets. Japan [at the time of writing] was an example of a country in which defence spending is exceptionally low and whose productivity is high. The patient was trapped by a defensive dilemma which affects both individuals and nations facing the arms race. She could either retreat into a massively defended state of isolation or emerge to be swamped by the horror of the nuclear threat. Both positions immobilised her. These two extremes are not uncommonly seen in people's responses to the arms race. Some are unconcerned and indifferent, while others inhabit a nightmare world of apocalypse and holocaust. A possible role for the medical profession is to alert the public to the great dangers of nuclear war without falling into either hysteria or complacency.

The second point centres on the notion of envy. The patient's hidden memory was of her attack on her baby cousin. In trying to understand this recollection, to find a reason for her apparently unprovoked aggression, she was helped by the idea that it may have sprung from envy. She remembered how she felt excluded by the admiration that this baby aroused, and her secret wish for revenge, to feel her power over the baby. She had felt at the mercy of her parents' whims: now the tables were turned. There is great mutual envy between the superpowers, and both perhaps have in common an envious attitude towards Europe, towards its cultural history and hegemony. For the USA, this is towards the parent culture while, for the USSR, Western Europe is like an older sibling with whom one can never quite catch up. For both there is an attitude of contempt and a primitive wish to destroy the envied rival.

The opposite of destructiveness and aggression is creativity. This leads to a final point. The patient's problem was triggered by questioning her most basic creative capacity: the ability to bear and love a child. Only when she was less frightened by her imagined destructiveness could she begin to trust her creative impulse and not abort it, as she had done before. In a similar way, the issue of disarmament is more and more linked up with the need to abolish world poverty and hunger. The Brandt report suggests that if there were general disarmament many of the 15 million children who die each year from starvation might be saved. There are psychological as well as economic reasons why it is unlikely that real progress will be made towards lessening the rich–poor gap until the arms race is halted. We are haunted in the West by the ghosts of Hiroshima and Nagasaki – just as the patient was in the grip of her guilty past. Awareness of guilt alone was useless – it merely made her depressed and inactive. Only when she could forgive herself did she change. While we live in the shadow of our own destructiveness it is unlikely that we can trust or believe in our capacity to create and preserve life.

Conclusion

The inbuilt biological response to fright is flight, fright, or freeze. There are two situations in which we can neither run away nor fight and win. The first is when the threat is internal. That is the problem for neurotics, who in the end cannot escape from themselves even though they frequently try to do so. The second is when the threat is all-pervasive. That is the case – at least in the northern hemisphere – with nuclear weapons. We may run the risk of destroying ourselves with them, but we cannot run away and hide. The threat can be dealt with initially by projection. The problem was eliminated for the patient by externalising her aggression, projecting it on to a threatening world; in the arms race it is done by locating the threat entirely in the 'enemy'. This works for a while, but not for ever. Eventually the repressed aggression returns, becomes a persecutor, incapacitates. We are becoming socially and morally incapacitated by the arms race. At this point there is only one solution: to face the reality of the threat. As in the legend of the Medusa, the defensive shield has to become a mirror. By reflection, the Gorgon's head can be removed. This is dangerous enough. The risk of failure is greater: to be burned and blasted and irradiated to stone.

PSYCHODYNAMIC PSYCHIATRY

This section consists largely of two extended surveys, written a quarter of a century apart but compatible in spirit. Both attempt to situate and validate the role of psychodynamics within psychiatry. Chapter 6 formed part of a long introduction to my clumsily named compendium *A Textbook of Psychotherapy in Psychiatric Practice* (1991), now, sadly, out of print. (I have since discovered how vital good titles are in selling books.) This was my first effort at editorship, and I assembled a group of friends, colleagues and former teachers aiming to cover the range of psychotherapies as applicable to the major psychiatric disorders. Chapter 10, reprinted here with the kind permission of my co-editors Sid Bloch and Stephen Green, is also from a multi-author book, *Psychiatry: Past, Present, and Prospect* (PPPP, aka GGG – The Good, the Great and the Grey), in which senior psychiatrists of differing persuasions look back on the state of their art and where they think the discipline is going. These bookends encompass three diagnostically oriented pieces: an attachment-oriented attempt to integrate interpersonal and biological approaches to depressive illness; a plea for narrative-based medicine and psychiatry; and a review article rebuttal of radical anti-psychiatry, arguing the case for integrative approaches to psychosis. An appendix to the first of these is a contribution to the *BMJ* series in which patients describe their experience of illness. In this case a patient of mine, Jackie, kindly invited me to write about her depression from the doctor's point of view.

PSYCHODYNAMIC PSYCHIATRY

CHAPTER 6

PSYCHOANALYTIC PSYCHOTHERAPY

This chapter is divided into three parts. The first stakes out the definitions and philosophies which inform the psychodynamic approach. The detailed study of case histories lies at the heart of psychotherapeutic work; the second part consists of two paradigmatic psychiatric cases presented from a psychotherapeutic point of view. Based on these cases, the third part considers the contribution of psychoanalysis to psychiatry, looking at assessment, formulation and diagnosis from the viewpoint of psychoanalytic psychotherapy.

The relationship between psychiatry, psychoanalysis and psychotherapy is one of continuing debate and exploration (Pedder, 1989; Wallerstein, 1989). Psychoanalysis took North America by storm in the 1920s and 1930s and, despite recent redefinitions, remains firmly within the mainstream of American psychiatric culture. The acceptance of psychotherapy within British psychiatry has, by contrast, been much more cautious. This is partly a result of the militant empiricism of the dominant Maudsley school, whose legitimate scepticism about the wilder claims of psychotherapy has turned at times into destructive dismissiveness (Will, 1984). This resistance has been mirrored by a reluctance on the part of psychoanalysis to integrate with psychiatry, for fear of being assimilated or marginalised.

The climate of mutual suspicion has abated in recent years. In the background have been sociological and economical changes which have affected psychiatry and psychotherapy alike. A purely medico-biological approach in psychiatry is no longer acceptable: patients also need and expect the understanding and interpersonal skills which psychotherapy can offer in response to their distress. Another important change has been the development of community psychiatry, which means that psychiatrists are no longer in a position of hegemony but share their power and influence with psychologists, community nurses, general practitioners and social workers, all of whom need psychotherapeutic skills and understanding if they, and their clients, are to survive the fragmentation of the post-institutional era. At the same time, psychotherapy can no longer afford to remain insulated from scientific evaluation. In an era of limited resources and rising expectations, the pressure for widely applicable, cost-effective and briefer forms of therapy grows ever more insistent.

The distinction between the biological and psychotherapeutic approaches in psychiatry can be traced back to the two great strands of European thought: those represented by the Enlightenment, with its valuation of reason, order and stability, and Romanticism, with its emphasis on individuality and the importance of the emotions and of change. Psychotherapy is perhaps closer to the romantic impulse in its valuation of individual experience and biography, its recognition of the power of the imagination, and the need to find a meaning and purpose in life (Holmes & Lindley, 1997). But there have been changes in philosophical perspective that blur these once clear demarcations between reason and imagination, science and art. It is clear, as Freud believed, that scientific methods can be brought to bear on human problems without necessarily being reductionist or dehumanising. It is also accepted that science itself is a system of meanings that cannot be value-free or absolute in its approach to the truth and, when reduced to scien*tism*, becomes a way of avoiding rather than revealing reality. A biomedical approach which sees depression simply in terms of an illness for which the appropriate drug should be prescribed, and ignores the part played by adverse life experience, is as obtuse as a psychotherapy which denies the relevance of genetics to schizophrenia. The emphasis in contemporary philosophy of science is on the *duality* of disease-causative and biographical-teleological models (Wallace, 1989). Rorty (1989) argues for tolerance and pluralism, seeing science and poetry as 'alternative modes of adaptation to reality'. Given the dominance of science in contemporary culture, this duality is inevitably unequal; psychotherapy has gained some measure of acceptance but is often relegated, as Freud (1926) anticipated, to 'one of many forms of treatment in psychiatry'. One aim of this book is to redress this imbalance.

Classification and definition of psychotherapies

The plea for pluralism is equally applicable within psychotherapy itself, which has at times been riven by conflict between competing models and techniques. This lack of unity has itself contributed to the marginalisation of psychotherapy. The author is firmly wedded to the view that only the full *range* of psychotherapies can meet the varying needs of psychiatric patients, and that the psychotherapies themselves can only benefit from mutual influence and cross-fertilisation. Once the plurality of psychotherapies is accepted, two problems arise. Firstly, an overall definition of psychotherapy is required that encompasses the great variety of approaches; secondly, there is a need for a classification that will differentiate and distinguish the main psychotherapeutic schools.

A possible overall definition of psychotherapy is as follows:

> Psychotherapy is a form of treatment based on the systematic use of a relationship between therapist and patient – as opposed to pharmacological or social methods – to produce changes in cognition, feelings and behaviour.

The advantage of this definition is that it emphasises the essentially *interpersonal* nature of the psychotherapeutic relationship, from which much of its power derives; technique, although of no less importance, can only be effective if a good therapeutic alliance is established. This definition is also wide-ranging enough to include most of the varieties of psychotherapy currently practised. Given this overall definition, the psychotherapies can be classified according to *theory, technique, setting, mode, length* and *level*, although none of these distinctions is entirely clear-cut.

Classification according to *theory* distinguishes between the Analytic, Behavioural-Cognitive, Systemic and Experiential-Humanistic approaches, but even within these broad categories there is much common ground. Most psychotherapies contain ingredients from more than one theoretical approach; a good example is Cognitive Analytic Therapy, which combines psychoanalytic and behavioural theories in a novel way.

Table 6.1 The psychotherapy 'matrix'

Theory	Technique	Mode	Setting	Timing	Level
Psychoanalytic	Interpretive	Individual	General practice	Very brief	Self-help
Behavioural	Directive	Group	Outpatient	Brief	'Level 1': counselling
Cognitive	Expressive	Couple	Day hospital	Time-limited	
Systemic	Supportive	Family	Inpatient	Indefinite	'Level 2':
'Humanistic'	Paradoxical				non-specialist psychotherapy
				> one/week	'Level 3':
				weekly	specialist psychotherapy
				< one/week	

Therapists' interventive *techniques* can be divided into those that are directive, interpretive, supportive, paradoxical, challenging and expressive; most therapies contain a combination of techniques, although the proportions vary greatly. Psychotherapeutic *settings* also vary widely from inpatient units to mental health centres and day hospitals, from psychotherapy departments to general practitioners' surgeries. Therapy can be in individual, group or family/marital *mode*. The *length* of psychotherapeutic treatment varies from one or two sessions to several years, although the average therapy within the National Health Service takes probably no more than a few months. Finally, classification by *level* of training and sophistication of the practitioner (which arouses much passion among therapists about their position within the psychotherapeutic pecking-order) ranges from the 'level 1' of basic counselling, through an intermediate 'level 2' practised by many psychiatrists, social workers, psychologists and nurses, to specialist 'level 3' treatments such as psychoanalysis (Pedder, 1989).

Psychotherapeutic psychiatry

This chapter is predominantly focused at 'level 2' practitioners – that is, at psychotherapeutically minded psychiatrists and other mental health workers who wish to bring psychotherapeutic methods and ideas to bear upon the patients and problems encountered in general psychiatric work. Psychotherapeutic esotericism is eschewed, but the difficulties posed by attempting psychotherapy with the mentally ill are not underestimated. My aim is to describe a *psychotherapeutically informed psychiatry*, or a *psychiatric psychotherapeutics*, relevant to the patients who are treated in psychiatric departments and to those who work in such units.

Psychotherapy has a dual role within psychiatry, both as an overall approach which takes account of the interpersonal and psychological aspects of any clinical situation and as a set of specific methods of treatment: psychotherapy in its adjectival as well as its substantive form, with being psychotherapeu*tic* as well as practising psychotherapy. It is just as important for a psychiatrist to understand the psychotherapeutic implications of routine practice – prescribing drugs, compulsorily detaining patients, or even making referrals for psychotherapy – as it is to be skilled in specific psychotherapeutic techniques. From this perspective, psychiatry should be practised psychotherapeutically always, should use psychotherapeutic methods as an adjunct often, and provide formal psychotherapy whenever necessary.

Outcome and the 'matrix paradigm'

Does psychotherapy *work*? Critics have claimed that psychotherapy is no more than, or no more effective than, placebo treatment and that psychoanalysis in particular is a non-scientific closed system of thought. The details of these charges and their rebuttal are exhaustively discussed elsewhere (Holmes & Lindley, 1997; Lambert, 2003; Roth & Fonagy, 2006). Their value has been to sharpen the debate and to force psychotherapists to examine their work more critically.

Psychotherapy research is a difficult and uncertain field; nevertheless, certain conclusions can confidently be stated. Firstly, psychotherapy is unquestionably effective. A standard method for evaluation of therapies is the measurement of 'effect size'; this is a comparison of the treatment and control group means on standard outcome measures. The method of meta-analysis, based on averaging large numbers of studies, has consistently shown that the effect size for psychotherapy is around 1 standard deviation (SD) unit. This means that the average psychotherapy patient does better than do 85 per cent of control subjects. Put another way, 70 per cent of psychotherapy patients improve significantly, while 30 per cent do not; 30 per cent of controls improve spontaneously, while 70 per cent remain the same (Roth & Fonagy, 2006). These figures are comparable with the results for anti-depressant therapy, where the effect size is also around 1 SD.

Secondly, these outcome studies are based on a 'drug metaphor' (Stiles & Shapiro, 1989) which, although useful, can be overplayed. Placebo psychotherapy can never be delivered blind as it can be in a drug trial. Psychotherapy is concerned with people, not physiologies, so expectations and assumptions make an inescapable contribution to outcome. It is important to note that 'placebo' treatments *do* produce change (with effect sizes of around 0.5), supporting the view that 'non-specific factors', as well as specific techniques, are important in psychotherapy.

A third conclusion concerns the differences between varying therapeutic approaches. The meta-analytic studies combine the results of many different types of therapy – behavioural, cognitive and analytic. On the whole, no consistent differences in outcome have been demonstrated for the different therapies, although some studies (e.g. Shapiro & Firth-Cozens, 1987) suggest slightly better results for cognitive-behavioural than for analytic methods, which may partly reflect the greater ease with which treatment goals can be specified in cognitive-behavioural therapies. This apparent equivalence of outcome between therapies has led to Luborsky's (Luborsky *et al.*, 1989) celebrated 'dodo-bird' verdict: 'Everybody has won and all must have prizes.'

The discrepancy between different techniques yet similar outcomes has been called the 'equivalence paradox' (Stiles, Shapiro & Firth-Cozens, 1988), for which a number of different explanations have been put forward. Frank (1986) emphasises the common factors in all therapies. These include 'positive involvement' with a therapist who possesses empathy, genuineness and non-possessive warmth; the development of new perspectives on previously intractable problems, leading to 'remoralisation' and a new 'assumptive world'; and the opportunities for exploration and trial-learning made possible by the security of the therapeutic situation. Ryle (1990) has suggested elegantly that, since behaviour is organised hierarchically, from basic assumptions through phantasies and plans to overt behaviour, with reciprocal feedback between different levels, change at one level will eventually produce effects at all the others and should therefore lead to similar outcomes. A third possible explanation for the equivalence paradox is that it is a research artefact, produced by averaging large numbers of therapies, therapists and patients, and that, if teased out, different therapeutic methods would indeed be found to be effective for different clinical problems.

This latter possibility can be related to Paul's (1986) idea of a 'matrix paradigm' in psychotherapy. Paul suggested that for each clinical situation the therapist should ask the question: '*What* treatment, by *whom*, is most effective for *this* individual, with *that* specific problem, and under *which* set of circumstances?' This might be adapted for psychiatric patients as follows: 'What form of psychotherapy, delivered by which member of the multidisciplinary team, is most effective for this personality, with that specific disorder, and in which setting?' Paul's paradigm suggests that an open-minded, even-handed attitude is needed within psychiatric psychotherapy if the full range of patient characteristics and difficulties is to be met; this patient with schizophrenia needs a skilled family therapist if he is not to relapse when he returns home; this patient with an acute episode of depression will do better if he is offered cognitive analytic therapy as well as anti-depressant drugs; this patient with recurrent relationship difficulties and episodes of self-harm needs an analytic approach if her life is to take a more positive turn and the negative pattern is to be broken.

The indications for different psychotherapies: eclecticism

If every psychiatric patient can benefit from some form of psychotherapeutic consideration and intervention, the question of the indications for psychotherapy becomes not *whether* the patient can benefit from psychotherapy but, rather, *which type* of psychotherapeutic intervention is likely to be most appropriate, and at what *level* (see Table 6.1).

Various attempts have been made to refine criteria for the different modes and models of psychotherapy. Malan's criteria for brief analytic therapy (Malan, 1979) include good initial motivation; evidence of reasonable previous adjustment; the absence of exclusion criteria, such as psychosis, substance abuse or acute suicidal feelings; and the capacity to respond effectively to a trial interpretation. These criteria have been confirmed and extended by subsequent studies, showing that good outcomes from *all* forms of psychotherapy are associated with three main factors: a strong therapeutic alliance, in which the patient sees the therapist and the therapeutic process in a positive light; some degree of educational achievement; and evidence of motivation, as shown by the ability to remain in therapy for at least ten sessions.

Despite Malan's finding that severely disturbed patients could achieve good outcomes in brief psychotherapy, there is undoubtedly a research trend suggesting that, the less severely ill and less socially disadvantaged a patient is, the more likely he is to benefit from therapy of whatever type. As much as 50 per cent of the variance in psychotherapy outcome is related to patient characteristics such as these, rather than to features associated with the type of disorder or the personality of the sufferer (Karasu, 1986). Modifications of technique are necessary if the undoubted benefits of psychotherapy are to reach the more severely ill and the socially disadvantaged (Holmes & Lindley, 1997).

Paul's 'matrix paradigm' implies an ideal in which psychotherapeutic intervention is matched with patient need, in terms of both illness and personality. Proven examples of this include the efficacy of family and behavioural interventions in schizophrenia; of cognitive therapy in depression; and of brief therapy, analytic and behavioural, in anxiety/depression (Abbass *et al.*, 2008). Research tends to confirm the clinical impression that introverts do better with analytic forms of therapy, while extroverts fare better with behavioural treatments (Bloch & Crouch, 1985). Despite these certainties, the application of the matrix paradigm remains elusive. Most treatments contain a variety of therapeutic elements and are broad-spectrum rather than highly specific, and most studies have failed to find major differential outcomes between the different therapies. Certainly, a narrow-minded or sectarian psychotherapeutic stance will never be adequate to meet the range of client needs (Roth & Fonagy, 2006).

Most psychotherapists, however, are by training and persuasion wedded to a particular school or approach. This raises a fundamental dilemma within psychotherapy: despite the clinical need for even-handedness, in order effectively to conduct (or perhaps even to write about) psychotherapy, a particular theoretical viewpoint and technical stance is required. Eclecticism is beneficial to the patient in the sense that no one form of psychotherapy can possibly meet all psychotherapeutic needs; but eclectic approaches in clinical practice can be confusing, and therapists, while retaining flexibility, get better results by practising one clinical method in depth rather than trying to master them all. It is better to be able to play one instrument in all keys than to play many instruments in only one. Variety within psychotherapy is inevitable on practical grounds, but also for the theoretical reason that the individuality which psychotherapy aims to foster cannot result from a Procrustean therapeutic stance.

Drugs and psychotherapy

If psychotherapy is to establish itself as an integral part of psychiatry, it will, in the present climate, have to be justified on economic grounds. Cost-effectiveness will have to be demonstrated to those responsible for 'third-party payments' (the state or insurance companies). A balance sheet for psychotherapy can be drawn up comparing 'offset costs' resulting from successful psychotherapy – reduction in drug use, fewer ineffective psychiatric and general practitioner contacts, reduced dependence on welfare payments, the economic benefits resulting from a return to work – with the cost of providing the therapy.

But the rationale for psychotherapy cannot be based on economic grounds alone. Anti-depressants and psychotherapy produce roughly similar effect sizes (around 1). The now classic NIMH study of depression, which compared anti-depressants, 'general psychiatric management', and two forms of psychotherapy, Cognitive and Interpersonal (Elkin *et al.*, 1989), showed that all three were equally effective in mild depression, and that a differential effectiveness for drugs *or* psychotherapy over placebo-type general management emerged only for the more severe cases. Psychotherapists claim that psychotherapy produces *qualitative* improvement in patients' lives, such as increased autonomy, greater integration and maturity, which, although hard to measure, may significantly reduce relapse rates, as well as being in themselves ethically desirable (Holmes & Lindley, 1997).

In clinical practice, many psychiatric patients receive a combination of psychotherapy and drugs. There is a naive view that drugs and psychotherapy are mutually incompatible, because drugs 'dampen' emotions while therapy evokes them. This can be refuted both theoretically and practically. Psychotherapy requires the patient to become more open to feared or unwanted feelings, whether this comes about through transference or de-sensitisation. While this process is impossible if feelings are completely inaccessible, it is equally so if they are over-whelming. For psychotherapy to work, there has to be an intact 'observing ego', detached enough to report on feelings, understand them and, where necessary, modify or accommodate to them. Drug therapy (or even ECT) can help restore this observing ego.

This theoretical argument is supported by empirical studies which show, for example, in depression and heroin withdrawal, that psychotherapy and drug therapy together produce better results than either alone. Nevertheless, drugs are frequently prescribed inappropriately or excessively, often in response to dynamic pressures such as the patient's demandingness or the doctor's counter-transferential anxiety or aggression; these pressures need to be understood rather than acted upon.

The organisation and delivery of psychotherapy

The availability of psychotherapy, within both statutory services and the private sec-tor, is very variable. Psychotherapy is provided by psychologists, by psychotherapy departments led by consultant psychotherapists and some psychotherapeutically minded psychiatrists, and by private psychotherapists, as well as in a number of social service and voluntary agencies. For a particular patient with a particular prob-lem, the type of therapy offered (if any) is likely to be determined as much by geography, income and the availability of therapists and trainings as by clinical need. To some extent, this diversity is healthy, and is consistent with the emphasis in psy-chotherapy on the variety and uniqueness of individuals, but it conflicts with the view that people have a right to an equitable provision of psychotherapy services, no less valid than their right to medical, psychiatric or social provision (Holmes & Lindley, 1997).

The UK Psychotherapy Faculty of the Royal College of Psychiatrists has con-sistently advocated policies – on *manpower, training* and *service* – aimed to overcome this uneven and inequitable distribution. Firstly, it has argued that there should be at least one full-time consultant psychotherapist for every 200,000 of the population, approximately one for each health district. Secondly, it has estab-lished guidelines for the psychotherapeutic training of general psychiatrists, although, unlike the situation in Australasia, these were at the time of writing not yet mandatory; it is still possible to qualify as a psychiatrist in Britain with little or no psychotherapeutic knowledge or skill. Thirdly, it has described possible models for a psychotherapy service within the National Health Service (see Table 6.2).

Although these patterns vary greatly according to local conditions and the size of population served, all contain three basic elements: a specific treatment service for particular groups of patients: training and supervision for psychiatrists and other members of the multidisciplinary team: and a liaison service which includes consultation and staff support for mental health workers.

Clinical biography

At the heart of psychotherapy rests the individual, with his own unique biography or 'case history', forming the bedrock upon which all theorising and psychothera-peutic practice is based. As examples, two patients suffering from severe depressive

Table 6.2 Organisation of psychotherapy services

Level of organisation	Population	Description	Level of training	Staff numbers	Organisation/structure
Health centre/ community	Fewer than 50,000	1 Based in primary care 2 Offering counselling and some other therapies, e.g. behaviour therapy of simple phobias; bereavement counselling, etc., often as an adjunct to other treatments 3 Refer difficult patients to district	1 GP-practice-based counsellors, CPNs 2 Additional training and supervision available from district psychotherapy team 3 Some district staff working on sessional basis	1 Number variable and determined by local circumstances 2 Sessional input 3 Close links with voluntary and local authority sectors	1 Informal, dependent on local circumstances 2 Advised as necessary by district planning team for psychotherapy
District	150,000–300,000	1 A wide range of therapies offered, including individual short- and long-term dynamic psychotherapy, plus group, family and marital therapies 2 Part of departments of psychiatry/psychology 3 May be based in day hospital	1 Specialist staff mainly full- and part-time 2 Supported by non-specialist staff	1 Specialist staff approx. 5 WTE, e.g. 3 full-time plus 20 further sessions 2 At least one of 'core' teams should be a consultant psychotherapist	1 Multidisciplinary organisation with 'core staff group' 2 District planning team for psychotherapy
Region (sub-regional)	1–4 million	1 Specialised service to own district plus care of some 'difficult cases' from other districts 2 Offering a wide range of types and levels of training for the region	1 Multidisciplinary specialist team covering all major methods of psychotherapy	1 Specialist staff from psychiatry, psychology 2 Staff for basic district plus additional regional staff 3 At least two consultant psychotherapists	1 Regional planning group for psychotherapy 2 Advise districts and regions 3 Co-ordinate training service and other needs, e.g. library
National		1 Academic and training resource 2 Specialist provision of library and training resources			

Source: Based on Grant, Margison & Powell, 1991.

illnesses – both psychiatric rather than purely psychotherapeutic cases – will now be presented. In one, failure to appreciate psychodynamic issues may have contributed to a tragic outcome while, in the other, psychotherapeutic understanding may have made a significant contribution to recovery.

Case study 1: Depression and the dynamics of non-compliance

Mr A, a 40-year-old teacher, became profoundly and suicidally depressed in the face of, as he saw it, mounting pressure at work and 'an inability to cope with the demands being made of me'. He was strongly suicidal and was admitted to hospital, where anti-depressants were started. In hospital, he made himself useful to the nurses and spent much of his time looking after the other, more helpless patients. His depressive symptoms apparently then lifted, and after leaving hospital he discontinued his anti-depressants, saying that he wished to solve his own problems and not to be drugged and befuddled. He was offered psychotherapeutic sessions which were characterised by long intellectual battles between him and his therapist. After a while, he discontinued these too, saying that he preferred to seek co-counselling where he could work more collaboratively on his problems.

He was an only child; when he was eight years old, his father developed a progressive and crippling illness. Mr A admired his father's fortitude in the face of this illness, and felt that he could never possess similar courage. Because of the family difficulties, he was sent away to boarding school, where he dealt with his feelings of loneliness and exclusion by deciding to 'go it alone' rather than bother his already burdened parents with his anxieties. He experienced his mother as rigid and controlling and had never felt particularly close to her. He married a warm and supportive woman whom he idealised but whom he felt he was letting down by his illness, as he did his eight-year-old son. Some weeks after his discharge from hospital, despite close supervision from his general practitioner and psychiatrist, at a time when he was apparently doing well and preparing to return to work, he killed himself. It was clear from his notebooks that he had been planning suicide for several months.

This history illustrates how important it is to grasp the dynamic aspects of a case as part of general psychiatric management. Just as Mr A had felt alone in his teens, had felt that he *had* to be self-sufficient, that his own needs were insignificant in comparison with those of his father, just as he experienced his longing for intimacy and holding as shameful, so in his illness he experienced 'help' as humiliation, admission to hospital as a punishment analogous to being sent away to boarding school, and having to take medication as controlling rather than helpful. Consciously, he felt that he should be able to cure himself, meet his own needs, as he had done in his teens; unconsciously, this avoidant man felt deep unsatisfied longings, and rage when they were not met.

While some of this was apparent to the psychiatric team, much was not. This was particularly true of the relationship with his mother, which was *enacted* rather than *understood* by the staff, as they tried vainly to insist that he took his medication and stayed in hospital, rather as his mother had insisted that he wear warm clothes as she packed him off to boarding school. Had the staff appreciated this, a management strategy might have been devised that took more account of the fragility of his sequestered inner world, so at variance with his external show of competence, and they might perhaps have been more alert to the ever present possibility of suicide.

This sad case illustrates how psychodynamic forces are inevitably brought into play in any psychiatric encounter. Through *transference*, the patient's day-to-day relationship with the hospital staff is coloured and shaped by earlier relationships of which he and they are often unaware, in this case experiencing them as controlling and contemptuous of what he felt to be his 'weakness'. Under the *regressive* effects of illness, the normal balancing effect provided by the ego is lost, and the influence of false assumptions becomes exaggerated. If transferential forces are not appreciated by the staff, they are likely, under the sway of counter-transference, to enact them in a way that may be counter-therapeutic.

The next case shows how an understanding of these process can lead to dynamic change and contribute to recovery.

Case study 2: Depression and the need to regress

Ms B was a 20-year-old who left home for the first time to work as a nanny in a distant town. There she met a young man of whom she become very fond. Their relationship was platonic; she spent a lot of time 'mothering' him – washing his clothes, cooking for him and helping him with his career. Her profound depression was precipitated by the discovery that he already had a girlfriend. She felt deeply ashamed of her 'mistake' and returned home to her parents, unable to continue with her job. She became more and more depressed, mute and retarded, while her parents – especially her mother, who had herself experienced depression while Ms B was young – became frantic with worry. She was treated with antidepressants, mood stabilisers and phenothiazines with little improvement. Admission to hospital for a course of ECT was considered, and the suicide risk seemed very high. Her parents, especially the mother, were opposed to hospital admission and felt that the hospital staff could never offer the level of vigilance and concern which she had achieved, her mother having given up her job to be with her daughter 24 hours a day. Any suggestion that separation from home might be beneficial was met with intense anxiety and anger in the mother, who felt that she was being criticised and judged. Meanwhile, the psychiatrist who was seeing the patient for supportive therapy felt increasingly worried and hopeless, that his contributions were irrelevant, and that all important communication was between the patient and her mother, and not with himself.

Eventually, the patient was admitted briefly to hospital for a course of ECT, and then started to attend as a day patient. There was a perceptible though slight improvement, but the situation remained stuck and worrying. With the help of a family therapist, a new formulation and management plan was made. The patient's depression could be seen in terms of separation-individuation. Separation from her family had activated feelings of defective self-esteem and negative assumptions about herself, possibly linked to her mother's depression when she was young; she lacked an inner sense of inexhaustible value and importance. Her awakening sexual feelings and the rejection confirmed her feeling about herself as unacceptable, mirroring her feelings about the inaccessibility of her very hard-working and slightly emotionally aloof father (described by his wife as 'absolutely brilliant at everything – except psychotherapy!'). Under the regressive influence of a depressive illness the patient returned to a symbiotic state of fusion with her mother, the ultimate expression of which were her suicidal wishes (dead, she could at last merge with the universe/mother). In addition to the patient being seen individually, the family was offered family therapy sessions in which, rather than trying unsuccessfully to separate mother and daughter, their intense mutual involvement was encouraged, on the principle of *reculer pour mieux sauter*. The mother was seen as a necessary 'auxiliary ego' and was offered 'supervision' in her vital work of keeping her daughter alive. At the same time, the importance of the parents as a couple was emphasised through discussion about their courtship and life before becoming parents. Evidence of differences between family members was encouraged, aimed at helping them to see how it was possible to remain together yet healthily separate.

The patient began steadily to improve, and material emerged in the individual sessions which seemed to confirm both psychodynamic and systemic formulations. Encouraged by the therapist, the patient remembered a favourite fairy story. This was Hans Anderson's 'Little Mermaid', who fell in love with an earthly prince and was allowed to leave her watery home and join him in return for abandoning the power of speech. Eventually, he tired of her silence and sought a wife. Overcoming her murderous jealousy, the little mermaid returned to the sea. But she had lived on earth so long she was now unable to swim: neither fish nor flesh, her only hope was death. This fairy tale seemed to encapsulate Ms B's experience of falling in love; the perilous transition from water to land which went so wrong symbolised all her own fears and inhibitions about moving from attachment to her mother to finding a man, from being a child to being a woman. Later, as her improvement continued, she dreamed of an older man who was trying to provoke her and her family into anger, while a depressed girl who was almost out of sight watched from afar. Her associations to the dream were that her father was sometimes obstinate and her relief that the depressed part of her was now almost out of sight. Following this dream, she said that a most unusual family row had broken out at the dinner table, in which, to her surprise, she had joined in. The row came to a successful end when the family started to think of what the neighbours would say about all this noise coming from a normally quiet house, and at this they all dissolved into helpless laughter.

Finally, 18 months after her breakdown began, she was fully recovered and ready to leave home once more. At her last session, she described an incident from the start of her illness in which she had been driving home with her mother in the dark. Due apparently to her mother's carelessness, the car engine had suddenly blown up. Her father rescued them, but 'it took him a very long time to get the engine clear and working again', she said, wiping away a parting tear.

In this case, a common enough psychiatric occurrence – a patient's refusal to come into hospital – was understood in terms of an unassuaged wish to remain symbiotically linked to her mother, and the therapeutic arrangements took account of her further need to negotiate an 'Oedipal' (three-person: male–female) stage of development by offering individual and family therapy, and by seeing the mother *and* the 'official' therapist as of equal importance in her treatment. The transferential references to the therapist as an 'obstinate' father, who took a long time to get things clear, were noted but not interpreted. These cases illustrate the three levels at which psychotherapy can contribute to psychiatry. Firstly, it provides a general framework for understanding the patient and her illness. Secondly, it can act as a guide to the management of the patient, taking into account not just the illness itself, but also the reactions of the staff and the milieu in which treatment is conducted. Thirdly, it is a specific mode of therapy, either on its own, or in collaboration with other forms of treatment.

The analytic contribution

At its most simple, the psychoanalytical approach consists of a theory of *personal meaning* and a theory of *development*. As Frank (1986) has pointed out, in one sense *any* theoretical conception of illness or personal difficulty, including the purely biomedical, contains a theory of meaning. Even if depression is viewed as merely a disturbance of cerebral amine metabolism, this attributes meaning to previously inchoate experience and is both valid and valuable to the patient. Mr A's guilt towards his wife and son was partially relieved by understanding that his perceptions were distorted by his illness. Much of the practice of biological psychiatry contains informal cognitive challenge and restructuring of this sort. The psychoanalytical viewpoint is qualitatively different from this in that it seeks a *personal* meaning for the illness in terms of individual biography, and because it assumes a level of *unconscious* meanings which influence the behaviour of both patients and therapists. Mr A's guilt could be linked with his experience of feeling let down by his parents, due mainly to his father's illness, when he was at a similar age to that of his son. He was aware of the guilt but not, apparently, of the feelings of anger and disappointment which lay beneath it or of the *transfer* of these feelings into his relationship with the staff: they in turn were unaware of their enactment of the role of a coercive but ineffectual mother. Seen in this light, the psychotherapeutic task consists of decoding personal, often unconscious meanings (cf. Rycroft, 1985). This interpretive viewpoint can be traced back to Freud's method of formulating symptoms, like dreams, as a compromise between a wish and a defence, a covert message whose meaning needs to be unravelled (Freud, 1905).

Seeing psychotherapy as a hermeneutic or narrative (Strenger, 2013) discipline whose aim is to help the patient make personal sense of his problem or illness leaves open the question of how the *truth* of any particular interpretation or meaning is established. At a clinical level, this is usually based on the affective response of a patient to an intervention (Malan, 1979), but the fact that an interpretation feels 'right' does not establish its external validity: false beliefs may, at least in the short run, be as satisfying as true ones. The scientific underpinning of the psychoanalytic viewpoint lies in its account of psychological growth and development (Bowlby, 1988). The meanings that are established in psychotherapy are often arrived at intuitively, but not arbitrarily; they are based on a theory of psychological maturation – of attachment, loss, differentiation, the establishment of an inner world – no less real than that of physical development. Ms B was vulnerable to depression because of hypothesised developmental difficulties in her early years. Her mother had herself been depressed and may possibly have been unable fully to respond to her daughter's emotional needs. This may have left Ms B with an internal 'depressed mother' rather than a 'mother who delights in my mere existence' (Holmes, 2013), and therefore with a fragile store of self-esteem. She remained emotionally dependent on her mother at a point in her life cycle at which separation was expected. So long as she remained emotionally close to her mother, the internal shared 'depressed mother' remained concealed. The move away from the mother entailed in the 'Oedipal shift' towards the father was inhibited, so avoiding the experience of rivalry and ambivalence and anger, all of which are needed later for the establishment of autonomous relationships and object-choice. These themes then became realised as phantasies (or, in CBT terms, 'automatic thoughts'): 'My father does not want me, he really belongs to my mother', 'My boyfriend belongs to his proper girlfriend', 'The hospital can't look after me properly, they are so weighed down with the other patients.'

The analytic contribution to psychiatry comprises three distinct elements. Firstly, it contains of a series of speculative hypotheses about the *aetiology* of psychiatric disorder, about how early environmental influences, together with biological factors, predispose to illness in later life. Secondly, it provides a language for *understanding* mental life that, by taking account of the internal world, makes sense out of the experience of mental illness, whatever its scientific explanation. Thirdly, it consists of a *method of treatment*, which in some forms is of proven effectiveness. These could be seen as the *scientific, ethical–hermeneutic* and *pragmatic* dimensions of psychotherapy.

The models of mental illness used by psychotherapists can be thought of in terms of at least three causative hypotheses. Firstly, there is a simple 'linear' theory, in which adverse childhood experience is internalised and predisposes to breakdown in later life. This simple model is applicable to the sequelae of severe trauma, but needs to be supplemented by more complex interactional 'circular' models. Here adverse childhood experience, rather than being seen as 'causative', is activated by illness – whether biological or interpersonal in origin – and so colours and shapes the content, but not necessarily the form, of the illness. Thirdly, intrapsychic and interpersonal factors may produce either 'deviance amplification' (Hoffman, 1981) or resilience in the face of adversity. Psychotherapeutic intervention has an impact at a number of different points. It may reduce the amplification of illness by providing appropriate support; it may offer the patient methods of combating illness, as in cognitive therapy, where the patient learns to ward off negative assumptions and thought patterns; or, in analytic therapy, it may, through the therapeutic relationship, offer a new experience in which early adversity can be reworked and modified, while previously warded-off painful feelings are assimilated into a more integrated personality structure.

Lines of psychoanalytical thought

The *object-relations* approach (Greenberg & Mitchell, 1983) sees the individual as fundamentally object-seeking (as opposed to pleasure-seeking) and views action, thoughts and phantasies, including symptoms, as taking place within an inner 'representational world' containing the self and his objects. Four distinct lines of psychoanalytical thought will now be considered, each of which, although overlapping with the others, has made its own unique contribution and is relevant to a particular set of clinical problems. They will be considered in decreasing proximity to the mainstream of Freud's ideas.

Ego psychology: adaptation and defence

Ego psychology is particularly associated with the work of Freud's daughter Anna and with the American psychoanalyst Heinz Hartmann. It is derived directly from Freud's 'structural model' of the mind (Freud, 1923), in which the ego is seen as mediating between the demands of the instincts, on the one hand, and the restrictions imposed by reality and enforced by the internalised parents or 'critical agency', the superego, on the other. This model evokes a picture of accommodation, adaptation, compromise and dynamic equilibrium that is compatible with common-sense notions such as that of coping mechanisms. It can be compared with medical metaphors like that of cardiac decompensation occurring in a susceptible individual when faced with the increased circulatory demands imposed by pregnancy or infection. Perhaps because of these parallels, the ideas of ego psychology, especially that of defence mechanisms, have been quite widely accepted within psychiatry.

Valliant (1977) has systematised the analysis of defences, dividing them into three main groups: immature (e.g. splitting, projection), neurotic (e.g. repression, intellectualisation) and mature (e.g. sublimation, humour). According to this model, personality structure can be understood in terms of the habitual use of defence mechanisms to maintain equilibrium in the face of internal or external threat. Mr A tried to defend against feelings of failure, anger and emptiness by using the obsessional defences of intellectualisation, isolation and control. Illness results if defences are too rigid or inflexible (Reich's 'character armour') or stress is too overwhelming for equilibrium to be maintained.

Many patients suffering from neurotic depression or anxiety face problems in their relationships of ambivalence, rivalry, anger, fears about separation, and feelings of sexual inadequacy and failure. Freud tried to relate these to the Oedipal stage of development, in which the child needs to be able to love the parent of the opposite sex and at the same time tolerate feelings of rejection and anger associated with the realisation that this parent is not his exclusive property, but has to be shared with the same-sex parent (with whom identification has to occur despite this rivalry) and with siblings. In an era in which children are increasingly growing up in one-parent families, these ideas need modification. The contemporary child's deepest longing is often for an intact mother–father couple rather than the exclusive possession of one or other parent. Split families may still be understood in Oedipal terms, however, and the trauma of a 'reality which confirms the phantasy' (Symington, 1983) makes such family disruption doubly painful. Ego psychology also recognises that healthy development requires a balance between a nurturing intuitive 'feminine' aspect and a boundary-setting, protective 'masculine' function. This applies just as much to looking after patients as it does to bringing up children. Pedder (1989) has discussed the damaging separation between a 'feminine' intuitive psychotherapy and a 'masculine' scientific psychiatry; one of the aims of psychodynamic psychiatry is to overcome this stereotype.

Kleinian theory: splitting and containment

Despite its relevance to psychotic states, the impact within psychiatry of the work of Melanie Klein (1948, 1969) and her followers, such as Bion, Rosenfeld and Steiner, has been limited. Nevertheless, Kleinian theory has a great deal to offer in psychiatric practice. It provides a convincing account – whether or not it is an accurate reflection of the mental life of infants, upon which it is supposedly based – of the envy, destructiveness and splitting which characterises the behaviour and inner world of the psychotic and borderline personality-disordered patients who form a major part of psychiatric work. Also, through the theory of psychological *containment*, as opposed to physical restraint, it provides a basis for the therapeutic response needed to help such patients which is relevant to the era of community psychiatry. The concept of *projective identification* and the Kleinian emphasis on counter-transference illuminates the difficult feelings engendered in mental health workers by disturbed patients, and shows how these feelings can, if understood, be put to good therapeutic use.

Seen from a Kleinian perspective, Mr A had split his world into a good, caring, but unattainable 'mother-wife' and a controlling, dominating woman towards whom he felt intense anger. This split was repeated in relation to himself: an over-conscientious self and a secret, hateful self who planned his suicide. The apparently inexplicable anger which some staff members felt when in contact with him, despite their liking him as a person and their otherwise professional attitudes, was an example of projective identification: unacceptable or feared aspects of the self are projected onto those with whom the person is in contact, who then experience those feelings as if they were their own. The staff's anger and feeling of being controlled were reflections of *his* unacknowledged anger and powerlessness. The acceptance by the staff of the patient's decision to leave hospital and to stop anti-depressants – to 'go it alone' – confirmed the patient's sense that his fear and anger could not be contained, and so transmuted or detoxified, but had to be 'sent away'.

Attachment theory: security and loss

The work of John Bowlby (1988; Holmes 1993/2013) is notable for its combination of rigorous empiricism with a psychoanalytic perspective emphasising the importance of early childhood experience for subsequent health or illness. For Bowlby, the origin of healthy development is the secure and responsive attachment of the infant to the primary care-giver, usually the mother. This enables the infant to explore both his own feelings and the outside world and forms a basis for self-confidence and curiosity in later life. *Anxious attachment* may result if the mother is physically or emotionally unavailable, and this in turn predisposes to subsequent dependency and anxiety. The premature loss of a care-giver may make an individual vulnerable to later depression, especially if grief is unexpressed.

Parkes (2006) has studied the role of unexpressed grief in psychiatry, and Brown and Harris (1978) have used Bowlby's ideas in their model of depression, vulnerability to which depends partly on childhood experience of loss, and partly on the presence or absence of attachment-figures with whom an individual can confide when faced with pain or difficulty. Pedder (2010) has combined these ideas with an object-relations view of an inner world in which, as development proceeds, the physical attachment to the parents is replaced by an internal 'good parent' providing feelings of security and self-esteem. The breast is lost but is 'reinstated in the ego' (Klein, 1957); the individual achieves autonomy but can receive nurturance from within and without when needed. Where this internalisation of the good object is impaired, the individual will be vulnerable to depression, as may have happened with Ms B. The task of therapy then becomes that of providing a secure attachment from which healthy separation can eventually, and with appropriate grief, take place; all being well, the patient will have built up a reservoir of good therapeutic experiences on which to draw when faced with subsequent difficulties and losses.

The interplay between attachment, loss and grief continues throughout life, and one advantage of Bowlby's ideas is that they are applicable to the whole life cycle, rather than infancy and childhood being viewed as the sole determinants of later events. Influenced partly by Bowlby, and also by the ideas of Erikson (1965), psychotherapists now see adulthood as a continuing developmental process, a series of stages and crisis points, each with its own potential for growth, stasis or breakdown (Nemiroff & Colarusso, 1985).

Self-psychology: Kohut, Winnicott and others

The term 'self-psychology' is usually associated with the American psychoanalyst Heinz Kohut (1977). It is also relevant to a rather disparate group of British analysts, notably Winnicott (1971, 1972), Rycroft (1985), Laing (1960), Symington (1983) and Casement (1985), whose work is characterised by an emphasis on an experiencing self rather than a mechanistic ego; a reaction against the obscurities of psychoanalytic jargon, which Bettelheim (1982) claims is based on mistranslation; an emphasis on meaning rather than metapsychology; and an insistence that the real relationship with the therapist is as important as his technical skill. Both Winnicott and Kohut are concerned with how the developing infant 'comes alive' psychologically through the creative nurturance of the mother. The basis of this, for Winnicott, is the mother's capacity to act as a temporary container for the infant's fears and hatred until the child is mature enough for them to be reintrojected and integrated into his developing self. Winnicott describes a 'transitional space', an overlapping realm that is not-quite-baby and not-quite-mother, in which the infant learns to play and to develop a sense of creativity and relational autonomy. Transitional space is inhabited for Winnicott by transitional objects such as teddy bears and security blankets, but the mother herself can also be 'transitional' in this sense. Kohut (1977) proposes a similar view of the mother and later care-givers (including therapists) as 'self-objects': neither self nor objects, but an overlapping combination of both, extensions of the self without whom the individual feels depleted and lacking in self-worth.

These ideas have several important implications for psychiatry. Firstly, they help in the understanding of certain schizoid individuals who, behind the carapace of a false self, lack an inner sense of aliveness and creativity. Secondly, the emphasis on the real presence of the therapist as a curative factor in therapy links with research showing how Rogers's (1951) common factors in therapy, such as genuineness, empathy and warmth, contribute significantly to good therapeutic outcomes. Thirdly, Winnicott's emphasis on therapy as 'learning to play' links with active therapies which emphasise creativity and child-like exploration as legitimate and valid therapeutic activities. Ms B was helped by remembering the little mermaid fairy story that so poignantly encapsulated her situation in late adolescence – a fish out of water – which, like a transitional object, both provided some distance from her overwhelming feelings and was a creative expression of them.

Diagnosis and assessment in psychotherapy

According to Osler's aphorism, it is more important to know what kind of patient has a disease than to know what kind of disease a patient has. This contrast between disease and individual lies at the heart of the problem of diagnosis and formulation in both psychotherapy and psychiatry. A medical diagnosis implies the assignment of a set of symptoms to a disease category that reliably predicts pathology, response to treatment and prognosis. A psychotherapeutic formulation also attempts to summarise and systematise a set of disparate phenomena, to indicate appropriate treatment and to have prognostic value, but it differs from medical diagnosis in a number of significant ways. Firstly, it almost always contains theoretical assumptions, for example, about the influence of childhood experience on adult life, while psychiatric diagnosis tries to be theory-free. Secondly, it focuses on interpersonal themes and relationship difficulties rather than symptoms alone. Thirdly, it concentrates on the *particular* circumstances of the patient and his unique biography rather than on general classes of disease. Finally, it is arrived at partly by intuition, based on the therapist's subjective response to the patient, rather than relying exclusively on objective data.

A diagnosis – whether medical or psychodynamic – is a tool and cannot be divorced from its purpose. The discussion that follows will consider, firstly, the psychodynamic formulation as part of the general understanding of any psychiatric patient; secondly, the systematisation of these formulations into diagnostic schemata; and, thirdly, the use of these schemata to indicate and guide different psychotherapeutic treatments.

The assessment interview

The word 'assessment' contains two very different etymological implications. One derives from *assidere*, to sit beside, with its warm overtones of empathy and intuition. The other is associated with the idea of fiscal investigation for the purpose of taxation: a cold reckoning of assets, debts and deficiencies. The psychodynamic assessment combines both elements. Consider this account by the psychoanalyst Robert Stoller (1984):

> Let us imagine we are with a patient who we sense is sad. You cannot deny there are circumstances when the patient's welfare and what we do next depend on our distinguishing whether he is sad, very sad, regretfully sad, agonizingly sad, tragically sad, deeply sad, sad/dreary, sad/dull, sad/troubled, sad/strong, bitter/sad, bitter-sweet/sad, sad/wretched, sad/rueful, genuinely sad, exhibiting sadness for masochistic effect, sad as the character structure remnant of a manipulating mother, glad to be sad, sad without grief, sad after a heterosexual loss, sad after a heterosexual loss mitigated by unconscious homosexual relief ... or depressed rather than sad. If you were the patient – even a back ward schizophrenic patient – wouldn't you hope your doctor could tell the difference?

The clinician uses his empathy and intuition to translate symptoms into interpersonal terms, based on the reactions evoked in him by the patient. Psychotherapeutic skill depends to a great extent on the capacity of the therapist to allow this internal resonance to take place, while at the same time remaining detached enough to observe the process as it happens. It is important to note the attention to detail implied in Stoller's account. The dynamically minded clinician is not content to be told that the patient is 'depressed' or 'anxious'; he wants to know what the feeling of depression is *like*, what thoughts come into the patient's mind when he feels depressed, what precise circumstances provoke depressed feelings, how he sets about combating them, whether they are felt to be located in a particular part of the body, and so on. In this, the psychotherapist is doing no more than any good clinician, a point encapsulated in Winnicott's (1971) aphorism 'psychoanalysis is an extended form of history-taking'.

A patient's expectations, assumptions and difficulties, both conscious and unconscious, will be manifest from the start or even before the start of the initial interview. Ms B, at her first appointment, was sitting very close to her mother in the waiting area and looked poignantly back as she was led away to the interview room – obvious evidence of her deep attachment to her mother. Less obvious were the feelings aroused by this in the therapist, who unwisely suggested that the best thing would be for her to go back to work as soon as possible; here he was enacting (rather than understanding) the patient's feeling that men would threaten to separate her from her mother and expose her sense of vulnerability and inadequacy.

Psychotherapy is not all softness and empathy. Information about unconscious mental life is elicited by conventional history-taking, including enquiries about early memories, early and current daydreams, dreams and phantasies. There will be an attempt to assess the quality of significant relationships in childhood, any major separations, losses or traumata, and a detailed account of the patient's psychosexual development. The circumstances of the onset of the illness are important, because they reveal the precipitating factors and point to an underlying dynamic constellation evoked by the precipitating stress. Mr A's depression was partly triggered by his son's learning difficulties, for which he felt responsible, just as he had felt responsible for his father's illness when he was a child. Ms B's unhappy love affair triggered feelings of shame and inadequacy that could be understood in terms of her inhibition of anger and unresolved rivalry in childhood.

Diagnostic systems in psychotherapy

The most widely used diagnostic systems in psychiatry are ICD and DSM, both currently in the process of revision. ICD presents considerable shortcomings for the psychodynamically minded clinician, being a uni-axial, atheoretical set of categories. DSM is more relevant, in that it is multi-axial, emphasising not just psychiatric diagnosis (axis 1) but also personality (axis 2) and stressors (axis 4). However, the concept of personality embodied in axis 2 is that of personality *disorder* rather than personality *organisation*, which the psychodynamic formulation tries to encapsulate. An axis was originally proposed for DSM defining 'defence or style', but was eventually dropped due to lack of general agreement among psychiatrists about how this could be defined.

There are several systematised diagnostic methods currently used by psychotherapists, mainly for research or teaching rather than routine clinical practice; none is without methodological shortcomings. Four will considered.

Defence style

Valliant's hierarchy of defences provides an obvious starting point for a dynamic diagnostic system. Their validity is supported by a 40-year follow-up (Valliant, 1977), in which mature defence styles were correlated with good subsequent adjustment. Defence styles can be realiably assessed by questionnaire and correlate well with other general measures of 'neuroticism', but attempts to link particular defences with particular psychiatric diagnoses – e.g. splitting and projection with Borderline Personality Disorder, undoing and isolation with obsessive-compulsive disorders – have proved unsuccessful (Andrews *et al.*, 1989).

Level of object-relations

Freud, and later Abraham (1924), proposed a developmental schema of libidinal maturation. Psychiatric disorder was conceived as correlating with developmental arrest at, or regression to, a particular level. Schizophrenia was associated with auto-eroticism, hysterical disorders with the oral phase of development, obsessive-compulsive disorders with the stage of sphincter control, and neurotic disorders, such as anxiety and panic, with the Oedipal stage of castration anxiety.

This simplistic model has been superseded, partly for lack of objective evidence, and partly because libido theory has generally been replaced with an object-relations view of development (Greenberg & Mitchell, 1983). The notion of levels or stages of development remains, however, and at least three can be defined:

> *Level 1: symbiotic stage* This is the symbiotic phase, where the patient is not fully differentiated as a person and seeks relationships characterised by merging and adhesiveness. He lives in a solipsistic world, seeing others as extensions of himself whose primary function is to meet his needs. Anxieties associated with this phase are those of primitive dread, fear of non-being, and disintegration.

> *Level 2: part-object stage; 'paranoid-schizoid position'* Here, the individual is more aware of others but relates to them as 'part-objects' rather than whole persons. This corresponds to the Kleinian paranoid-schizoid position, where the world is split into good and bad, and in which unwanted parts of the self are expelled into others by projective identification. Anxieties associated with this stage are those of abandonment and loss of control.

> *Level 3: whole-object stage; 'depressive position'* This is the Kleinian 'depressive position', or Winnicott's 'stage of concern', in which the individual inhabits a three-person world of separate, caring and cared-for objects, but is subject to rivalry, competition and doubts about sharing and acceptance. Fears associated with this stage are those of inadequacy and loss.

The attempt to assign a person to any one stage of development is difficult, especially as, under the regressive pull of illness, earlier and more primitive levels may be uncovered. Ms B revealed in the depths of her depression a level 1 symbiotic link with her mother; as her recovery progressed, level 2 issues of intense self-criticism (projected into others whom she saw as despising her) emerged; later, level 3 questions of comparison of herself with others predominated.

Conflict analysis

Freud's dynamic view of neurosis was based on a conflictual model in which illness arises when contradictory wishes or impulses become irreconcilable – for example, feelings of aggression towards those upon whom one depends, or between sexual wishes and fears of rejection. Ryle (1990) systematised this approach into a series of statements ('traps', 'snags' and 'dilemmas') which encapsulate such conflicts. For example, a common dilemma is that of 'too near – too far': 'Either I get too close in relationships and feel smothered or trapped, *or* I get too far and feel lonely and unwanted.' Traps are of the 'if but ...' type: 'If I am more independent my husband won't like it', or 'If I do what I want I run the risk of failing.' Snags are circular snares of the type: 'I feel unacceptable, so I placate; placation leads to exploitation; exploitation makes me feel angry; anger is unacceptable; therefore I placate, etc.' Patients can readily identify with pre-existing statements of this sort, which form a basis for therapy in which the assumptions that underlie them are examined and challenged. Luborsky (Luborsky *et al.*, 1989) has developed a similar research tool, the Core Conflictual Relationship Theme, which assigns patients' problems to a predetermined list of wish–fear–consequence themes. An example would be 'I wish to feel attractive; I fear rejection; therefore I feel inadequate.' These themes are repeated in the patient's everyday life and in the transference and, it is hypothesised, occurred also in childhood. To this extent, conflict analysis overlaps with the next category, dynamic focus.

Dynamic focus

The idea of a dynamic focus around which therapeutic efforts should be concentrated is particularly important in brief therapies (Malan, 1979), but Thomä and Kächele (1986) see psychoanalysis itself as a focal therapy with an ever shifting focus. The concept of focus is an extension of Strachey's (1934) idea of a 'mutative interpretation', which brings together at one nodal point the external relationship difficulty, the transference, and the hypothesised underlying childhood constellation. An important feature of focus derives from Freud's dictum that an interpretation should be aimed just near enough the surface of consciousness for the patient to able to grasp it, but far enough below to enable the overcoming of a resistance (Freud, 1911–15).

The dynamic formulation

The dynamic formulation consists of a summarising statement that starts with the *psychiatric diagnosis*; proceeds to consider the *dynamic precipitant* of the illness, the *maintaining factors*, and the *childhood origins* or vulnerabilities. It considers the patient's *strengths and weaknesses* and *defence-styles*; proposes a *focal theme* which brings together the preceding elements; and goes on to suggest a possible form of *therapeutic intervention*, including a *prediction* about issues likely to arise in therapy, and possible outcome.

As an example, we will take Ms B. The psychiatric *diagnosis* was severe depression with endogenous features. The *precipitant* was the failed relationship and the resulting feelings of shame and inadequacy. The *maintaining factor* was the symbiotic relationship with the mother and the illness itself, which made further exploration or social contact problematic. The *childhood origins* included possible difficulties in infancy, perhaps associated with her mother's depression and her sometimes rigid and inaccessible father. The assessment interview suggested a strong theme of loss and separation: several deaths were preoccupying the patient, and there was a counter-transferential pull to separate her from her family, either by sending her back to work or by admission to hospital. The *focal theme* thus concerned the difficulty in making an Oedipal 'move' from mother to father without feeling that what she had left behind was irretrievably lost. Her *strengths* included good academic achievement, her *weaknesses* inhibition of assertiveness and aggression. Her *defence styles* were predominantly mature-neurotic: sublimation, altruism, repression and intellectualisation. The severity of her illness, together with her tendency to intellectualise and the close involvement of her family, meant that the chosen methods of *treatment* were drugs and ECT, supportive individual therapy and family therapy. *Predicted themes* were those of dependency on the therapist and repressed anxiety and anger about separations and breaks in treatment.

Conclusion

In 1954, Dennis Hill, later to become professor of psychiatry at the Maudsley, wrote: 'My wish is to see a psychiatry which is one and undivided and … which is fundamentally psychologically oriented' (Hill, 1954). Then, as now, that wish may have been utopian. Since it was written, there have been enormous developments in both the biomedical and psychological aspects of psychiatry. Molecular genetics is beginning to make visible the biological substrate of psychiatric disorder, while psychotherapy, no longer confined within a narrow psychoanalytic or behaviourist credo, has established the psychobiological reality of an inner world based on attachment, exploration, loss, grief and belief.

As differentiation and specialisation have proceeded, the tension between the biological and psychological approaches has decreased. Hill's call for unity seems a less necessary idealisation. There is a movement away from a paranoid-schizoid era, in which opposing sides belittle and dismiss each other, to a climate more akin to the depressive position, in which each recognises the other's value and where rivalry is a stimulus to greater understanding rather than destructiveness. The tensions between the different branches of psychotherapy can also now more easily be contained, leading to creative competition and clarification. This unity of opposites can be seen metaphorically in terms of male and female (Pedder, 1989), 'left' and 'right' brain functions, or the entwined strands of a DNA helix. At each nodal point within psychiatry and psychotherapy, there are rational and intuitive elements; the creative tension between them often generates the most fruitful progeny.

Psychiatry at its best is a vigorous hybrid, combining science and art, reason and imagination, the biological and the psychological. The central reference point for psychotherapy is the individual, with his unique intrapsychic, familial and social experience. While psychotherapy remains part of a wider psychiatric whole, that pivotal vision will not be lost.

CHAPTER 7

AN ATTACHMENT MODEL OF DEPRESSION

Integrating findings from the mood disorder laboratory

Introduction

After two decades in the wilderness, psychoanalytic therapies for depression are making a muted revival (Abbass, 2006; Lemma, Target & Fonagy, 2010), based in part on recent research in the basic science of mood (cf. Luyten & Blatt, 2011). This paper examines psychoanalytic approaches to depression and its treatment in the light of current findings in the fields of attachment, genetics, neuro-imaging, neuro-endocrinology and child development. It attempts to develop a model of mood disorder that does justice to both brain *and* mind and to encompass the experiential phenomenology of depression. The aim is to highlight the specific psychoanalytic contribution to the understanding and treatment of depression, and to claim its place as an equal therapeutic player, alongside CBT and pharmacotherapy.

In the spirit of clinical relevance, let us start with an unremarkable – yet nonetheless poignant – example of depression as one might encounter it in the clinic.

> Jane, 47, a married business woman with two children, was referred for psychoanalytic therapy by a physician because of medically unexplained abdominal pain. She had a near full-house of Major Depressive Disorder symptoms, including weight loss, sleep disturbance, panic symptoms, low mood, poor concentration and a feeling of hopelessness. An obvious precipitant was the death of her mother some eight months previously, but as the story unfolded it became clear that many of her symptoms predated this.
>
> During the assessment phase of her therapy she mentioned, as though in passing, that she had also developed panic attacks after an 'unwanted pregnancy' at the age of 18.
>
> 'Unwanted by whom?', I asked.
>
> 'Oh, my boyfriend at the time was dead set against it.'
>
> 'And you …?'
>
> 'Oh, I was longing for a baby, but he wasn't having it …'

'Indeed it was you, not he, who was "having" it. I suppose what he "had" was his way; you were left with the unmourned grief of a child that never was.'

Then came bitter tears, as though the loss had been yesterday.

We'll return later to Jane, to the childhood relational constellations which predispose to depression in the face of loss, and the ways – including picking up on linguistic ambiguities – in which therapy can help overcome 'affect phobia'.

Psychodynamic-attachment models of depression

Nearly a century after its first appearance, 'Mourning and melancholia' (Freud, 1917) remains the seminal psychoanalytic text on depression. With significant modifications, it is still relevant to current understanding. In the section which follows I shall interweave Freud's views with Bowlby's (1980) attachment-derived theory of depression, which both influenced, and was influenced by, social psychiatry research in the 1970s (Brown & Harris, 1978).

The Freud–Bowlby story of depression contains five main themes.

1 Loss and the 'two circuits'

As his title suggests, Freud starts from parallels between the phenomenology of mourning and depression. In both there is a 'profoundly painful dejection, cessation of interest in the outside world, loss of the capacity to love, [and] inhibition of all activity' (Freud, 1917, p. 244). Both, he observes, may arise in 'reaction to the loss of a loved person, or to the loss of some abstraction which has taken the place of one, such as one's country, liberty, and ideal, and so on' (p. 243).

Depression follows actual or symbolic loss, both of which activate feelings of failure and lack of efficacy. But, for Freud, the reaction to loss in depression is often both obscure and disproportionate:

> one cannot see clearly what it is that has been lost, and it is all the more reasonable to suppose that the patient cannot consciously perceive what he has lost either ... even if the patient is aware of the loss ..., but only in the sense that he knows *whom* he has lost but not *what* he has lost in him ... melancholia is ... related to an object-loss which is withdrawn from consciousness, in contradistinction to mourning, in which there is nothing about the loss that is unconscious.
>
> (Freud, 1917, p. 245)

Freud moves here from the outer to the inner world – from the world of psychiatry, one might say, to the world of psychodynamics. He goes beyond external loss to the *internal* sense of impoverishment characteristic of depression, confidently stating that in depression the loss is necessarily 'withdrawn from consciousness'? But is this invariably so? Let's go back to Jane.

Jane knew she had 'lost' her mother. But what was it about that loss that felt so irretrievable, made her feel so 'lost'? At one level she was fully aware of what was gone from her life. Her mother, who had lived next door, was her constant companion, her confidante and her 'best friend', the person she could turn to whenever things were difficult – in this case when she developed abdominal pain. As a child she recalled playing out in the back yard, and the panic feelings she experienced when she looked up in search of her mother's face at the kitchen window, normally ever available for safety and reassurance, and, preoccupied with a chore, she wasn't there.

Her mother had been at the apex of her attachment hierarchy, with her husband, for all his good qualities, definitely at number two or below. Thus when, on her honeymoon, she become temporarily deaf after a plane journey, her husband was dismayed that she rang her mother for reassurance rather than turning, as he had expected, to him. Her mother's absence now left a vacuum of which Jane was painfully aware whenever she felt in need of succour.

A further a twist emerges from the history. Jane had, she said, been abruptly weaned aged three months, when her mother had to attend to *her* mother (Jane's grandmother), who became seriously ill at that time. One might postulate that Jane's vulnerability to separation and fear of abandonment had their origins in this developmental trauma and its sequelae.

Jane's case is perhaps atypical in that depression and bereavement were in her case intertwined. But we can still ask of Freud's theory: in what sense was Jane's loss hidden from consciousness? A moment in our work together illuminates this.

Jane felt that my probings about her relationship to her mother somehow carried the implication that she was making a great fuss, and that she should have 'got over' her grief by now.

'I wonder how close *you* were to your mother', she declared. 'Perhaps you just don't understand what it is like to have had such a loving and intimate relationship with one's Mum.'

My slightly defensive reply went: 'On the contrary, my feeling is that, although you are depressed and feel the physical pain from your stomach, you still haven't yet allowed yourself to experience the full force of the mental suffering entailed in loosing such an all-important person in your life.'

At this Jane burst into powerful sobs, going on to describe how for the first few months she had been unable even to look at her mother's house, and still now could not enter it to do the necessary sifting and disposal of her possessions.

What was 'hidden from consciousness' was not the *fact* of her mother's death but its emotional import, the associated affect. This she kept literally at arm's length in her avoidance of exposure to any experience which might bypass the fragile defences she had built against feeling the loss. Her transferential anger gave a glimpse of the inner cauldron of misery and rage that she was fighting so hard to keep at bay.

Psychodynamics

The discussion at this point requires a brief diversion into a contemporary account of psychodynamics. The term predates Freud (first used in 1874), but usually refers to an intrapsychic psychoanalytic model in which the various forces considered to make up the psyche – conscious and unconscious, or id, ego and superego – are in a state of dynamic equilibrium.

Based on attachment research, a contemporary model of psychodynamics can be envisaged, now comprising two interlocking dynamic circuits.

- 'Circuit 1', the intrapsychic, corresponds to the classical account, in which the basic affective mesolimbic primary processes (Panksepp & Watt, 2011) – panic/ grief, rage, care, seeking, lust and play – are subject to continuous appraisal and regulation (mentalising) by cortical functions.
- 'Circuit 2', the interpersonal, links these cortical functions, especially in the right hemisphere, to emotional interchange with significant others, actual (parent, spouse, 'buddie') or symbolic (i.e. an internal representation of the other) in an individual's environment (Schore, 2003). A large body of evidence now supports the view that, at least in infancy and early childhood, intrapsychic equilibrium is moderated by this interpersonal environment. No man – or woman – really is an island.

Recent studies by Mikulincer, Shaver and colleagues (reviewed Mikulincer & Shaver, 2008; Mikulincer *et al.*, 2009) are consistent with this model. Attachment styles are often thought of as fairly stable traits. Their experiments illustrate how these can be altered by appropriate environmental 'priming'. In one study subjects were exposed to a traumatic story in which a child was killed in an automobile accident, and levels of compassionate responses towards the bereaved parents were then rated. As might be expected, insecure subjects' empathic responses were limited and inhibited compared with those of their secure counterparts.

The experiments were then repeated, but subjects were now 'primed' with positive or neutral stimuli, either subliminal (flashing words such as 'love' and 'support' onto a screen so briefly that the subjects did not consciously register them) or supraliminal (asking the subjects to think about a loving or supportive relationship, or showing them a picture of a mother cradling a baby). The outcome was that insecure subjects, when exposed to positive but not neutral stimuli, then responded in ways indistinguishable from their secure counterparts.

The importance of this research is that it suggests a dynamic interaction with internal objects and current here-and-now experience, and that thoughts, feelings and behaviours are best seen as the result of the interaction between these two circuits. When the external relationship is lost, or withdrawn from, internal and often archaic (transferential) representations become more salient.

An attachment perspective suggests that in normal psychological functioning there is an actual or symbolic Other in the mind whose soothing and regulating role can be evoked when stress, exhaustion or illness prevail (Holmes, 2010). This secure base function provides a background below-consciousness awareness of one's own and the Other's state of mind, providing a sense of security and allowing exploration (including of one's own painful feelings) or 'seeking' (Panksepp & Watt, 2011) to proceed. As an adult one can be 'alone in the presence of the other', either literally, as different members of a family or community go about their daily tasks, or symbolically, in the presence of one's internal 'guardian angel' or good internal object, or perhaps simply in the knowledge that support is at hand when needed.

Loss (continued)

This interplay between the intrapsychic and the interpersonal is disrupted in depression. Without her mother, Jane had lost the secure base she needed when faced with the threat which her stomach symptoms represented. The fact that Jane had never built up a secure *internal* mother, perhaps due to her premature weaning experience, made her particularly vulnerable to post-bereavement depression. The circuit between inner need (to work through the painful feelings associated with irreversible separation) and outer response (the necessary holding needed while internal adjustment took place) had been severed.

Jane's avoidance of anything associated with her mother exemplifies '*affect phobia*'[1] (McCullough *et al.*, 2003) as a central a feature of depression. Helping to overcome affect phobia is a key therapeutic aim for a psychodynamic approach. Affects evoke phobic avoidance when the means to *regulate* them are lacking (Schore 2003). A circuit is broken, this time in the inner world, between the emotion, with its physiological components, and its verbal representation in the conscious mind. Affect phobia is clearly different from classical psychoanalytic repression, but nevertheless contains the idea that people avoid experiencing certain feelings (which are therefore to a greater or lesser extent 'withdrawn from consciousness'), not necessarily because they are forbidden by a punitive superego (see below) but because they are, in the absence of secure base, simply too painful to bear on one's own.

This suggests a link and mutual feedback between the two broken circuits, the inter- and intra-personal. Jane was in physical pain and felt 'depressed', but in depression there is often an *absence* [2] of feeling – no pleasure, no excitement, no hope, just a sense of deadness. For Jane to *experience* real sadness she needed to feel safe enough in the therapeutic setting to do so, including trusting the analyst to tolerate her resentment at his lack of understanding. Jane's paradox – which therapy's job was to help unravel – was that the one person who could have provided the safety to think about her loss was the mother whose death provoked the need to think about it in the first place.

2 Self-preoccupation

There is a 'narcissistic' aspect to depression in that, as in mourning, the sufferer withdraws into herself. Loved ones are by definition invested with special significance. When the loved one is gone, 'The object cathexis ... [is] withdrawn into the ego' (Freud, 1917, p. 249). But, unlike in normal mourning, in depression the sufferer becomes mired in a state of self-absorption, unable to find a new object, to reinvest the world with meaning. The self now becomes the arena where relationships are played out. In mourning the bereaved person's initial reaction is often one of denial: 'My loved one is not irretrievably gone, just lost, away on a long journey, will soon return, is asleep, not dead', etc. Then, through a period of painful 'reality testing', the sufferer comes gradually to accept the actuality of the loss.

In depression this interplay between reality and the inner world is compromised (disrupted 'Circuit 2'). The external world feels emotionally inaccessible. There is no helping relationship with which to explore the painful feelings of loss. Jane's pain was now more 'real' to her than her connection to her husband and children. We shall see later how Freud's account of this depressive self-absorption is confirmed by findings from neuro-imaging research.

3 Identification with the lost object

The third tenet of psychoanalytic depression theory centres on Freud's famous phrase 'the shadow of the object':

> Thus the shadow of the object fell upon the ego, and the latter could hence-forth be judged by a special mental agency, as though it were an object, the forsaken object. In this way an object-loss was transformed into an ego-loss and the conflict between the ego and the loved person into a cleavage between the critical activity of the ego and the ego as altered by identification.
>
> (Freud, 1917, p. 249)

The 'shadow of the object' theory suggests that in depression the loss is initially mitigated by its transposition from the external to the inner world. This protects the individual from the vagaries of fate, but a price has to be paid. The inner world is no longer 'fed' from its connection with loving others. The pain of the outer actual loss is now replaced by guilt and inner emptiness, in which one part of the self attacks another. As restoration of the lost object seems impossible, despair, which Bowlby (1980) identified as the nadir of grief, takes over. 'Seeking' (Panksepp & Watt, 2011) is inhibited and the individual becomes locked into a depressive cocoon.

There are several other points to be noted here. First, Freud's language is poetic – the use of the word 'shadow' evoking the darkness of the death-shades with which depression sufferers struggle. This is not a merely aesthetic point. Freud is moving from an explanatory model – testably linking depression with loss – to a hermeneutic one in which the *meaning* of depression is subject to exegesis: the reason depressed people become self-absorbed is because they see through a glass darkly.

In this hermeneutic world we are beginning to *make sense* of experience rather than provide an external 'scientific' account of it. In Freud's model the sufferer has suffered an external loss, but deals with this by transposing relationships into the inner world where the missing loved one lives on, albeit at the expense of external relationships. Every time Jane touched her painful tummy it was as though she were touching the pain of her missing mother.

In addition to emphasising the shift from an outer loss to a 'loss in the ego', Freud picks up on *conflict* between the self and its objects as a central theme in depression. People become depressed, this view suggests, because (a) they have been, or feel, abandoned, (b) they experience rage and outrage about this, (c) they protect the object from their rage by identification, taking the battle – in Jane's case with the mother who wasn't there when she needed her – into the self, but (d) this anger towards the object arouses guilt, and depression then becomes a punish-ment fitting to the crime. Finally, (e) if, in the 'depressive position' (as opposed to the paranoid-schizoid world of depressive illness) one can 'reinstate' the whole object in one's inner world, in both its loving and its abandoning aspects, then one is inured to further loss. If, through the transpositions and transferences of therapy, Jane could find, lose and reinstate a good internal mother, forgivable despite hav-ing let her down through absence, she would be able to transcend her pain, physical and mental, and her locked-in inner battle with depression.

It should be noted that the 'shadow of the object' concept is a crucial starting point for the Klein–Bion model of the inner world. Young psychiatrists are taught the Kraeplinian doctrine that, compared with schizophrenia, 'where there's depression, there's hope'. But the Klein–Bion model offers a different sort of hopeful spin on depression (Taylor, 2009). By valuing the 'depressive position' as a state of psychological maturity, it positively connotes the struggle to acknowledge and contain ambivalent feelings towards the lost object.

4 Role of childhood trauma

The next aspect of Freud's theory is the emphasis on childhood trauma as the developmental precursor of adult depression. In the passage quoted, Freud takes conflict between ego and object as inherent in the trauma of the Oedipal situation. We are now more likely to see childhood trauma as a result of an actual event – neglect, abandonment, or physical and/or sexual abuse. Freud notes that in many cases of depression there is no obvious loss, or the loss seems relatively trivial. But we now know from the work of Brown and Harris (1978) and Paykel (Paykel & Herbert, 1989), and more recently (e.g. Artero *et al.*, 2011), that loss does indeed play a very significant role in depression. At least 70 per cent of depressed women have experienced a significant loss event or chronic difficulties in the year preceding the onset of the depression, as compared with around 25 per cent of non-depressed people. Nevertheless it is possible to become depressed without obvious loss, and it is possible to experience major loss without becoming depressed. A probabilistic or 'cascade' model (including genetic vulnerability, a 'kindling' model, as well as life events; see below) is needed adequately to account for illness in any particular case.

Brown and Harris (1978) showed that vulnerability to loss depends on both current factors (lack of employment; having more than three children under 15; lack of a supportive relationship) and antecedent ones (early separation from or loss of mother). Parker (1979) showed that, as compared with controls, depressed women are more likely to view their mothers as having offered 'low care and high overprotection'. Recent studies of depressed patients combining pharmacotherapy and psychotherapy (Zobel *et al.*, 2011) suggest that early adversity is an important variable in predicting outcome, and that those with adversity (around 50 per cent in the Zobel study) benefited more from psychotherapy and anti-depressants than if treated with pharmacotherapy alone.

Freud's model suggests that a pre-existing 'ambivalence' predisposes to depression. Early childhood trauma – whether through neglect, abuse or insensitive parenting – can predispose to depression when faced with loss in adult life. Adverse experiences evoke in the child a mixture of hurt and hate, re-evoked by comparable experiences in adult life. Hurt would normally trigger attachment behaviours and lead the sufferer to seek proximity to a comforting parent. But if that person is also the *source* of the hurt, and therefore liable to evoke in the child the wish to inflict retaliatory pain, the sufferer is in an impossible dilemma. Turning the hate against oneself, seeing oneself as unlovable and 'hateful' ('full of hate', as well as 'hateable') becomes the uncomfortable compromise.

5 'Primal emotions' in depression: attachment perspectives

This leads us to Freud's account of self-hatred in depression:

> The melancholic displays ... an extraordinary diminution in his self-regard, an impoverishment of his ego on a grand scale. In mourning it is the world which has become poor and empty; in melancholia it is the ego itself. The patient represents his ego to us as worthless, incapable of any achievement and

morally despicable; he reproaches himself, vilifies himself and expects to be cast out and punished. He abases himself before everyone and commiserates with his own relatives for being connected with anyone so unworthy.

(Freud, 1917, p. 246)

the piece that behaves so cruelly ... comprises the conscience, a critical agency within the ego, which even in normal times takes up a critical attitude towards the ego, though never so relentlessly and so unjustifiably.

(Freud, 1921, p. 52)

This idea flows from plank three of his theory, that in depression the lost and ambivalently regarded object is, through identification, instated in the self. The depressed person's psychical self-attack[3] is thus, in Freud's view, a displacement of revenge which properly belongs to the lost, abandoning or unloving object.

This ingenious twist is certainly not the whole story. True, irritability and anger are often evident in depression, and in some cases this is indeed turned against the self, most obviously in suicide. But there are more plausible ways of conceptualising this. For Bowlby (1980), loss was best seen as irreversible separation. Separation from a secure base exposes the individual to risk; risk evokes fear. Anger at separation can be seen as a negative reinforcement schedule designed to reunite the separated one with the secure base – whether this is the baby crying blue murder for her mother or the parent reprimanding the child for risky behaviours. The lack of an answering response to these angry outbursts gradually persuades the bereaved person that the separation is irremediable and paves the way for despair.

But not everyone suffering from depression manifests the quasi-psychotic self-reproaches Freud's theory addresses. Insecure attachment is a risk factor for depression (Murray, 2009). Blatt's (2008) dichotomous division of depression into 'anaclitic' (object-leaning) and 'introjective' (self-absorbed) patterns maps well onto attachment theory's two forms of 'organised insecurity' – hyper- and hypoactivating (Mikulincer & Shaver, 2008). Those with hyperactivating attachment patterns are oversensitive to separation and therefore prone to 'anaclitic' depression. Hypoactivation, where psychic pain is damped down in the service of security, renders its sufferers more prone to introjective ruminative patterns of depression.

Thus ruminative self-reproach is a salient feature of introjective depression. The more obsessive depressive – perhaps exemplified by Freud himself – will have had developmental experiences in which feelings were damped down ('hypoactivated') in order to remain protected by a stressed or rejecting mother (Ainsworth *et al.*, 1978). Turning protest in on the self is a way of staying safe without running the risk of alienating the secure base. Freud developed the idea of the harsh superego from observing this self-critical 'agency': in many depressed people there is a gulf between real self and ideal self; narrowing this discrepancy is a major therapeutic target (Kuyken *et al.*, 2005).

But in the dependent, 'anaclitic' type of depression, self-attack and anger are generally far less prominent (Blatt, 2008). For these sufferers the predominant feature is anxiety at impending separation. Jane's intimate relationships illustrate anxious attachment – the 'ambivalent' or 'hyperactivating' variety. Her attachment pattern was one of clinging adhesion to an inconstant object rather than mature dependency. This was played out in the transference, as she tried to manoeuvre the therapist into making life-decisions for her, especially when it came to taking antidepressants, the thought of which evoked in her an irrational fear.

'Please tell me whether I should take those pills or not', she pleaded.

The therapist's response was: 'The psychiatrist in me thinks it would be a really good idea to give them a try; but as a psychotherapist I believe it's vital for you to find the freedom to make decisions for yourself (and anyway, they're unlikely to work unless you do!).'

Jane saw herself as helpless rather than worthless. Lacking a secure 'internal mother' who could see her through moments of misery and doubt, she needed the physical presence of an external mother/therapist in order to feel safe. Jane's hyperactive attachment pattern meant that she recruited an external 'transferential' circuit of security, compensating for her depressive impairment in mentalising when stressed (Lemma, Target & Fonagy, 2010).[4]

Self-attack as diverted aggression thus cannot be taken as a general account of depressive experience. A more nuanced picture, taking into account individual differences, is needed. There remains, however, value in the idea of sadism, rage and revenge – i.e. 'primitive' or 'primal' emotions – holding sway in depression, whether these be stimulated by a fight or flight response, overwhelming fear, helplessness or overwhelming despair. As we shall see, a contemporary model of the disruption of brain function in depression suggests that the normal regulation, modulation and mitigation of these primal emotions is disrupted.

In sum, despite some limitations and aberrations, the psychoanalytic model of depression remains highly relevant to today's clinical practice. Against that psychoanalytic background, the remainder of this paper will juxtapose recent sociological and neurobiological findings in depression in an attempt to build bridges between these seemingly disparate realms of discourse.

Evolutionary psychology

Given the ubiquity and obvious fitness-reducing aspects of depression, a fundamental and in a sense preliminary question to be considered is what its evolutionary *function* might be (Nesse, 2005). I shall mention three possible approaches.

The psychoanalytic-attachment model proposed above is consistent with Simpson and Belsky's (2008) 'psychic pain hypothesis'. Sensitivity to physical pain is an essential protective mechanism for living organisms. Analogously, in the interpersonal environment, the capacity to experience psychic pain on separation ensures that no effort is spared to maintain the attachments essential for security and ultimate reproductive success. The capacity to become depressed in response to irretrievable loss is the dark side of the life-enhancing virtues of intimate attachment. Those that feel no psychic pain on loss may be protected from depression but risk deprivation through the superficiality of their attachments. Proneness to depression is the price paid for propensity to attachment.

A second popular idea derives from 'rank theory' (Nesse, 2005). Again the argument centres on the vulnerability associated with attachment – epitomised in Francis Bacon's view of a spouse and children as 'hostages to fortune'. But, as Tennyson (who suffered from depression when his beloved friend Hallam was drowned at the age of 24) famously puts it – ''Tis better to have loved and lost than never to have loved at all.' Attachments are essential; but they inevitably will sometimes be lost. In social groups where rank and dominance hierarchies prevail, loss lowers rank, rendering the sufferer vulnerable to reduced access to resources – food and reproductive opportunities. In depression one's needs are adaptively restricted (loss of appetite, libido, etc.), and, by being temporarily *hors de combat*, the sufferer is no longer seen as a threat and so can be allowed to recover in peace.

This perspective is consistent with recent studies showing a strong relationship between social disadvantage and the incidence of depression (Pickett & Wilkinson, 2010). Generally the poor have higher levels of mental illness; this makes sense in terms both of the incidence of adverse life events (unemployment, housing difficulties, divorce and separation, death, illness rates) and the availability of mitigating support (high divorce/separation rates again, access to good medical services, including talking therapies). But the issue is not simply a matter of absolute poverty. Pickett and Wilkinson have studied the impact of income *differentials* in advanced societies. They show that, the greater the inequalities, the greater the levels of indices of social difficulty, including mental illness rates. They link this with the 'affluenza' concept (James, 2007): inequality fosters 'rank anxiety', in which envy is rife; therefore people are more prone to see themselves as 'failures' or 'losers' (a linguistic link with loss and depression) compared with more egalitarian and socially cohesive societies. Other evolutionary anthropologists see cooperativeness as an alliance of the weak against the strong, an antidote to dominance hierarchies, which, as the rank hypothesis suggests, can be breeding grounds for depression.

A third evolutionary view is the so-called niche change hypothesis (Watson & Andrews, 2002). Here depression is seen as a necessary moratorium (to use Erikson's (1950) word for adolescence) – an opportunity to review one's situation, change direction if needs be, and generally *reculer pour mieux sauter*. Clearly this is highly relevant to the work of psychotherapy.

While positively connoting depression may be clinically helpful, and while depression in minor forms may be adaptive, the gross and severe forms that are psychiatry's business are perhaps better seen as 'dysregulation' of these more adaptive depressive responses to loss. The purpose of therapy might then be to help the patient to get back on a productive rather than a self-defeating depression track (Gilbert, 2006) or, to return to Freud, to help replace neurotic misery with everyday unhappiness.

Social psychiatry

As we have already seen, some of the most important findings in mood disorders in the second half of the last century came from social psychiatry research, especially the work of George Brown and his colleagues (Brown & Harris, 1978). These have continued with the 'Newpin project' (Lederer, 2009), an intervention study of the impact of befriending on depressed mothers in a deprived area of East London. Harris and her colleagues have shown that recovery from depression is fostered by the combination of befriending and a favourable 'new beginning' event, such as getting a job or starting a new relationship – an important reminder that life events can be antidotes to depression as well as precipitants. A neuroscience perspective (Panksepp & Watt, 2011) would see these new beginnings in terms of activating 'Seeking' and 'Playing' affective modules, as opposed to 'Rage' or 'Panic'. In addition to adventitious 'new beginnings', the facilitating presence of the Other, including the psychoanalyst who, if Winnicottian, will see the process of therapy as 'learning to play', will play a crucial role here.

Epigenetics

Epigenetics, a cutting-edge branch of biological science, is the study of heritable changes in the phenotype transmitted by non-genomic means, but it is often more widely referred to as the study of developmental pathways. Epigenetics helps reconcile the sterile nature–nurture debate whose psychiatric manifestation is the divide between 'organic' and psychotherapeutic psychiatry.[5] In the terms of this paper, the epigenetics of developmental psychobiology can be summarised by the 'equation' Phe = G x E squared.[6] A given phenotype (Phe) is determined by genetic makeup (G) times the environment (E) 'squared'. Squared because, given the 'two circuits' theory of psychodynamics, 'E' comprises Ec (the current environment) and Ed (the developmental environment), both of which influence gene expression. Developmental neurobiologist Champagne (2010, p. 564) puts it thus:

> there is emerging evidence that changes in gene expression both within the brain and in peripheral tissues are associated with differences in the quality of the early environment and that these developmental effects are maintained by epigenetic mechanisms that control the activity of genes involved in disease risk and behavioral variation.

This takes us to 'Circuit 3', the temporal circuit linking early developmental experiences with adult function. For female rats, maternal care in one generation directly influences the ability of those pups to care for their infants in the next. Epigenetics shows how, contrary to Darwinian dogma, acquired characteristics can be heritable. This is because DNA sequence is only part of the developmental story. DNA is tightly bound in the cell to histone proteins. DNA is only available for transcription by mRNA into protein if the binding is sufficiently loose, and environmental influence impacts directly on histone binding in certain tissues, including the psychobiologically relevant hypothalamus.

In addition, different environments switch promoter genes on or off, thereby determining varying phenotypic manifestations. Champagne's experimental model is maternal grooming behaviour in rats. (Champagne, 2010; for reviews, see also Polan & Hofer, 2008; Goldberg, 2009). 'Good' rat mothers show a high degree of 'LG' (licking and grooming) behaviour with their pups, who in turn, when compared with offspring of low LG mothers, typically show less fear when presented with novelty as adults.

The subtle interplay between gene expression and current and developmental environment is illustrated by a study in which rats were put into one of three rearing environments, designated enriched, impoverished or neutral (Champagne, 2010). Those in the impoverished environment did not develop high LG behaviours even if they had a high LG mother; those in the enriched environment developed them even if their mothers had been low LG. Only in the neutral environment did LG 'breed true' so that low LG mothers had low LG offspring and high LG mothers high LG offspring. It was in those environments that high LG mothers, when rearing offspring of low LG mothers, could transmit high LG to the children and grandchildren of those fostered pups, presumably by epigenetic mechanisms. Significantly (see below), the low LG offspring showed accelerated sexual maturation compared with the high LG reared group. This suggests that the environment plays a crucial role in enhancing or suppressing genetic potential, and that this operates both distally (impoverished or enriched) and proximally (maternal licking behaviours).

As mentioned, the biochemical basis for these effects involves DNA methylation, which, by affecting gene-protein transcription rates, can alter the glucocorticoid receptor responsiveness in the hippocampus. Rodent data suggests that perinatal environmental conditions can result in long-term silencing of promoter genes through DNA methylation and that this epigenetic modification results in changes to HPA responsivity that persists into adulthood (Weaver *et al.*, 2005).

These studies are relevant to human psychopathology because we now know that, in humans, exposure to abuse in infancy is associated with altered levels of DNA methylation in hippocampal tissue (McGowan *et al.*, 2009). Oberlander *et al.* (2008) found elevated neonatal GR promoter methylation levels in infants born to depressed mothers. The methylation of the neonatal GR promoter predicted increased salivary cortisol levels of infants – a measure of 'stress' – at three months.

This epigenetic variability in response to stress, in both humans and rodents, can be conceptualised as adaptive. The harsher the environment, the more short-term survival strategies take precedence over the comparative 'luxuries' of nurture and exploration. In adverse environments, high reactiveness (adaptive misperception: 'take any unexpected sensation as potentially threatening') and early sexual maturation (when life expectancy is reduced) become priorities.

This overall conceptual framework applies equally to the seminal and much quoted work of Caspi *et al.* (2003) on the role of the serotonin (5-HTT) transporter gene polymorphism in depression. Possessing one or both copies of the s ('short') allele in itself predisposes to depression in relation to stressful intercurrent events compared with those with the l ('long') allele. The combination of childhood maltreatment/low care and possession of one or both short alleles is a quantitative predictor of depression in adult life (Artero *et al.*, 2011).

Here too the immediate reactivity that poor care elicits may be adaptive, in that such infants need to be able to latch onto whatever care is available and be self-protectively hyper-reactive to adverse experiences, even if this stores up future trouble. The recent finding that insecurely attached girls at one year have earlier menarche compared with their secure counterparts underscores this point (Belsky, Houts & Fearon, 2010).

However, it should be noted that there are a number of studies which fail to replicate the Caspi *et al.* findings (Risch *et al.*, 2009), and Fonagy (2009, p. 277) has claimed that 'no significant interaction effect between genotype and stressful life events on depression has been thus far found.' Given the suggestive animal findings, this non-replicability presents a challenge to psychodynamic clinicians and researchers to elaborate more subtle ways of measuring environmental influences and the possible relationship between them and the neurobiology of mood disorders.

Meanwhile, Steele and Seifer (2010) have studied another epigenetic locus, DRD4 polymorphism, known to represent a risk for attachment disorganisation (in which depression is also often a feature). Interestingly, DRD4 is also a marker of high responsiveness to a therapeutic intervention designed for toddlers with aggressive behaviour problems. Thus it seems that the same genetic polymorphism that represents risk may also confer protection:

> The DRD4 allele may indicate an increased biological sensitivity to context with potential for negative health effects under conditions of adversity (e.g., unresolved mourning regarding past loss or trauma in the mother) and positive effects under conditions of support and protection.
>
> (Steele & Siefer, 2010, p. 63)

The general conclusions for the psychodynamic clinician from these epigenetic studies can be summarised as follows:

a)　We need to think in terms of cascading *developmental trajectories* in which the interplay of genes, the social environment, both proximate and distal, and the part played by mitigation, reversibility and compensatory factors are all taken into account.

b)　In addition to the intersecting interpersonal and intrapersonal circuits promoting or protecting against depression, a third, temporal 'circuit 3' links infancy with later functioning.

c)　Suboptimal parenting in infancy can epigenetically increase depression vulnerability in the next generation via decreased exploratory behaviour and heightened reactivity. These features may be transmitted to the third generation and beyond.

d)　There may be a paradoxical but benign relationship between vulnerability/ reactivity and responsiveness to psychotherapy. This is a welcome reversal of Hart's (1971) 'inverse care law', which states that, the more an individual needs care, the less likely they are to receive or benefit from it, a problem which has been particularly applicable to psychotherapy.

e)　Epigenesis suggests that early childhood adversity is potentially amenable to psychotherapeutic intervention, but this may need to be at a relational and prolonged level (rather than brief and cognitive) if permanent changes to HPA axis reactivity is to be achieved.

Neuro-imaging and functional brain architecture

For Freud, psychoanalysis was 'psychodynamic', in that the mind was conceived as a *system* in which the flow of energy and the various impediments thereto were the determinants of health or illness. This model is consistent with the emerging picture of the dynamic inter-relationships between different brain areas which the new technologies of neuro-imaging suggest. As Mayberg puts it:

> Depression is ... a system-wide disorder, in which interruption at specific sites or 'nodes' within a *defined functional circuit* or network linking many brain regions can result in depressive symptoms ... [due to] failure to appropriately *regulate* activity in this multi-region circuit, under circumstances of cognitive, emotional, or somatic stress.
>
> (Mayberg, 2009, p. 717; author's emphasis)

Structural areas implicated in depressive illness include: the dorsolateral pre-frontal cortex (DLPFC), cingulate cortex, basal ganglia, amygdala and hippocampus (Mayberg, 2009). Three sets of findings stand out as particularly significant from the perspective of the psychodynamic clinician. First is the well-replicated consensus that there is *decreased dorsolateral pre-frontal cortex (DLPFC) activity* in depression (Wang *et al.*, 2008), as measured by blood flow and glucose metabolism. This relationship is quantitative, in that there is an inverse relationship between severity of depression and prefrontal cortex function (Brody *et al.*, 2001).

Second, ventral prefrontal cortex (VPFC) and amygdala *hyperactivity* has been consistently reported, especially where depression is associated with anxiety and obsessionality (Osuch *et al.*, 2000). The amygdala, fully developed at birth, and functionally connected to the hippocampus, is at the centre of the fear regulation system and is particularly involved in implicit as opposed to episodic learning of intense, emotionally charged experiences (LeDoux, 1994). The significance of this will be developed below.

A third region relevant to the genesis and treatment of depression is the subcallosal cingulate gyrus, and in particular area Cg 25. Severe depression is associated with excessive neural activity in this region, as are sad mood states in normal subjects (Mayberg, 2009). Responders to SSRI anti-depressants show reductions in blood flow in Cg 25 as their depressive symptoms remit (Mayberg *et al.*, 2000).

The temptation to make a coherent 'story' out of this assemblage of findings is hard to resist (cf. Carhart-Harris *et al.*, 2008):

1   Decreased DLPFC activity is consistent with the clinical observation of depressive disengagement from the world (psychoanalytic tenet 2 above) and the move from an Object Relations to an intrinsic, 'narcissistic', Default Mode Network (Carhart-Harris *et al.*, 2008), in which external Self–Other circuits are replaced by endogenous Self–Self circuits.

2   Hyperactivity in the basal ganglia and amygdala can be seen as reflecting 'damming up' of feelings arising from limbic system centres; there is a failure to subject them to rationality and, via reality-testing, bring them into play in the interpersonal field and thus 'discharge' them. Hence the salience of 'primitive emotions' in depression (psychoanalytic tenet 5 above).

3   Cg 25 can be postulated as a primary repressive agency, attempting to damp down and keep at bay impulses from lower centres (Carhart-Harris *et al.*, 2008) which threaten to overwhelm the under-functioning higher centres such as the DLPFC (cf. Mayberg, 2009). The Cg 25 centre acts in a 'superego'-like fashion, punitively self-persecuting as Freud postulated, vainly attempting to maintain a degree of psychic equilibrium.

4   Given that the amygdala matures prior to the hippocampus, and given amygdala hyperactivity, implicit (as opposed to episodic) memories of childhood trauma may be revived in depressive states (cf. Renn, 2012). The salience of these ingrained procedural memories may make sufferers with a history of childhood trauma less amenable to short-term therapies (Zobel *et al.*, 2011).

This model predicts that recovery from depression will entail a normalisation of the DLPFC, Cg 25, VPFC, and amygdala dynamic balance. Depressed people who respond to anti-depressants do indeed show concomitant increases in PFC activity and decrease in Cg 25 blood flow (Mayberg *et al.*, 2000). However, the converse is found in CBT responders, who show *decreased* DLPFC blood flow as they get better. Viewing brain function as a dynamic system makes sense of such apparently paradoxical effects. CBT encourages patients to use their rational cognitive capacities to re-evaluate the primitive emotions that dominate in depression (Kuyken *et al.*, 2010). It is likely therefore that, after an initial burst of PFC activity, they will move from high to low PFC blood flow as equilibrium is restored.[7] This would be particularly true for Blatt's 'introjective' group, where successful treatment will need to reduce the tendency to rumination and may entail long-term therapy (Leichsenring & Rabung, 2011).

An integrative model for depression

I shall now suggest a psychoanalytic-attachment model of depression which incorporates the above findings and offers some possible mechanisms of action for psychoanalytic psychotherapies.

a)   In a *normal resting state*, the individual and her/his attachment figures are in dynamic equilibrium, in which the security and responsiveness of the environment facilitates exploratory mental function (including exploring one's own and others' mental states, i.e. 'mentalising'; Lemma, Target & Fonagy, 2010). The neural substrate for this entails interacting intersecting feedback loops between the DLPFC and the external environment ('interpersonal circuit'), on the one hand, and the 'intrapersonal circuit', i.e. the 'lower' centres, including the amygdala. The architecture of the latter is the product of the 'temporal circuit' via the establishment of the emotional system during child development. Primal emotions, evoked by external relationships, are filtered through the 'gateway' of the Cg 25 and processed – regulated, moderated, mentalised – by the DLPFC.

b)   The establishment of a *'good internal object'* is the result of repeated cycles of loss and repair throughout childhood. This leads to an internalised emotion-processing attachment circuit analogous to the external one that has been lost.

c)   The system of intersecting circuits is disrupted by significant *loss events*, whether actual, e.g. loss of an attachment figure through death or divorce, or symbolic, e.g. loss of self-esteem following a career setback. This leads to a turning inwards towards the intrapersonal circuit. In the normal grieving process, however, there is sufficient 'ego strength' for the sufferer to replace the lost external relationship with an internal 'good object', enabling the primitive emotions of mental pain, anger, guilt, etc., generated in the lower centres to be processed. Adaptive repression plays a part too: under the aegis of Cg 25, pain is modulated and dealt with in manageable quanta. In addition, the supportiveness of the environment and the availability of potential new attachment figures, once grieving is accomplished, significantly influence outcome.

d)   *Depressive illness rather than normal grieving* may result following loss, depending on developmental factors:

   i)   an insecure rather than a secure attachment relational disposition;
   ii) a history of childhood trauma or neglect which 'sets' the HPA axis in ways that lead to excessive reactivity to loss and potential for triggering of early trauma by current loss events.

e)   *Dysregulation* following loss will follow different patterns depending on the individual's attachment style. In the hypoactivating (avoidant attachment) type the subject withdraws from the environment and tries to deal with primitive emotions by repression. Here excessive activity in Cg 25 leads to an 'introjective' pattern with typical self-reproaches and rumination, as elaborated by Freud. In the contrasting hyperactivating (ambivalent attachment) pattern the depressed person becomes 'anaclitic', seeking reassurance, becoming overly dependent and attempting to use the clung-to other as an auxiliary ego as a means of processing the primitive emotions with which she is flooded.

f)   *Therapy* helps move the depressed individual back onto a less dysregulated pathway, and to restore normal responses to loss and setback, in a number of ways:

i) offering a stable secure collaborative object relationship which temporarily takes over some of the functions of the lost object;

ii) fostering the cognitive processing of emotions and thereby overcoming affect phobia. In the introjective pattern the intrapsychic dynamic is opened out, lessening the repressive grip of the superego/Cg 25 (cf. Cathcart-Harris *et al.*, 2008), allowing feelings to be 'felt' and processed with the auxiliary help of the therapist;

iii) in the anaclitic pattern the therapist gradually returns projected feelings back to the sufferer, re-empowering her/his DLPFC's autonomous capacity to regulate her/his emotions.

iv) the intensity of primitive emotions 'from below' is reduced. This can happen in a number of ways, including the gradual processing of implicit memories of trauma in psychodynamic therapy; anti-depressant therapy; and meditative techniques in MBCBT (Kuyken *et al.*, 2010). In each case there may be a gradual resetting of the HPA axis, with reduced glucocorticoid sensitivity, and perhaps thereby enhanced skilfulness in using cognition to modulate emotion.

g) Finally, there is the instantiation of *hope*, the possibility of a new beginning. The lost object is restored to the inner world, which is thereby strengthened in parallel with a renewed interest in external reality. 'Hope' can be equated with the relinquishment of self-absorption and a renewed trust that exploration ('seeking' and 'play'; Panksepp & Watt, 2011) will yield fruit, bolstered by the knowledge that security will be available if loss or threat once more supervene.

Practice points

In this survey I have deliberately avoided a focus on outcome research and the relative merits of different therapeutic approaches.[8] Nevertheless, the model proposed above has significant implications for psychoanalytic practitioners.

First, depression needs to be seen as a heterogeneous condition (Blatt, 2008). A stepped care model (NICE, 2005) seems appropriate, in which CBT's combination of a good therapeutic relationship and reactivation of cognitive function in the DLPFC may in many cases suffice to restore psychological equilibrium. Where there is a history of early trauma or neglect, the prognosis tends to be less good and the indications for a psychodynamic approach correspondingly greater (Zobel *et al.*, 2011; Leichsenring & Raybung, 2011). It is important to bear this heterogeneity in mind within the psychoanalytic paradigm as well, in that the standard psychoanalytic model of depression of 'anger turned against the self' seems more applicable to introjective than to anaclitic patterns.

Psychoanalytic practitioners need to consider what the unique contribution of their discipline might be in the treatment of depression. Three points stand out. The first, while not specifically psychoanalytic in itself, is length of treatment. It may well be that, in severe cases, prolonged treatments are needed if the biological substrate for depression is to be re-set in less pathogenic ways. Lessening the strength of primitive emotions, reducing the need for excessive repression, decreasing the reactivity of the HPA axis, and fostering the capacity of the mind to regulate and process painful feelings all take time.

Secondly, psychoanalytic approaches can help transmute and modify implicit memory systems which are likely to be awry in individuals who have experienced trauma or neglect in early childhood. Therapy entails a degree of new experience in which sensitivity, responsiveness and the capacity for reflection gradually come to replace confusing, disorganising and controlling interpersonal patterns of relating. Becoming aware of these ingrained patterns, as well as providing a setting in which they can be changed, is central to the mechanism of action of psychoanalytic therapy (cf. Fonagy, 1998; Renn 2012).

This leads, finally, to psychoanalysis' unique contribution to psychotherapy practice – working with the subtleties of transference and counter-transference. Let us return to the case with which we began.

> The presence of affect phobia was signalled in Jane by a verbal ambiguity. The double meaning of 'he wasn't having it' exemplified how repressed primal emotions make their presence felt and the therapist's role in identifying these markers of repressed meaning. The implicit message from the therapist and therapeutic situation was: 'Your painful feelings are present; you aren't consciously aware of them, but they manifest themselves in your speech patterns and perhaps in your somatic symptoms; it is now safe to feel those feelings in the secure presence of a therapist.'
>
> Closer to transferential home, as described earlier, Jane was in a dilemma about taking anti-depressants. The vacuum left by her mother's death meant that she found it difficult to make decisions for herself and tried to push the analyst into deciding for her, which he initially resisted. At the end of one session, stung by her indecisiveness, and probably in a minor enactment, he found himself encouraging her to stop vacillating and give them a try.
>
> She returned the following week admitting that she still hadn't been able to bring herself to start them. Her demeanor seemed shamefaced and guilty. The analyst pointed this out. 'Oh, I thought you'd be really cross with me', she replied. While noting his counter-transference of mild exasperation, the analyst then explored with the patient a possible parallel between the sense that Jane felt she had to please him, that he would be annoyed if she didn't take her pills, and the way she and her mother had related. Jane expanded, and for the first time ambivalent feelings about her mother surfaced. Yes, mother was her best friend, *but* she could be demanding and difficult at times and, if Jane crossed her in any way, she would sulk. Then Jane would feel utterly wretched and abandoned and would feel compelled break the ice and say she was sorry.
>
> The minutiae of transference led to a formulation as follows. Jane's relationship with the therapist revealed a picture of anaclitic depression arising out of the hyperactivating pattern of insecure attachment. Jane's maternal caregiver was inconsistent: sometimes she was available or even over-available, sometimes mysteriously absent and rejecting. This set up a pattern of clinging attachment in which Jane's self-composure was dependent on proximity to her object. When her mother died this was not just a present loss, but revived earlier feelings of abandonment when her mother had withdrawn her love if Jane stepped out of line, and possibly procedural residues of premature weaning and her mother's anxieties about the loss of *her* mother. Jane's resentment about this had transmitted itself counter-transferentially to the analyst.
>
> For Jane to benefit from therapy (anti-depressants aside) she would need to co-create a pattern of relationship in which the analyst was available but not

controlling, and to be able to express disagreement and resentment towards him without feeling that would lead to rejection. Strengthened in this way, she would be more resilient to the stresses and losses which the future might bring.

Implicit in the above is the idea that the neurobiology of transference in depression depends on hypofrontality of the DLPFC. Instead of the normal interlocking of two mutually exploring minds, the sufferer's appraisal functions – of both self and other – are inhibited, so that 'primal emotions', including implicit procedural memories, biologically inscribed via epigenesis, are either projected onto or into the therapist (anaclitic pattern) or sequestered within the pressure cooker of the psyche (introjective pattern). In both cases the therapeutic task is to reactivate the DLPFC and thereby reduce affect phobia. In the anaclitic pattern difficult feelings are gradually returned from therapist to the sufferer for reappraisal; in the introjective pattern the therapist encourages the patient to mentalise and modulate the hitherto warded-off mental pain and rage.

Conclusions

In moving from an external loss to its meaning and significance in the inner world, Freud was moving from psychiatry to psychoanalysis, from explanation to meaning. It could be argued that, in exploring the biological and scientific, as opposed to the existential, dimensions of depression, as we have done here, an essential aspect of the psychoanalytic project has been lost. As Lear (2003, p. 146) puts it:

> We can learn much about the brain that is of value in alleviating human suffering ... but none of this can answer the subjective question: what is it *for me* to become a person? Psychoanalysis is a process by which I come to take responsibility for hitherto unconscious aspects of myself. I thereby deepen myself as a subject.

The thrust of this paper has been to suggest, to the contrary, that the more we understand ourselves as biological beings, and the more conscious and objective we are of both brain and mind and how they dovetail one with another, the deeper and more responsible our subjectivity can become.

POSTSCRIPT: CHRONIC DEPRESSION – A COMMENT ON A SUFFERER'S ACCOUNT

A long-term patient of mine, Jackie, published an account of her illness in the British Medical Journal, and I was invited by her and her GP to write a 500-word commentary. This is what I said.

Our patients are our best teachers. During my tutelage with Jackie I have learned a huge amount about major depression: what it feels like, its impact on sufferers' and their loved ones' lives, and what does and what doesn't help.

I have witnessed the toll taken by this ubiquitous disease, no less devastating in its impact than other chronic conditions such as diabetes or rheumatoid arthritis. Jackie, an able and enthusiastic student, could barely finish her course at university, her employment prospects have been blighted, her social life has been restricted, and her capacity for pleasure and fulfilment curtailed.

I have grasped how, at their worst, psychiatric services reinforce sufferers' feelings of isolation, stigmatisation, inferiority and powerlessness. I say this not just to distance myself from old-style mental hospital regimes, but also about my own initial attempts at working psychotherapeutically with Jackie. I painfully discovered that my assumed opacity and efforts to 'interpret' her depression in terms of unexpressed anger and childhood trauma (for which there was much evidence) merely reinforced Jackie's feelings of failure and her conviction that she, the victim, was to blame for her illness. What she needed was validation, confirmation that the world does really treat the mentally ill differently, and understanding that to be depressed is at best to live only partly. It was only when I decided to move into a more supportive therapy mode that I felt that Jackie began tentatively to trust me. At times I am sure that she resisted and resented me and what I stood for. I have learned to respect and acknowledge that resentment and its legitimacy, despite knowing that such strong feelings are coloured by a depressive world-view. Painfully, Jackie has taught me how corrosive the 'division of suffering' between patient and doctor can be. By acknowledging our own vulnerability we can lessen the need to project our disturbances into our patients.

Staying the course with Jackie has shown us both how favourable life events form the new beginning that can be the starting point for recovery from depression. The uncompromising devotion of Jackie's husband and the delighted witnessing of her daughter's flourishing, unscathed by her mother's illness, have made a huge difference. Watching Jackie gradually emerge from the darkness of her depression into a sense of light-heartedness and possibility has been a privilege and a relief. The frequency of our sessions over the years has been gradually attenuated. We are now more likely to meet at the local train station than in the consulting room! A long-term therapeutic relationship can provide a secure base where illness can be explored, accepted and sequestered, helping the sufferer to live with a degree of normality in the outside world. I suspect – unless this be rose-tinted nostalgia – that the current fragmented and episodic psychiatric services, for all they avoid Jackie's early mental hospital horrors, may militate against this. If so, psychiatry – and maybe its patients – is the poorer.

Notes

1   Affect phobia has the advantage of being a bridging concept between psychoanalysis and cognitive-behavioural conceptions of depression.
2   Paralleling the absence of the loved one.
3   Which can perhaps be compared with the physical self-attack of auto-immune illnesses, where at a somatic level self–other differentiation goes awry.
4   The complementary 'hypoactivating' pattern means that avoidant people find it difficult to draw on external support when it is needed.
5   Bowlby always maintained that attachment theory, rooted as it is in evolutionary biology, was no less 'organic' than psychopharmacology.
6   This tongue-in-cheek formula is based of course on the rhyme scheme of e=mc squared.
7   This argument is in some ways is comparable to apparently contradictory conceptualisation of defence mechanisms. The concept of reaction formation accounts for both the excessive passivity that may betoken aggression and the aggression concealing latent fear and vulnerability.
8   But note, among others, Shedler (2010) and Abbass (2006) for robust evidence for psychoanalytic treatments for depression.

CHAPTER 8

ANTI-PSYCHIATRY AND THE PSYCHOTHERAPY OF PSYCHOSIS

I hate to admit it, as one of those psychiatrist bad-guys who are the main target of its invective, but Bentall (2010) has written an excellent book. The main theme is the malign and ineffective impact of psychiatry on mental illness, focusing on psychosis and in particular schizophrenia. Bentall's thesis runs roughly as follows. Today's psychiatric patients are little better off than they were 200 years ago when medicine first took over the care of the mentally ill from religion. Attempts to see schizophrenia as a genetically determined illness have generally failed. To the extent it is legitimate to talk about schizophrenia at all, its causes are to be found in the environment, and in particular in the emotional abuse and trauma which such people have undergone in childhood. Psychiatric diagnoses are myths, based on pseudo-medicalisation of human distress. Psychotic symptoms are found throughout the population, and those called mentally ill are merely those who have had the misfortune to fall into the hands of psychiatry. Patients suffer, to be sure, but what they have is valid complaints, not reified artefactual symptoms. Psychiatric so-called treatments, drugs, ECT, and – horror of horrors – psychosurgery (and its contemporary progeny, Deep Brain Stimulation), are at best useless, at worst destructive of mind, body and soul. The medicalisation of mental distress serves the interests of the big pharmaceutical companies and the doctors who are in their pocket, but not their patients. What the mentally ill need is warm, accepting, autonomy-promoting friendship from clinical psychologists, not cold, coercive, paternalistic psychiatrists peddling side-effect-producing drugs and depriving sufferers of their liberty through involuntary hospitalisation.

Sound familiar? From one perspective Bentall is merely echoing what was said half a century ago by those venerable pioneers of anti-psychiatry R. D. Laing and Thomas Szasz. Of course, the fact that something has been said but not heard before does not necessary mean that it is untrue. And Bentall certainly brings a new set of skills to the debate. His is, or at first blush looks like, an evidence-based set of factual propositions rather than polemic, poetry and scientifically questionable case-examples.

But, sadly, Bentall's use of evidence is tendentious. He uncritically quotes studies which support his thesis while subjecting those whose conclusions contradict it to nit-picking exactitude; if the results are against him (as, with reservations, they are on the polygenetic theory of schizophrenia), he will say that they are 'unclear'. Equally, where there is doubt, he speculates within his chosen parameters alone, without considering other options. To take one example, his psychological account of paranoid delusions rests heavily on the dopamine hypothesis. Raised dopamine levels increase people's expectations of anticipated pain or reward, and therefore make them more likely to attribute salience to neutral environmental stimuli. He claims that raised dopamine levels must in some way be related to childhood trauma. In reality we simply don't know what their origin is, much less why this particular condition often manifests itself in elderly females, often with no previous history of illness. Negative capability – the capacity to tolerate doubt – and, indeed, clinical humility feature minimally in Bentall's repertoire.

That said, there is much that is valid and important here. Unfortunately Bentall cannot resist overstating his case. Yes, it is true that no simple genetic basis for schizophrenia has been found; but there is good evidence that an accumulation of small genetic predispositions (so-called copy error transcriptions) do indeed make people more liable to develop psychosis. Yes, psychotic symptoms are not confined to people diagnosed with schizophrenia, but that does not invalidate the diagnosis, any more than the fact that a lot of people get pains in their joints rules out the reality of rheumatoid arthritis. Yes, psychiatry's history is chequered, and bad things have been done, and perhaps are still being done, in its name. But would one want to discredit the entire profession of gastroenterology because, until the discovery of helicobacter, peptic ulcer was treated with surgery, thereby inflicting unnecessary suffering and in some cases death on its subjects?

Similarly, childhood adversity probably does play a part in the evolution of schizophrenia, but the majority of people exposed to such adversity do not become psychotic (which is not to say they don't suffer in other ways), and a significant subgroup of people with schizophrenia have developmental anomalies that are independent of life-experience. Environmental causes may rest as much in maternal malnutrition, influenza or vitamin D deficiency as in parental malevolence or neglect. And, yes, there is a group of people who suffer from schizophrenia (about 40 per cent) who do not seem to get better despite all psychiatry's best efforts. But 60 per cent do improve, and it seems likely that the modern armamentarium of mental health – early intervention, low-dose medication, befriending, cognitive therapy and environmental provision (sheltered housing, employment, social groups) – really does help.

Finally, the very concept of schizophrenia, while shaky in comparison, say, with that of diabetes, in that no unique biochemical or structural abnormality has been identified, does have validity. It can perhaps be compared with the diagnosis of 'congestive cardiac failure' (CCF), a condition in which the lungs become filled with fluid as a result of the heart's inability to pump blood efficiently through them. There are many causes of CCF – cardiomyopathy, ischaemic heart disease, fibrosis of the lung, disease of the heart valves, etc. – but they all produce a recognisable clinical picture. The same is true of schizophrenia, which is probably made up of a number of sub-patterns and etiologies, including exacerbation by cannabis, minor degrees of intellectual impairment, and trauma, both physical and mental.

How can such an intelligent and eloquent author as Bentall be so seduced by the partiality of his arguments and the evidence? Well, who would not want to be on the side of the angels? For Bentall, 'badness' is firmly located elsewhere – in the doctors, the drug companies, the abusers, but never in the human condition itself. This is a message the world wants to hear, and that includes not just the literati who adorn the cover of his book but the sufferers themselves. The symptoms of schizophrenia are generally terrifying, confusing and painful. To feel that they are all the fault of the doctors is comforting and helps counteract the horrible stigma attached to mental illness. Who would want to feel they were suffering from an illness whose origins we don't fully understand and from which they might make at best a very partial recovery?

Ironically, Bentall is prisoner of his own black-and-white world-view. His rigid distinction between the organic and the psychological, the medical and the psychological, between genes and the environment, is simply outdated. Gene–environment interplay is where the action is. Thus long allele versions of the serotonin transporter gene protect children from the deleterious effects of environmental adversity, while the short variety renders them vulnerable to depression in later life. Environmental conditions have a major impact on the way in which genes are expressed. For example, cannabis smoking (especially the high THC varieties such as 'skunk') is almost certainly related to the development of schizophrenia by affecting some genetically predisposed individuals and not others. In addition, epigenesis – i.e. non-genomic inheritance – means that environmental conditions, via affecting methylation rates, directly affect future generations. Similarly, in the arena of treatment, pitting pharmacology against psychotherapy is counter-productive and old hat. Generally, in severe mental illness the combination of medication and psychotherapy gets better results than either alone. Current sophisticated thinking about schizophrenia brings together multiple genes, gene–environment interaction, and acknowledgment of the role of social and psychological factors into a cascade hypothesis that is a long way from simplistic dichotomising.

One danger of Bentall's polemic is that it may not be about what it purports to be at all. Psychosis and mental distress are realities and exist in all societies so far studied. Understanding why this might be so is potentially a neutral value-free scientific enterprise. But, thanks to the ambiguity of the manifestations of mental illnesses, and the relative powerlessness of patients, psychosis sufferers can be a convenient vehicle for the projection of personal and social conflict. The power of the professions is under scrutiny: let's leave surgeons alone – we might need them for an operation sometime – and concentrate our firepower on psychiatrists (memorably once described by a distinguished psychiatric professor in a public meeting as 'half as intelligent as clinical psychologists and paid twice as much'). The instrumentalism of contemporary life is a cause for concern: why not focus that worry on the supposed reification of people's problems in psychiatric diagnoses? Childhood neglect and abuse is horribly common – why not nail one's outrage to the banner of the misunderstanding of the mentally ill? Many social groups – students, journalists, clinical psychologists even – feel marginalised, that their authentic voice is not being heard. Why not champion the heard and unheard voices of schizophrenia as a safe displacement from one's own sense of disempowerment?

Despite these caveats and disagreements, as far as the biology–psychology battle goes, the debate will continue, and Bentall's approach is one strand in what I hope will be an eventual rapprochement. Clinically, there is plenty of work to go round for psychiatrists and clinical psychologists both; with severely disturbed patients it is only multidisciplinary teams that can provide the containment and multifaceted approach needed. As for professional rivalry, envy and mutual disparagement, these are no doubt inevitable, and should perhaps not be taken too seriously.

In sum, as a work of science this is a stimulating albeit one-sided account: its marshalling of the evidence is as much prejudicial as it is authoritative. As a book of politics it is a fine polemical essay. Psychiatry and psychiatrists deserve to be scrutinised, even if Bentall's targets are mostly easy game and his remedies anodyne. If it serves to raise the profile of psychiatry, to highlight the intellectual and moral challenges it presents, and to draw attention to the sufferings of its patients, it will have done a fine job.

CHAPTER 9

NARRATIVE IN PSYCHIATRY AND PSYCHOTHERAPY

The evidence?

For every thesis there is an antithesis. The current ascendancy of evidence-based medicine (EBM), for all its power and beauty, has created disquiet among some clinicians and researchers. Are randomised controlled trials (RCTs), practice guidelines, national service frameworks, and protocols really the end of the story, or is there still a place for clinical judgment, the importance of the doctor–patient relationship and the traditional emphasis on individual meanings and case histories? Evidence-based medicine has thrown up a counter-movement, less organised and influential perhaps, whose voice is still uncertain, but which nevertheless holds onto narrative and story as a bedrock of clinical practice. The purpose of this chapter is to review aspects of narrative-based medicine (NBM) as they impact on psychiatry and psychotherapy, to consider research aspects of narrative, and to look at ways in which EBM and NBM can complement each other both for the benefit of the individual patient and more widely.

Evidence-based medicine argues that medical practice should model itself on scientific method and that all interactions with patients should be guided by the falsifiability principle: only those interventions which have been shown by rigorous tests to be effective should be implemented; thus will the health of the population benefit and the costs of health services to the public purse be justified. In itself this approach is unexceptionable – who could reasonably disagree? – and yet many health workers feel that something vital to medical practice is left out in this uncompromising position.

The limitations of evidence-based medicine

The narrative critique draws on a number of different empirical and philosophical strands. First, there is the uncomfortable gap between efficacy and effectiveness: many doctors prescribe treatments which do not meet the rigorous criteria of EBM and, conversely, fail to deliver treatments which have been shown to work. In schizophrenia, for example, there is a continuing failure to deliver psychosocial interventions, and especially family therapy, despite two decades of strong evidence for their efficacy. Doctors need more than published results of RCTs to change their practice: acquiring psychosocial skills for themselves, treating patients and their families, and seeing the resulting changes that can come about (and those that cannot) are all necessary. Only when the evidence is backed by a story of a successful treatment which the doctor can see with his or her own eyes is it likely to be incorporated into day-to-day practice. We learn by doing, and doing involves a self-generated narrative in which we are active agents of change, shaping, and being influenced by, the results of our activities. For MacIntyre (2013), we *are* our narrative: our sense of self is inextricably bound up with our life-stories and the meanings they have generated. Narrative is thus synonymous with training and learning.

Advocates of narrative argue that, with all the huge advances of modern scientific medicine, there has been a loss of 'meaning' in our work and in what has been offered to the patient. But what do we mean by meaning? According to Quine (Gibson, 2004), meaning arises out of connectedness – we look up a word in the dictionary and are offered another set of words to which that word is connected, and they in turn are linked to another set of words, and so on, until we reach a web of meanings that comprise an entire language. This is also described by the philosopher/psychoanalyst Cavell as 'meaning holism' (Cavell, 2006). Meaning in this sense can be linked to both metaphor and story. Metaphor is a fruitful collision or connection between apparently unrelated phenomena. Many of the metaphors that arise in psychiatry and psychotherapy connect bodily experience to the external world. For example, a middle-aged man whose business had failed and who becomes depressed might describe himself as 'gutted' as he spoke about looking round his empty warehouse. The clear link between the external event and his feelings, however painful, give meaning to his pain and help him cope with it. Meanings in this sense are affect-regulatory. Similarly, stories are series of linked intentions and actions which create a sense of connection and agency: first this happened, then I did that, and the result was the other.

Evidence-based medicine is often described as 'instrumentalist', in that it applies the scientific method within a given reality but does not consider the historical and sociological forces which shape that reality. For example, resistance to the implementation of psychosocial interventions in schizophrenia arises in the context of a pharmaceutical industry which invests large amounts of money in order to influence doctors to prescribe its neuroleptic treatments, with psychosocial interventions coming in a very poor second in the list of priorities. The instrumentalist perspective of EBM posits the doctor as a scientific agent of change, offering his validated treatments to a passive patient. In NBM, doctor and patient together are 'co-constructors' of a shared reality in which the history and expectations of each play significant roles in determining outcome. For example, we need to know what our patients' *attitude* towards medication are – whether they are 'anti-pills', have tried homoeopathy or have specific spiritual beliefs, tend to be forgetful, are obsessional, etc. – before gauging the likelihood of compliance with our prescriptions. These attitudes are all embedded in the patients' individual experience and encoded as a series of stories – a grandmother, say, who was given aspirin, developed a gastrointestinal bleed and died, or a religious teaching which fosters a passive acceptance of 'fate' – which comprise their personal narratives. Critics of EBM argue that modern medicine tends to downplay these vital aspects of medical practice, while the traditional skills of history-taking and listening suffer in the face of the drive to examine, investigate and intervene. Good practice requires a blend of evidence-based and narrative approaches, in which scientific knowledge is adapted and tailored to fit with the particular circumstances, biography and personality of each individual patient.

Narrative and causality

Supporters of EBM might be happy to concede the points made so far but argue that what is being said is both obvious and trivial – *of course* we need to take histories carefully and respect patients and their beliefs, but the cutting edge of treatment remains based on evidence, not narrative. 'What about Down's syndrome?' they might suggest. The narrative approach held sway until the discovery of trisomy in 1956: mothers of Down's syndrome babies were asked about adverse physical and emotional events during pregnancy and were found to have a much greater incidence of trauma than mothers of non-affected babies. Here a narrative explanation stood in the way of the 'real' evidence: the overwhelming need to make sense of experience led these mothers to connect the trauma of their abnormal baby with previous trauma, whereas in reality there was no such link, and presumably mothers of normal babies had had equal amounts of unhappiness whose significance faded once their babies were born without blemish.

The argument here is essentially about causality. Bolton and Hill (1996) distinguish between 'intentional' and 'non-intentional' causality – the former implies agency of some kind, while the latter is outside the realm of human intention. Garland (1998) similarly distinguishes trauma that has a 'man-made', intentional aspect from traumas that are outside the realm of human agency. Down's syndrome turned out to be a 'non-intentional' story about chromosomes, not human agency. But if we take Down's syndrome as a paradigm we will miss much that is central to medical and especially psychiatric practice – the interplay between intentional and non-intentional causality is where most problems lie. As a counter-example, if we simply collude with patients who attribute their depression to a 'chemical imbalance in the brain' (which is not to deny that such 'imbalance' exists), and fail to take account of the ways in which their illness arises out of their life-story, we will miss the role of loss and the associated grief which Brown and Harris (1978) have shown to be causative factors in the origins of depressive illness, and which may also play a role in the *expression* of a genetic vulnerability to schizophrenia. Furthermore, however much Down's syndrome is a product of 'non-intentional causality', there remains a story to be attended to about how a family copes with the advent of a handicapped child.

The uses of narrative in clinical practice

What is the role of narrative in clinical practice? Narrative methods are central to history-taking and formulation, to engagement, and to several aspects of psychotherapy.

History-taking and formulation

Psychiatric patients often present to services in bemused and de-contextualised states. A patient arrives in casualty after an overdose. A young person who has been behaving strangely is dragged along by anxious relatives. Someone known to be psychotic refuses to let his community worker into the house. The clinician's task is to find a story into which this fragment of inexplicable or worrying behaviour can be fitted. A story is always about the interplay of intention and context – or, to put it the other way round, when we have found a human agent acting within a context, then we have a story. In a clinical context, a story is a sequence of events centring on a suffering patient. It consists of alternating episodes of 'what was done to me/what I felt' and 'how I reacted/responded/felt about it in return'.

We often ask a patient on first meeting: 'What's the story?', or 'How did you land up here in this room talking to someone like me?', or 'How did it all begin?' The aim is to reconstruct a narrative chain out of an apparently disconnected series of events, ending with the here and now, this patient talking to this doctor, in this room, on this day, about this subject – the story so far. By proceeding in this way we begin immediately to encourage the patient to become the author of her own story – to consider what has happened to her, how she has reacted, and what she was and is feeling about it. We start from a feeling of puzzlement, akin to embarking on reading a novel or listening to a story – 'Why did so-and-so meet so-and-so on such-and-such a day?', 'What is going to happen next?', 'How will it all end?' – and do not rest until we have a picture of what the overall shape of the story might be. At first glance this will probably be fairly familiar: the overdose that followed a row with a boyfriend, the young man who has been smoking too much cannabis, the patient who has stopped taking his medication. But stories are infinite: each one leads on to another. Why did she react to a row in that way? Why did the row occur in the first place? Is this an example of separation anxiety in someone whose parents split up when she was a child? What led him to retreat into cannabis? Had he lost his job or his girlfriend? Did the cannabis make him depressed, or was it the other way round? Why did he stop his pills? Was it the side-effects? Or did the hallucinations tell him to? Perhaps he only believes in homoeopathy? Is that a valid or a delusional belief? And so on. Thus a narrative approach to history-taking and formulation leads the listener deeper and deeper into the causal chain of events – both intentional and non-intentional – which underlie the presenting problem, and can be used to help patients put their illness in a context which helps give meaning to their apparently meaningless pain.

Engagement

'Engagement', or therapeutic alliance, is the backdrop to the mutual commitment of doctor and patient to the understanding and tackling of the problem which the patient brings for amelioration. In psychotherapy the quality of the therapeutic alliance is the single best predictor of good outcome for treatment. A narrative approach can be a powerful method of engaging the patient, who encounters a clinician who genuinely wants to know how things look from his, the patient's, point of view, who wants to hear *his*, or at the very least *his side of*, the story. Every good psychiatric clinician is driven by a fascination with the phenomenology of patients' experience, by the ramifications of their delusional system, the minutiae of their everyday lives – by a wish to understand this particular person's story, to get to the heart of her suffering – and accords this enterprise equal importance to the need to understand the mental or biochemical mechanisms involved. In working with psychotic patients, EBM will tell the clinician which antipsychotic drug is likely to be effective; but listening carefully to the details of the patient's psychotic experiences, and trying to draw out a narrative pattern in his story, is a precondition for successful prescription. Without the engagement which this implies, the patient is far less likely to take his medication or to trust the clinician in other ways.

Narrative and supportive psychotherapy

A significant part of the effectiveness of psychotherapy is attributable to 'common' or 'non-specific factors' which form part of the therapeutic process, whether psychoanalytic or cognitive. Supportive psychotherapy relies on this phenomenon for its usefulness. A basic technique in supportive psychotherapy consists simply of encouraging patients to tell their story and to 'ventilate' their feelings about the events of their life. Winnicott described psychoanalysis as an 'extended form of history-taking'; offering patients a supportive relationship sustained over many years similarly comprises a significant part of the work of the consultant psychiatrist. The narrative stance requires a consistent curiosity on the part of the doctor, who always wants to hear more, and who learns to cultivate a creative puzzlement about aspects of the patient's story which do not seem to make sense.

The importance of this emergent 'autobiographical competence' has been supported by a study which showed that even physical illness can benefit from narrative activity. Patients with rheumatoid arthritis and asthma were asked to write about stressful experiences in their lives. Compared with controls who did not write, or simply wrote about neutral topics, their symptoms improved over a six-month period on a variety of objective measures. It is intriguing to speculate about the possible mechanisms which might explain this finding. One possibility is to think of writing or telling one's story as representing a form of surrogate relationship, albeit with oneself, with the anxiety reduction and possibility for processing mental and physical pain that that entails. Narrative activity helps create an internal sense of a 'secure base'. The objectification of feelings involved in the writing task helps the sufferer to distance herself from her pain. In addition, relationship implies connectedness and an escape from the narcissism which chronic illness, whether physical or mental, can foster.

Narrative and attachment

This links with the concept of 'reflexive function' (RF), or mentalising, which has emerged from attachment research, suggesting that people who are able to 'represent' and so reflect upon their experience in words, however problematic or painful, are more likely to be able to form secure attachments than those who lack such capacity (Fonagy *et al.*, 2002). For the purposes of our discussion, this self-reflexive capacity is important in three ways.

First, because it is exactly what psychotherapists aim to foster in their patients, whether they be cognitive therapists working with automatic thoughts and assumptions or analytic therapists with their motto 'Where id is, there ego shall be'. Ego is the psyche's story-teller. Second, in a general practice context, the very existence of a general practitioner (GP) and a surgery gives a message to the patient that his pain and difficulties can be 'represented' – first talked about and then acted on so as to reduce suffering. Third, RF and narrative style generally have been shown to be linked with early relationship patterns. Longitudinal studies have shown that children who are securely attached in infancy are more likely to have a coherent and 'free-autonomous' narrative style when talking about themselves in early adulthood compared with insecurely attached children, whose narratives tend to be either over-elaborated and confused (linked with ambivalent attachments) or sparsely dismissive (linked with the avoidant attachment pattern). The ways in which people talk about themselves reveal fundamental relationship patterns.

This insight into narrative styles can enhance the quality of listening with which we approach patients and guide our interventions in 'story-making' or 'story-breaking' directions. Patients with self-sufficient, unelaborated, dismissive narratives need to be encouraged to break open their defensive stories and consider other possibilities. Those who seem unable to find a narrative thread and to be drowning in the chaos of their experience need to be helped to find a shape and a pattern which helps fit things into place. Narrative style, in other words, can be a guide to diagnosis, pointing to particular relationship patterns in childhood, and propensities in adult life.

Narrative and metaphor in dynamic psychotherapy

Dynamic therapy is redolent with metaphor. The words 'metaphor' and 'transference', although from Greek and Latin roots respectively, are etymologically the same, referring to carrying something across and therefore, by extension, to the making of connections. Hobson's (1985) Conversational Model, or Psychodynamic-Interpersonal Therapy, explicitly encourages patient and therapist to explore feelings using metaphor. A metaphor is a fundamental narrative device: a memorable image that gives meaning to the patient's difficulty, a 'third term' which helps a patient to begin to objectify her problems. It links together different aspects of the patient's life and is open to discussion, modification or elaboration by both patient and therapist. In a Winnicottian sense it lies 'transitionally' between patient and therapist, with a life of its own, and is not wholly the property of either. As a 'third term', a metaphor belongs to the 'Oedipal' stage of development, where the child has to cope with the triangle of mother, father and herself, but also gains the objectivity which being able to observe the parental couple from the outside brings. Metaphor thus simultaneously pulls patient and therapist together and separates them from the lure of narcissistic fusion or collusion.

As a fundamental narrative device, metaphor and simile can be compared with the scientific hypotheses of EBM. Both represent speculations which need to be tested against reality. For EBM, the criteria are objective; but, for NBM therapists, the main test of their metaphors is whether they 'feel' right to themselves and their patients. Unlike a scientific hypothesis, metaphor is always specific to a given situation – it upholds the uniqueness of the individual life-history. Its terms are not interchangeable in the way that in an equation, for example, the number 3 can always be substituted by the square root of 9 to give the same result. People are troubled by a fairly limited range of problems, centring on the biological fundamentals of relatedness – 'birth, copulation and death' (Eliot, 1986) – but one life-history is never exchangeable with another. We cannot create a composite Dickens novel by replacing Pip by Martin Chuzzlewit in *Great Expectations*. This is a basic difference between EBM, which is based on the behaviour of populations whose elements are equivalent, and NBM, which is always about particular cases. This is not to say, however, that therapeutic metaphors are *entirely* subjective. Psychotherapy research methods can measure the impact of therapist utterances in terms of patient speech patterns or emotional responses, and thus get some indication of the therapeutic impact of a metaphor.

The narrative thrust in dynamic psychotherapy is always patient-centred. The role of the therapist is as 'auxiliary autobiographer', helping the patient to clarify the contours of his own story and to make sense of it. A similar practice at the level of the family is to be found in systemic therapy. Here the effort is to track 'family scripts', the unconscious rules and expectations which shape family life across generations and which trap individual members in painful or self-defeating roles and behaviours.

Some family therapists go further than this and use story-telling and jokes as a therapeutic device in their own right. For example, if a couple is rowing in a session, the therapist might intervene with the well-known joke 'Is this a private fight, or can anyone join in?' Stories here are equivalent to the generalisations and laws of EBM – universal psychological truths which can help people cope with mental pain. The informal subculture of medicine abounds with such stories. 'Balint groups' for trainee psychiatrists are one way to legitimise doctors' need to look at their own stories when faced with the emotional impact of their work. In one such group it emerged that, as the junior doctors were lunching together, someone had proposed a competition for the most absurd form of deliberate self-harm encountered during the past six months; these ranged from attempting to gas oneself with carbon monoxide in an open cabriolet to hanging oneself using the emergency bell pull. While this was undoubtedly disrespectful to the patients concerned, it also expressed the tremendous strain which young doctors experience in the face of their patients' death wishes – a story in its own right, which also needs to be told. Here too NBM recognises and celebrates this aspect of practice, complementing, enhancing and helping to deliver effectively the many contributions of contemporary scientific medicine.

Stories we remember – true or false?

The recovered memory debate has raged furiously in psychotherapy and cannot be ignored in any discussion of NBM. There are those who claim that false memories can be implanted in suggestible subjects by unscrupulous psychotherapists, while on the other side there is much evidence to suggest that painful memories can be obliterated from memory, only to surface at times of stress or further trauma. The key issue for the discussion of narrative is that stories should not necessarily be taken at face value. Indeed, it is often a mark of an inexperienced therapist to attend too closely to 'content' and to miss the tone, context and interactive dimension of what is being said. Stories always exist in an interpersonal setting: there is a story-teller and a listener, and the story needs to be understood in terms of their relationship. Therapists should ask themselves why is *this person* telling me *this story*, in *this way*, on *this occasion*? They should also be able to tolerate the uncertainty of not knowing how true any particular story happens to be. While some issues are indeed matters of simple fact – was this person sexually abused or not? – more often memories are questions of tone and perspective. As already mentioned, some patients need help to create a coherent account of what has happened to them (story-making), others to consider possibilities other than the simplistic account to which they cling (story-breaking). In the course of treatment, people's view of themselves and their history will change. The past is reconsidered in the light of the present. The 'true story', to recapitulate, is a pattern of agency and context. The therapist's task is to help patients find a story that pays due attention to both – to what they have made of what they are made of.

Research in NBM

Although narrative-based medicine may not sit comfortably with conventional EBM methodologies, especially the RCT, narrative is far from unresearchable. In the course of this chapter, three approaches to systematic study of narrative have already been mentioned. Brown's studies of depression rely on narrative methods in which verifiable events are evaluated by researchers who then look at the interpersonal context of the sufferer and make judgments about how loss and difficulty have impacted on individual lives. The Adult Attachment Interview (AAI) (Main,

1995) is a quintessentially narrative instrument which takes transcripts of interviews and subjects them to structural and linguistic analysis, resulting in reliable
codings of narrative style, which in turn link with attachment patterns. Luborsky
et al.'s (1989) Core Conflictual Relationship Theme approach similarly relies on
interview transcripts to extract narrative episodes which are then classified according to predetermined interpersonal features. This measure of psychotherapy
process can then be used in a variety of ways, for example to look at correlations
between outcomes and, say, to focus on transference in the content of the sessions.

Conclusions: towards integration

I have tried to argue the case for NBM, both theoretically and as central to the
everyday practice of psychotherapeutic psychiatry. Conventional medicine has a
tendency to be conservative and to be at times self-serving. Evidence-based
medicine is a necessary spur which questions traditional assumptions and values.
There is no inherent conflict between narrative- and evidence-based approaches:
understanding the patient's story helps align scientific knowledge with the specific needs and predilections of individual patients. But in an ever accelerating
culture we run the danger of losing touch with historical and developmental
perspectives: the 'present' is always an evolution and mutation from the past. It
is simply not good enough for psychiatrists to seek for the symptoms of schizophrenia, prescribe the latest antipsychotic, and feel that the job is done. We need
to attend as closely to the patient's story and context as we do to the minutiae
of the mental state examination. Evidence-based medicine and NBM are complementary facets of a wider whole. Finding the ways in which they intersect is an
urgent task for the next generation of psychiatrists.

CHAPTER 10

PSYCHODYNAMIC PSYCHIATRY
Rise, decline and renewal

This chapter charts the varying fortunes of psychodynamic psychiatry (PP) from the halcyon days of the 1960s, through the sharp decline in the 1980s and 1990s 'decade of the brain', to retrenchment and revival in the twenty-first century. I start by exploring what is meant by the term 'psychodynamic', outlining some of the key psychodynamic ideas that have entered into everyday psychiatric thinking and vernacular. The discussion then shifts to a historical account of the rise and fall of psychodynamic psychiatry in the UK and the US, followed by a brief worldwide survey. Moving to a possible future role for PP, I consider its evidence base, its contribution to the treatment of the principal psychiatric diagnoses, and its role in the expanding fields of neuro-psychoanalysis, neurogenetics and developmental psychopathology.

What is psychodynamic psychiatry?

Prejudice is rife in psychiatry. Mental illness is stigmatised, as are its sufferers and, to an extent, its practitioners. Within psychiatry itself, psychoanalytic psycho-therapists are sometimes characterised as antediluvian 'Freudians', clinging to outdated ideas and impervious to evidence-based theory and practice. In the course of this chapter I shall hope to bust some of these myths.

Psychodynamic psychiatry must be differentiated from its parent discipline of psychoanalysis, although they are often mistakenly viewed as synonymous; here we shall be concerned with the role of psychoanalysis only insofar as it has impacted on PP. The term 'psychodynamics' predates Freud (first used in 1874) but traditionally refers to a multi-modular mind in which the various forces considered to comprise the psyche – consciousness and 'the' unconscious, id, ego and superego – are in a state of dynamic equilibrium. There is an implicit contrast with 'psycho-static', 'medical model' categories of mental illness with their specific aetiologies and treatments.

The brain/mind can be visualised as a dynamic system comprising two principal circuits, one intrapsychic, the other interpersonal. The intrapsychic circuit corresponds to the classical account, in which the basic affective mesolimbic primary processes – panic/grief, rage, care, seeking, lust and play – are subject to continuous appraisal and regulation (mentalising) by cortical functions. The interpersonal circuit links these cortical functions, especially in the right hemisphere, to emotional interchange with significant others, actual (parent, spouse, combat 'buddie') or symbolic (i.e. an internal representation of the other) in an individual's immediate and developmental environment. A large body of evidence now supports the view that, at least in infancy and early childhood, intrapsychic equilibrium is moderated by this interpersonal environment. It certainly is the case that no child is an island. This relational view found an early champion in the US in the Washington School of psychiatry, under the leadership of Harry Stack Sullivan, and in the UK through the group of psychiatrists and psychoanalysts associated with the Tavistock Clinic in London.

The umbrella term 'psychodynamic psychiatry' thus implies both a developmental and an interpersonal perspective on the origins of psychological distress and malfunction, together with specialist expertise in the psychotherapeutic treatments able to alleviate them. A number of PP concepts and approaches have been incorporated into the psychiatric mainstream. Here I touch on three.

First is the view that psychiatric symptoms – depression, anxiety, addiction, delusions, etc. – need to be viewed not as reified things-in-themselves but as manifestations of underlying dynamic processes, the resultant of the interplay between affects and the various defences mounted to modulate and regulate them. Thus a psychodynamically informed 'formulation' aims to tease out the precipitating loss events that triggered a depression, together with the pre-existing vulnerability dating back to childhood. The latter might be associated with a 'narcissistic injury' in which a loved parent became depressed herself and was unable to provide the validation and unconditional delight children need if they are to acquire the self-esteem necessary to mitigate life's later vicissitudes. Or, to take another example, deliberate self-harm might be viewed as a last-ditch attempt at self-soothing in an individual whose capacity for comfort when distressed is compromised, both at a physiological level following adverse early childhood experience and contemporaneously through social isolation and/or problematic relationships. Implicit in the above is an affect-defence model of psychic function. 'Depression' in the first example is itself seen as a defence against experiencing the unbearable pain of loss and failure; in the second, self-harm in a way circumvents a feeling of abandonment and rage at those who have let the sufferer down.

Defence mechanisms (a term originally developed by Anna Freud) have been studied and developed by George Vaillant (1997), who classified them as follows: mature (e.g. humour), neurotic (e.g. intellectualisation), immature (e.g. passive-aggressive) and pathological (e.g. denial and projection). Valliant's long-term follow-up studies of men classified originally under those four headings reveal that those with mature defences had better adjustment, happiness, job satisfaction and friendships, fewer hospitalizations, better overall health, and a lower incidence of mental illness. Conversely, presence of immature defences is related to poor adjustment, higher divorce rates and marital discord, less satisfactory friendship patterns, a higher incidence of mental illness, a greater number of sick-leave days taken, and poorer health generally. Implicit in this model of psychopathology is the idea that a person's character can be understood in terms of how they negotiate the psychobiological challenges of development – the need to be safe, to reproduce, to be part of a social network, to provide for and rear children, to cope with loss and trauma, etc. 'Defences' represent the often unconscious strategies and attendant compromises people arrive at as ways of balancing the internal, relational and social forces to which they are subject.

A second key psychodynamic theme for psychiatrists flows from the affect-defence model. People are liable to deploy defences in situations that arouse anxiety. The psychoanalytic notion of transference and counter-transference is relevant to psychiatric work in that people suffering from mental illness often perceive and react to mental health professionals on the basis of ingrained models of care-seeking/care-giving. These derive typically from childhood, and, since the majority of psychiatrically ill people will have had sub-optimal developmental experiences, problematic expectations will be 'transferred' onto the mental health system. Splitting and projection (e.g. 'this *wonderful* psychiatrist, that *appalling* one', or vice versa), avoidance (inability to comply with arrangements and appointments), clinging (entrenched dependent roles), risky behaviours (life-threatening or sexual) and angry outbursts (which trigger instant attention, albeit negative) are common occurrences in mental health work and betoken the emergence of primitive affect-defence patterns enacted in relation to the mental health system.

Psychiatrists need to be able to read and react to such turbulence in terms of transference rather than themselves being sucked into the maelstrom of primitive mental functioning. The pressure and anxiety of psychiatric work likewise may elicit counter-transference responses from mental health professionals. These may be manifestations of 'projective identification', i.e. the lodging of the patient's unwanted feelings within the psychiatrist, which, if correctly understood, provide a useful guide to the patient's state of mind. For example, if the psychiatrist feels frightened when interviewing a patient, it is likely that the patient will be terrified too, however overtly threatening he or she may seem.

The notion of counter-transference also captures the psychiatrist's own developmental history and how it may be activated in the clinical situation. Effective psychiatric work needs both a space and time for self-scrutiny, whether through staff groups, personal analysis, mindfulness training, or simply self-directed fostering of the capacity for reflection. However achieved, without such self-knowledge the psychiatrist himself may act out in counter-therapeutic ways – becoming a 'compulsive carer'; overworking; being frightened to take the risks needed to empower the patient to take responsibility for their own lives; or, in a species of unconscious aggression, subtly blame and undermine patients for their perversity or failure to improve. A key PP premise is that interactions between mental health professionals and their patients will be coloured by prior developmental experience. Awareness of these processes – at individual and group levels – will militate against reproducing pathological relational (and thereby iatrogenic) patterns in clinical interactions.

A third general point flows from the fact that, compared with non-medical therapists, the psychodynamic psychiatrist is in a unique position to provide an integrative approach to the treatment of psychiatric disorders. The most obvious example is that psychiatrists are in a position both to prescribe and to undertake psychotherapy. But that combination presents particular challenges. The patient may project their anger and disappointment in the psychiatrist by focusing on the uselessness of the medication, or their requests for more pills may be a covert way of alluding to deprivation; the psychiatrist may alleviate his own sense of futility and covert narcissism by juggling with the patient's prescription. Prescribing is an action, and thus potentially runs counter to the atmosphere of 'as-if-ness' and free association the psychodynamic therapist wishes to foster; it can easily become an enactment of inner conflict rather than a rational and logical means to alleviate distress. None of these are insuperable obstacles, but the psychodynamic psychiatrist needs to be sensitive to them and be prepared to attend to the inevitable mistakes and moments of acting-out when they arise.

Another aspect of integration flows from the fact that 'standard' psychodynamic models, on the whole, are less effective in treating psychiatric disorders than tailor-made, disorder-specific treatments. Some of the specialist therapies which have now been developed for Borderline Personality Disorder (BPD), depression, anxiety, and eating disorders to be discussed below exemplify this. Rather than being an adherent of a particular psychodynamic approach – Kohutian, Kleinian, ego-psychological, relational, etc. – the psychodynamic psychiatrist aims to be a non-partisan integrative practitioner, bringing the full range of psychotherapeutic expertise to bear on the illnesses in ways that the evidence suggests is most effective. This applies also across psychotherapeutic modalities: for some conditions (depression and anxiety), CBT is the initial treatment of choice, followed by psychodynamic therapy for non-responders; for others (eating disorders), what is best is the combination of individual and family therapy; for yet others (BPD), long-term psychoanalytically informed group therapy supplemented by mindfulness training may be what is required.

In the next sections I shall look at the ways in which these general principles have played out in the specific historical conditions in various parts of the world.

Psychodynamic psychiatry in the UK

War is a potent catalyst for social change. The First World War raised the profile of psychiatry by drawing on the skills of such outstanding intellects as W. H. Rivers and Henry Head in the understanding and treatment of shell-shock. In the Second World War the UK military command needed to identify potential leaders from men outside the traditional officer class. A group of outstanding psychoanalytically trained psychiatrists and psychologists, including Winifred Bion, Jock Sutherland, John Bowlby and Eric Trist, was recruited to the task. They were seen as having expertise in assessing character and, rather than relying on academic or rank, devised methods of selection based on observing people's actual behaviour in group situations. Tapping into a person's psychodynamics in the here and now provides a better picture of their aptitudes than a consciously shaped interview performance.

Thus the period 1930 to 1960 saw an upsurge of interest in psychoanalytic approaches in the UK and, as we shall see, in the US. Even before the outbreak of war there had been an influx of psychoanalytic refugees from Nazi Germany to Britain. Freud arrived in London with his daughter Anna in 1938. Other UK asylum-seekers included Melanie Klein (invited by Ernest Jones, Freud's first biographer and pioneer of psychoanalysis in the UK), Hannah Segal and Michael Balint.

The Tavistock Clinic in London had been founded by Hugh Crighton-Miller for the treatment of shell-shock in the First World War. After the Second World War it became a centre of excellence, training a cadre of psychodynamically minded psychologists, psychiatrists and child psychotherapists, with Jock Sutherland, John Bowlby, Donald Winnicott, Wilfred Bion and Michael Balint among its luminaries.

From the point of view of PP, Balint's (1957) contribution was particularly significant. A Hungarian, analysed by Sándor Ferenczi, Balint was a pioneer in the then embryonic field of psychotherapy research, and recruited fellow analyst David Malan in the 1950s to undertake one of the first outcome studies of Brief Dynamic Psychotherapy. They found that six months of weekly therapy for people suffering from depression, anxiety and mild personality problems could produce significant benefits, sustained at two-year follow-up. Technical innovations came with time-limited once-weekly therapy: the 'active' therapist; a relentless focus on the presenting problem and its psychodynamic meanings; and preparing for termination from the outset, thereby bringing to the fore issues of loss and abandonment, so salient in the origins of neurosis.

Balint's enduring contribution was the development of the eponymous 'Balint groups'. These were originally conceived as a means of training GPs in psychodynamic thinking, enabling them to interact more sensitively and effectively with the psychiatric component of their caseload. The impetus behind the Balint group movement was the realisation that high-cost, highly labour-intensive psychoanalysis would be unlikely to make a significant impact on the mental health of the general population. Training front-line workers in psychodynamic thinking, and facilitating the 'small but significant' alteration in personality which flows from a psychodynamic approach, was, Balint maintained, the best way to change medical and psychiatric culture rooted in instrumentalism, paternalism and concrete thinking.

Balint groups are innovative in form as well as aim. A group of GPs meet regularly with a psychoanalytically trained facilitator. Discussion is based around case material brought by one or more of the participants. In contrast to the prevailing psychoanalytic mores, the role of the facilitator is neither pedagogic nor authoritarian. The participants are assumed to be the experts on themselves, their patients and one another. The facilitator's role is to set the scene, to maintain the boundaries of the group, and to widen and deepen the discussion where necessary, including encouraging reticent members while restraining the loquacious.

In the UK and other anglophone countries, trainee psychiatrists are required to attend a weekly Balint group facilitated by a senior psychotherapeutically trained practitioner. This provides an opportunity to examine the impact of working with highly disturbed and suicidal patients, and to begin to identify, respect and make use of the counter-transference reactions that such work evokes. Learning from one another's mistakes, successes, doubts and uncertainties is integral to the process.

Bowlby (1988; Holmes, 1993/2013), also based in the Tavistock Clinic, was one of the best-known and most influential psychoanalyst-psychiatrists of the second half of the twentieth century. He is credited with being one of the first clinicians to work directly with parents and children together, and hence is a founding father of family therapy. Bowlby's studies of the impact of separation of children from their parents when admitted to hospital, popularised by the films made by James Robertson, led to a radical change in paediatric medicine, with hospitals thereafter providing open access for parents. Family work in preventing relapse in schizophrenia can be traced to Bowlby's pioneering spirit.

Bowlby's development of attachment theory, while arising in part from his psychoanalytic roots, created a new psychological paradigm. His trilogy *Attachment*, *Separation*, and *Loss* represents the integrative potential of the hybrid discipline of psychiatry at its best. Attachment theory embodies the simple yet profound idea that psychological health depends on the availability of a sensitive and responsive care-seeker–care-giver relationship and that, when such relationships are rigid, insensitive, strained or severed, adverse psychological consequences follow. The relationship between loss and depressive illness is well established and flows from Bowlby's conceptualisations. Grief and bereavement and abnormal grief reactions were studied by Bowlby's colleague Colin Murray Parkes (1975), and represent another psychodynamic contribution to mainstream psychiatry.

The 1950s saw the establishment of a number of therapeutic communities using psychoanalytically informed individual and group methods for the treatment of mental illness. These were antithetical to the mental hospital set-up of the day, which they saw as eroding individuality, fostering passivity, and mired in a paternalistic philosophy where power was located around a hierarchically organised staff structure. Therapeutic communities encouraged patients to be active and to play a full part in maintaining the institution, both practically (washing, cleaning, cooking, etc.) and in planning and discussion. Group meetings ensured that support and challenge from fellow sufferers was as important as professional expertise. A key part of the philosophy was the trust placed in mentally ill individuals to find their own solutions, placing professionals in a facilitating rather than a controlling role.

One of the champions of social psychiatry was R. D. Laing, who achieved international renown in the 1960s, especially with his first book *The Divided Self* (1960). Published when he was only 28, it was based on his experiences as an army psychiatrist and trainee psychoanalyst, first in Scotland and then at the Tavistock Clinic. Far removed from the stereotypical psychoanalytic mould of a Jewish émigré or an upper-middle-class Bloomsbury Grouper (although sharing with both a degree of 'outsider-ness' integral to psychoanalytic culture), Laing came from humble Scottish origins to take the psychiatric world by storm. He introduced British readers to Harold Searles (1965) and Fromm-Reichman's (1959) US psychoanalytic models of psychosis, as well as European existential philosophy. *The Divided Self* was on the bookshelf of every would-be 1960s radical. Sadly, Laing's meteoric rise was short-lived; he was soon burnt out by alcoholism, psychedelia and success itself.

However, Laing's long-term influence should not be underestimated. He drew attention to the inhumane condition and culture of mental hospitals, subsequently detailed by Goffman (1961) and Wing (Wing and Brown, 1970), leading eventually to their closure and replacement with acute hospital units and community-based services. Laing validated the inner world and experience of the severely mentally ill, seeing psychotic phenomena as covert communications, often about traumatic or painful experiences, rather than meaningless manifestations of a dysfunctional mind. He emphasised the family context of psychosis and, although wrong in attributing blame to the parents of psychosis sufferers (family mis-communication is as much a consequence of the stress of living with psychosis as it is a cause of illness), stimulated research which showed that lowering expressed emotion in families reduces the relapse rate in schizophrenia. Laing's work helped to de-stigmatise mental illness, presciently anticipating research showing that psychotic symptoms are relatively common in non-clinical populations, with the mentally ill representing the severe end of a spectrum of widespread non-rational ways of being and seeing.

During the 1970s and 1980s there was a rapid expansion in the numbers of PP psychiatrists in the UK. Consultant psychiatrists specialising in psychotherapy – almost all psychoanalysts – were re-designated as consultant psychotherapists. Their principal role was to train junior psychiatrists in the basics of PP and specialist trainees to become consultant psychotherapists. In addition, led by consultant psychotherapists, a small number of tertiary specialist units, such as the Cassel Hospital and the Henderson Hospital, provided day and in-patient services run along psychodynamic lines for severely disturbed, mainly personality-disordered patients. Being patient- rather than training-focused, these units were necessarily eclectic, employing large- and small-group therapies, art therapy and psychodrama. An influential paper from this period was Tom Main's 'The Ailment' (1989), describing the impact of 'difficult patients' on mental health services, the ramifications of institutional counter-transference and the need for fora in which to think about such dynamics.

This efflorescence was, however, short-lived. By the 1990s clinical psychology was beginning to emerge strongly as an independent profession, throwing off the shackles of its handmaiden role, no longer primarily producing psychological reports for psychiatrists, analogous to X-rays for physicians. Just as interventional radiology has replaced much of the work previously done by surgeons, so clinical psychologists began to become the primary providers of psychological therapies. Enthusiastically espousing the new psychotherapeutic discipline of CBT, their services were now seen by cash-strapped managers as cheaper and more comprehensible than those provided by consultant psychotherapists.

At a political level consultant psychotherapists were fatally handicapped by having no identified client group for whose care they were directly responsible. As the economic situation worsened, managers realised that psychotherapy services could be curtailed without any danger of protest from concerned patients or their families (in contrast, say, to those suffering from eating disorders or dementia).

Refusing to cut their cloth, to develop diagnosis-specific brief treatments, to engage in outcome research, or to embrace a variety of differing psychotherapeutic approaches, practitioners of PP became increasingly marginalised. Some resorted to ad hominem 'interpretations' of envy or psychological flawedness in their opponents as a way of bolstering their increasingly precarious status. PP ran the risk of being seen as a desirable yet dispensable luxury, concerned mainly with the so-called worried well rather than being an integral part of civilised psychiatric practice.

There were honourable exceptions to these self-defeating trends. Jonathan Pedder's *Introduction to psychotherapy* (co-authored with Dennis Brown, and later Anthony Bateman) remains an excellent introductory text. The Jungian analyst Robert Hobson (1985) (co-author with Russell Meares of the influential paper 'The persecutory therapist') developed his 'conversational model' (CM), a brief dynamic therapy emphasising the here-and-now relationship and the 'minute particulars' of therapist–patient interaction, in preference to putative childhood reconstructions.

CM was ahead of its time in using video recordings of sessions for both research and teaching, and became one of the first psychodynamic therapy models to be tested empirically. Thus David Shapiro and his colleagues (Shapiro *et al.*, 1994) in Sheffield showed the efficacy of the CM in a head-to-head 16-session study of CBT versus CM in mild to moderate depression, establishing the so-called equivalence paradox of equifinality of outcomes between the two techniques. Another CM researcher, Else Guthrie (Guthrie *et al.*, 1991), showed the superiority of CM over treatment as usual (TAU) in irritable bowel syndrome and deliberate self-harm.

Anthony Ryle, with his integrative model of brief integrative therapy, Cognitive Analytic Therapy (CAT), is another notable contributor. CAT entails a number of innovative features: the use of written communications in which the therapist offers the patient a formulation after four sessions and a 'goodbye letter' in the penultimate one; a collaborative milieu; an emphasis on the cyclical self-perpetuating aspects of neurosis and a focus on the search for 'exits' from such vicious circles; and homework tasks aiming to promote benign ones. CAT has been shown in its 24-session form to be a promising treatment for BPD.

Despite these more hopeful signs, two well-intentioned institutions set up by the UK Labour government (1997–2008) contrived to strike fear into the hearts of psychodynamic psychiatrists. The National Institute for Clinical Excellence (NICE) convenes experts who review research in specific topics, leading to 'guidelines' for evidence-based practice in all branches of medicine, including psychiatry. Laudable as this may be, nowhere does NICE advocate PP as a first-line treatment for psychiatric disorders. Currently, pharmacotherapy and CBT outshine psychodynamics when it comes to published evidence. While absence of evidence does not necessarily equate to evidence of absence, it has been hard for PP to challenge this bias, although a more balanced position is beginning to emerge.

Another related development has been the Increasing Access to Psychological Therapies (IAPT) programme. The impetus behind this innovation should have benefited PP. Impressed by the evidence from advanced countries that greater economic prosperity does not necessarily equate to increased happiness, the economist Richard Layard convinced the UK government that investment in psychological therapies would help raise the general level of happiness, as well as reducing the numbers of people suffering from chronic depression and somatisation disorders, often living on costly benefits. CBT was seen as the treatment of choice for these conditions, and training programmes were set up establishing IAPT therapists across the country. PP, once again, was out in the cold, although belatedly the IAPT board added a brief dynamic therapy, Dynamic Interpersonal Therapy, to its programme.

With CBT now the first-line treatment for common mental disorders in primary care, the focus and role of PP has shifted, perhaps appropriately, to complex and disturbed cases requiring long-term treatments. Anthony Bateman and Peter Fonagy (2004, 2008) have developed and tested a psychodynamically informed treatment for people suffering from Borderline Personality Disorder. Bateman's clinical base was a psychodynamic day hospital in a deprived area of North-East London. Determined to compete in the mainstream of psychiatry research, he and Fonagy undertook a randomised controlled trial outcome study, with long-term follow-up, in which a particular version of psychodynamic psychiatry, Mentalisation-Based Therapy (MBT), was compared with treatment as usual (TAU). Their methodology was impeccable and their results remarkable, leading to a series of acclaimed papers in the *American Journal of Psychiatry*. Bateman and Fonagy have shown that a two-year partial hospitalisation programme for BPD sufferers, in which they receive a combination of individual, group and milieu therapy, outperforms TAU on almost all the important criteria: days in hospital, episodes of deliberate self-harm, medication levels, and health and social service resources consumed. An important finding is that differences begin to emerge strongly only 18 months into the programme. Eight-year follow-up shows that these gains are maintained, although the quality of life of BPD sufferers still remains poor. The programme is based on intensive staff supervision and support and a coherent treatment philosophy. People suffering from Borderline Personality Disorder are seen as lacking the reflexive (or 'mentalising') skills needed to negotiate the world of interpersonal relationships ('to see others from the inside and oneself from the outside'), as well as being prone to states of easily triggered hyperarousal incompatible with mentalising. The core of the programme is to take everyday 'living/learning' (a therapeutic community catchphrase) experiences and to foster the participant's capacity to mentalise their own and others' actions and feelings in terms of beliefs, desires and intentions.

The significance of Bateman and Fonagy's contribution is that they have developed and tested a specific model of therapy for a defined client group for whom PP offers a positive outcome, in contrast to conventional psychiatry, which often leads to iatrogenic deterioration in BPD sufferers. The specific skills of the psychodynamic psychiatrist – able to prescribe when needed and to manage suicide and deliberate self-harm, as well as offering reflexive psychoanalytically informed therapeutic practice – suggest a future role for PP as the custodian of Axis II clients with complex and difficult problems.

Psychodynamic psychiatry in the US

Summarising the discussion so far, we can identify a number of themes: a significant wartime role for psychoanalytic psychiatrists; expansion led mainly by refugees from Europe fleeing facism; insularity and arrogance of PP practitioners militating against cross-fertilisation and research; medical elitism; the inexorable rise of CBT and of the psychology profession; and attempts to limit costs incurred by government and insurance companies in long-term therapies.

Despite the very different socio-political context of the US, we see similar forces in evidence. For at least two decades psychoanalysis was virtually the only game in town. Ignoring Freud's espousal of 'lay analysis', US psychoanalysts insisted that candidates for the profession be medically trained. In the 1950s and 1960s there was not a single head of a psychiatry department in the US who was not a psychoanalyst. Three-quarters of posts within the American Psychiatric Association (APA) were held by psychoanalysts. Personal analysis and psychoanalytic candidature were *de rigueur* for psychiatrists who wished to advance in their profession. There were of course tensions. Psychologists felt justifiably envious and excluded. Psychoanalysts of a liberal bent clashed with their more orthodox counterparts. There was nevertheless a sense of a psychoanalytic mainstream – in the mid-1950s Charles Brenner's *Elementary textbook of psychoanalysis* sold more than 1 million copies.

But in the mid-1970s things began to change. A number of factors came together to threaten and eventually to replace psychoanalytic hegemony. The oil crisis of 1973 meant that a period of unprecedented economic growth and stability in the US faltered. Cheaper, more effective, less opaque therapies were required. Insurance companies insisted that only treatments for defined medical conditions would be reimbursed. The IPSS (International Project for the Study of Schizophrenia) project found that American psychiatrists' diagnostic practices were far vaguer and more all-inclusive than those of other countries, including the UK (with the ironic exception of the USSR). The APA responded with DSM-III, which abolished overnight the psychoanalytic shibboleth of the neurosis–psychosis dichotomy in favour of specific diagnoses required to satisfy highly specific criteria.

The way was open for CBT to produce time-limited packages of treatment for DSM-defined conditions such as depression, anxiety, post-traumatic stress disorder and bulimia. This was in stark contrast to psychoanalysis' typically unfocused, ill-defined, intensive therapies of uncertain length. Psychopharmacology was also gathering momentum as a scientific force. The catecholamine hypothesis for depression and the dopamine hypothesis for schizophrenia, while not intrinsically antithetical to PP, shifted the focus from the psyche to the brain. Private insurance companies' 'managed care' paradigm increasingly favoured cheaper psychopharmacological treatments over psychotherapy. Another significant factor was the celebrated 'Chestnut Lodge' case, in which Raphael Osheroff, a neurologist suffering from Major Depressive Disorder, successfully sued the celebrated psychoanalytic in-patient unit when, after prolonged ineffective psychoanalytic treatment, his family arranged for him to be treated with anti-depressants and he recovered in short order.

Faced with this challenge, psychoanalytic psychiatrists responded in a number of ways. Some clung to a fundamentalist mentality, seeing brief therapies and psychopharmacology as manifestations of a fast-food, fast-therapy, degenerate society, with psychoanalysis as guardian of the true faith. Others shifted the focus of psychodynamics away from treating mental illness towards a secular quasi-religious exploration of the Self. Some abandoned psychoanalysis altogether and joined the biological opposition. Yet another group, notably Otto Kernberg and Robert Wallerstein and John Gunderson, belatedly realised that systematic evaluation was needed if PP was to re-enter the scientific mainstream, and so initiated programmes of painstaking research.

Another leading figure in the fightback was Glen Gabbard (1994), professor at the Menninger Clinic in Kansas (named after William and Karl Menninger, who occupied a dominant position in US psychiatry in the post-war period), itself a victim of the changing fortunes of PP, now relocated to Houston. Gabbard's *Psychodynamic psychiatry in clinical practice*, first published in the 1980s, remains a best-seller, now into its fifth edition. Gabbard is a vigorous critic of the funding imbalance between general medicine and psychiatry and between 'organic' psychiatry and psychotherapy, commenting, with characteristic aphoristic aplomb, 'It is not uncommon for insurance policies to pay in six figures for organ transplants but offer only nickels and dimes for psychotherapy.' In addition to psychoanalytic expertise, Gabbard exudes a persuasive mix of common sense, clinical wisdom, style and wit. The thrust of his approach is not to reject non-psychodynamic methods but to argue for an integrated approach in which psychopharmacology and various forms of psychotherapy, including psychoanalysis, work in concert. The common factor is the doctor–patient relationship; the central contribution of PP is its capacity both to theorise that relationship and to maximise its therapeutic efficacy.

Global perspectives on psychodynamic psychiatry

From a UK and US perspective, the situation of psychodynamics in the German-speaking world (Germany, Austria, Switzerland) appears paradisal. Psychotherapy, including psychoanalysis, is treated as a medical speciality, equivalent to physical medicine, and is covered by private and government insurance schemes for up to a total of 360 sessions. The historical reasons for this may lie in part in reaction to the shameful Nazi dismantling of the 'Jewish science' in the 1930s (which, ironically, led to the flowering of psychoanalysis in the UK and the US) and also to the fact that research in psychotherapy outcome was initiated in Germany in the 1950s, some 20 years before the need was felt in the anglophone world. Today Germany remains at the forefront of both outcome studies and process research, with Horst Kächele and his colleagues at Ulm leading figures in the latter.

Psychodynamics are similarly valued in the Scandinavian countries. In the 1970s there was an interesting development of 'shuttle training', in which a group of UK psychoanalysts and group analysts (including Pedder; see above) went regularly to Denmark to 'train the trainers' until a sufficient cadre was established for self-sufficiency. Similar arrangements have more recently been developed in Russia, Eastern Europe and now China, where, following the demise of communism, there has been a hunger for psychoanalytic ideas and therapies. With developments in electronic communication, 'Skype' supervision helps maintain a psychoanalytic culture in these hitherto deprived regions.

In Europe, France represents something of a special case. Psychoanalysis is divided between the Freudian and Lacanian schools. Many psychiatrists are psychoanalytically trained. Empirical approaches, including psychotherapy research, tend to be seen as an Anglo-Saxon aberration and are eschewed in favour of philosophical disputation and Freudian fundamentalism. In the francophone areas of Canada, however, the concept of mentalising has been developed, feeding into MBT as developed by Bateman and Fonagy.

As British ex-colonies, Canada and Australia have built on and improved some of the more positive features of the mother country. While not as intensive as in Germany, in both Canada and Australia limited psychoanalytic therapy is covered by insurance, and training in psychodynamic psychotherapy is a mandatory requirement for qualification as a psychiatrist. Both countries boast centres of psychodynamic excellence. Pre-dating Bateman and Kernberg, Russell Meares in Sydney integrated Heinz Kohut's self-psychology into an evidence-based treatment for BPD. In Canada, Allan Abbass extended Malan and Habib Davanloo's work into a model of Intensive Short-term Dynamic Psychotherapy (ISDP), showing it to be effective in treating depression, PTSD and BPD.

A burgeoning urban middle-class and a post-Catholic culture have made South America a fertile seedbed for psychoanalysis. The early leading figures trained in Europe and then returned to their countries to establish their own schools. The Argentinian Horacio Etchegoyen's *The fundamentals of psychoanalytic technique* is a masterly account of Kleinian psychoanalysis. Psychology is a popular undergraduate subject in South America, and the majority of psychotherapists are psychologists, not psychiatrists. Extending psychoanalytic approaches to the wider population remains problematic, although, intriguingly, Peru now has a pioneering indigenous psychoanalyst.

PP is more or less confined on the African continent to South Africa. For the non-white and rural population, mental disorders are treated largely by traditional healers, but there are now psychodynamically informed outreach projects in the townships, e.g. for victims of sexual abuse. An interesting development in Uganda has been an Interpersonal Therapy (IPT) outreach project in which a controlled study of group therapy for depression facilitated by locally trained therapists has been shown to be effective. Another development has been narrative therapy for victims of war trauma, where controlled studies have been successfully evaluated and found to be helpful.

In Asia, a number of non-theistic religions and psychological disciplines, such as Daoism, Shintoism, and Zen Buddhism, have been incorporated into professional treatment, raising the possibility of an authentic Asian psychodynamic approach to mental illness and its therapy. There are flourishing psychoanalytic institutes in South Korea and Japan. Takae Doi (1989) coined the term *amae* to describe a particular kind of mother–child intimacy unique to Japan, which has thrown new light on the kinds of intimate dependency PP can foster. Salman Ahktar (2012), an Indian psychoanalyst working in the US, has questioned the neo-Kleinian emphasis on negative emotions such as envy and destructiveness and has written about the positive influence of the psychoanalyst, illustrating how East–West dialogue in psychotherapy can become a two-way process.

Green shoots for a psychodynamic future

Can PP survive as a significant force within psychiatry? Or is it doomed at best to a role, comparable to osteopathy vis-à-vis mainstream medicine, of 'optimal marginalisation', at worst to be an esoteric backwater yearning nostalgically for a long-gone past? Has psychotherapy effectively been handed over to clinical psychology, with psychiatrists returning to their nineteenth-century role as neurologists and psychopharmacologists? In this concluding section, I survey some signs that psychodynamics may indeed yet recover some of its former glory and play a worthwhile role in the psychiatry of the future.

Neuro-psychoanalysis has captured the imagination of leading figures in both psychoanalysis and neuroscience. One of Freud's earliest essays was the unpublished 'Project for a scientific psychology', attempting to combine – misguidedly he later decided – the neurology of the day with his burgeoning psychoanalytic ideas. Over a century on, there has been a tentative rapprochement between psychoanalysis and contemporary neuroscience. Analysts, in search perhaps of scientific credibility, have been beguiled by the vivid imagery and circuitry of their neuroscience colleagues, who in turn have been fascinated by the psychoanalytic meanings that may underlie their brain mappings.

There are numerous areas of mutual interest. These include the distinction between the explicit/declarative memory system and implicit/procedural memories, and the ways in which the latter may encode early trauma with far-reaching but largely unconscious effects; parallels between Freud's conscious/unconscious dichotomy and the interplay between cortical and sub-cortical structures, especially the limbic system; 'mirror neurones' as the basis for empathy, in which watching others' actions and emotions trigger equivalent parts of the brain in the observer; neuroplasticity and thus the possible ameliorative impact of psychotherapy; and tracking changes in regional blood flow in response to therapeutic interventions. Unexpected support for a rapprochement between neuroscience and psychoanalytic approaches has come from the Nobel prize-winning neuroscientist and psychiatrist Eric Kandel (1999, p. 520), who argued:

> the whole is more than the sum of the parts. There is something wonderful and special about each person as a unique individual – a unique set of biological functions, if you will. The ultimate aim is to use reductionism, not only to take things apart, but to put them together again. You have to be a reductionist and a holist at the same time.

Another growth area revolves around potential links between developmental psychopathology and the science of intimacy. A developmental perspective is indispensable for understanding major psychiatric illness. Gene–environment interaction and epigenetic processes are cutting-edge research areas. A now classic example is Avshalom Caspi and colleagues' (2003) finding that only in the presence of the short allele version of the Serotonin Transporter gene does childhood adversity predispose to adult depression. A further relevant finding is that another epigenetic locus, the DRD4 allele, increases biological sensitivity to environmental context, with potential for negative health effects under conditions of adversity but positive effects when support and protection are available, the latter including psychotherapy.

Apart from a general validation of its emphasis on the importance of early environmental influence and of a developmental perspective, PP has a specific contribution to make to this field in that it focuses on the subtleties of interpersonal interaction that may trigger adverse or beneficial epigenetic processes. Thus the Adult Attachment Interview is a sophisticated instrument for studying the minutiae of intimate relationships whether parent–child, spousal or psychotherapeutic. An example is a study which tracks how, in the course of Clarkin and colleagues' (2007) Transference-Focused Therapy, BPD sufferers' capacity to articulate and reflect on their experience becomes more subtle and elaborated.

A continuing theme that has kept psychodynamics alive has been the acknowledgement that trainee psychiatrists, whatever their eventual orientation, need basic psychotherapeutic skills, as well as to be conversant with the theories and practical uses of psychodynamic approaches in the treatment of mental illness. A 'signed-up' case book recording supervised practice in a number of psychotherapeutic modalities, including long- and short-term psychodynamic therapy, is now a precondition for qualification as a psychiatrist in the UK, the US and Australasia.

Another notable recent development has been the establishment of departments of psychoanalysis and psychoanalytic studies within the universities. Rejected by the anti-Semitic culture within the universities of his day, Freud created his own institutions for training and promulgation of psychoanalysis. While this fostered free-wheeling creativity, it has also meant that psychoanalysis failed to keep step with many of the intellectual currents of the twentieth century: systems theory, observational child development, ethology, structuralist anthropology, linguistics and philosophy. In particular, psychoanalytic research was confined by Freud's conception of the primacy of the individual case study, important though that is, rather than subjecting analytic therapies to the statistical and probabilistic methods of mainstream science.

When University College London (UCL) established the UK's first chair of psychoanalysis in the 1980s, it was held on a short-term basis sequentially by John Bowlby, Joseph Sandler, and the French psychoanalyst Janine Chasseguet-Smirgel. Since the 1990s it has been permanently occupied by the psychologist, psychoanalyst, psychotherapy-outcome researcher and child development expert Peter Fonagy. Thanks to Fonagy and his colleague Mary Target, following incorporation of the Anna Freud Centre (AFC), UCL–AFC has become an international powerhouse for teaching and research in psychoanalysis and psychodynamic psychiatry. In addition to the Psychoanalysis Unit at UCL, there are now in the UK psychoanalytic departments at the universities of Essex, Sheffield, Birkbeck (University of London) and Exeter. A free-standing International Psychoanalytic University has been founded in Berlin, and the New School for Social Research in New York has a major psychoanalytic presence, as do a number of US universities. Such departments allow for cross-fertilisation between different disciplines (including such diverse areas as philosophy, literary and gender studies, and art history) and encourage psychoanalytic research in its widest sense. Exposing PP to the rigours of academia helps hone its strengths and blow away its anachronistic fustiness.

One of the ironies of psychiatry is that, although the majority of psychiatrists see themselves primarily as medical experts in diagnosis and prescription, the public consistently stress the need for talking therapies. But hard evidence is needed if governments and insurance companies are to be persuaded to fund psychotherapies. We have seen how PP quixotically gave CBT a 20-year head-start when it came to evidence of efficacy and effectiveness. But the merits of psychodynamic therapies are steadily emerging, and ways of overcoming the methodological difficulties in evaluating psychodynamic therapies are beginning to be developed.

In studying PP, blinding is impossible, randomisation undesirable, and funding for long-term therapy hard to obtain. A compromise is to compare active treatment with either 'treatment as usual' or reliance on pre-/post-measures. The second half of the 2000s saw a number of meta-analyses of PP in high-impact journals (e.g. Leichsenring *et al.*, 2004; Shedler, 2010), all of which pointed to similar conclusions. First, psychodynamic therapies produce large effect sizes (average 0.8 to 1.2), comparable to those achieved by both CBT and IPT and by anti-depressants. Second, gains tend to increase even after the period of therapy has finished, in contrast to non-psychotherapeutic treatments. Third, improvements in psychodynamic therapy subjects, although substantial, tend to reveal themselves towards the latter period of therapy, suggesting an initial period of psychological reorganisation ('pupation') before enduring change, butterfly-like, can emerge. Fourth, the longer the period of therapy, the greater the gains. This was important, since earlier studies claimed a negative logarithmic 'dose-effect curve', suggesting that effective psychodynamic therapy initiates, but is not necessary for, the perpetuation of benign cycles of action and reflection. Finally, psychodynamic therapy, despite being labour-intensive, is cost-effective in that, compared with controls, utilisation of health and social services post-therapy tends to drop dramatically.

Another relevant point concerns the mechanism of action of psychotherapies generally. Knowing that a given therapy 'works' in terms of symptomatic improvement and improved social outcomes says nothing about the mechanism of action of the therapy. There is some evidence that basic psychodynamic processes may apply to all effective therapies. Two key factors are the establishment of a secure, sensitive and interactive working alliance and the capacity of the therapist to facilitate the experiencing of previously avoided painful feelings. It seems that, even in CBT, these psychodynamic factors contribute significantly to the outcome variance.

Such claims for the efficacy of PP have not gone unchallenged. One criticism is that psychodynamic therapy outcomes have been measured with a heterogeneous collection of patients with a variety of diagnoses and problems. It is therefore difficult to determine the precise indications for psychodynamic therapies as compared with the diagnosis-specific therapies developed by CBT. Another is that head-to-head studies, where psychodynamic therapy can be compared with briefer, cheaper therapies, are lacking. A third objection centres on the tension between standard psychotherapeutic technique – which for BPD sufferers may either be ineffective or produce deterioration – as compared with diagnosis-specific treatments. There is also a need for real-world effectiveness studies which can encompass integrative approaches. These might well include packages comprising psychopharmacology, social measures and family therapy in parallel with individual PP.

Recent work has begun to address some of these questions. Anxiety disorders are typically seen as the preserve of CBT, so it is significant that Milrod (2009) has developed a psychodynamic therapy model for anxiety, concentrating particularly on the avoidance and denial of anger, which has demonstrated good outcomes in 21 sessions compared with controls, sustained over six months follow-up (a short period admittedly, but comparable to the CBT studies of which third-party funders are enamoured).

A number of evidence-based psychodynamic treatments have now been developed for depression. Brief PP has been found to be as effective as CBT, IPT or anti-depressants (Abbass *et al.*, 2008). An example is Dynamic Interpersonal Therapy (DIT) (Lemma *et al.*, 2012), which has managed to breach CBT's monopoly in the UK's Improving Access to Psychological Therapies programme (see above). DIT concentrates on the interpersonal aspects of depression: how recent losses trigger traumatic memories of early childhood separations and how these may be reactivated in therapy (transference reactions to therapist's absences); and fostering the capacity to think about ('mentalise') negative affects rather than being overwhelmed by them.

The complexity and difficulty of the problems posed by people suffering from BPD represent a major problem for psychiatric services. Patients often fail to engage with standard treatments and when they do, as we have seen, therapy may interfere with the natural tendency of BPD to remission. Two manualised modified psychodynamic therapies, Clarkin et al.'s (2009) Transference-Focused Therapy (TFT) in New York and Bateman and Fonagy's Mentalisation-Based Therapy (MBT) (Bateman & Fonagy 2004, 2008) in London, have both been shown to produce significant improvements for BPD sufferers compared with treatment-as-usual controls. As mentioned above, MBT combines attachment and psychoanalytic principles, seeing BPD sufferers as deficient in mentalising skills and therefore liable to recurrent interpersonal conflict without being able easily to learn from experience. MBT eschews 'deep' or infancy-oriented interpretations. The latter at best are incomprehensible to people who lack reflexive competence, at worst precipitate feelings of shame and humiliation. MBT, TFP and indeed non-psychodynamic therapies for BPD, such as Dialectical Behaviour Therapy, are optimally delivered in dedicated centres by specially trained and closely supervised and supported groups of therapists. This group of patients – for whom suicide and deliberate self-harm are an ever present risk – is best treated by psychodynamically sophisticated mental health professionals, among whom psychodynamic psychiatrists play a leading role.

Finally we turn to the controversial role of psychoanalytic approaches to schizophrenia, which illustrate in microcosm the rise, fall and tentative rebirth of PP charted in this chapter. 'Schizophrenia' and related psychoses were, since Freud's account of Judge Schreber's memoir, seen as legitimate subjects for PP, although Freud himself was sceptical about the possibility of analysis with such patients. Pioneering units such as Chestnut Lodge in Maryland were staffed by outstanding analysts, including Harold Searles (1965) and Frieda Fromm-Reichman (1959), who wrote freely about psychoanalytic therapy for psychosis (to be weighed alongside her many virtues, the latter was also responsible for the egregious misnomer 'schizophrenogenic mother'). Following Melanie Klein's accounts of manic-depressive psychosis, British analysts, among them Bion and Herbert Rosenfeld, similarly upheld the view that psychotic illness could be understood and treated psychoanalytically.

The turn away from PP began with the discovery in the 1950s of effective drug treatments for psychosis. It became clear clinically that many patients with schizophrenia failed to improve or even deteriorated when treated psychoanalytically. Eventually Tom McGlashan, a Chestnut Lodge staff member, published a much publicised follow-up study of schizophrenic patients, showing that psychoanalytic therapy was contraindicated, ironically in line with Freud's caution first expressed nearly a century earlier.

At this stage, it seemed that PP for psychosis was dead and buried. But gradually the picture has begun to change. In Scandinavia a 'needs adapted' approach to schizophrenia was developed, the components of which include recognition of the value of each patient and their individual life trajectory; minimal medication; intensive family therapy; and establishing a long-term relationship with a key worker. Such a relationship, containing elements of support and attachment, is not formally psychoanalytic, but there is also sustained work in helping the patient understand the nature and meaning of his illness and its origins rather than simply seeing it as a biologically determined 'disease'. Meanwhile, other research has revealed the widespread nature of psychotic symptoms and the role of childhood adversity and trauma as precursors to the development of psychotic illnesses, strongly suggesting that environmental factors such as the family and the wider social environment may crucially determine whether particular thinking styles become entrenched as psychiatric illnesses. While formal psychoanalytic therapy for psychosis remains ethically and practically questionable, psychodynamically informed therapy on a long-term basis, containing elements of support, symptom management and, where appropriate, interpretation, is now part of any civilised service for people suffering from schizophrenia and manic depression.

Conclusion

Had this essay been written ten years earlier, its conclusions about the future of PP might have been far more pessimistic. The ubiquity of neuropsychiatry, the dominance of CBT and psychology, the ascendancy of psychopharmacology, and the growth of multi-professionalism within mental health have increasingly combined to confine psychiatrists to a forensic and prescribing role. A decade later, the picture looks very different. PP has a significant contribution to make to mainstream psychiatry in four main areas. First, it is playing a big part in the development of diagnosis-specific therapies, particularly in the domain of complex personality disorder. Second, PP enables psychiatrists to understand the transferential and counter-transferential thoughts, feelings and enactments aroused by clinical work, thereby helping to avoid the ever present iatrogenic dangers implicit in psychiatric practice. Third, through greater understanding of the nuances of the therapeutic relationship, PP-oriented psychiatrists can empathise and communicate effectively with their patients, even when the focus of treatment is not primarily psychodynamic. Finally, PP has a vibrant contribution to make to the continuing intellectual challenge presented by the attempt to understand and help people suffering from mental illnesses. Leon Eisenberg famously quipped that psychiatry should be neither brainless nor mindless. This essay has argued that, as psychiatry becomes increasingly brain-minded, PP offers the most comprehensive clinical account of the mind and its disorders currently available.

PSYCHOTHERAPY
Integrative and attachment-informed

The papers in this section reflect my abiding clinical interest and standpoints – attachment-informed integrative eclecticism. 'Family and individual therapy' emerged from my simultaneous training in family therapy and psychoanalytic psychotherapy and argues that these apparently very different perspectives share many common features. In the following chapter I again look for points of overlap and rapprochement, this time between psychoanalysis and CBT. The integrative theme is continued in the next paper, which sets out how attachment theory and research provide a 'meta-theory' applicable to all psychotherapies, including psychoanalytic psychotherapy. This theme is continued in 'Superego', in which I deconstruct this enduring psychoanalytic concept and show that it is as much to do with security as with sexuality, also suggesting that positive features of the therapeutic relationships – encouragement, humour and validation – are as important as dissecting the negative transference. The final paper in this section considers relational psychoanalysis, the psychoanalytic perspective I find most congenial and compatible with my attachment preoccupations. It attempts to alert UK readers to this burgeoning movement in the US and elsewhere.

PSYCHOTHERAPY
Integrative and attachment-informed

CHAPTER 11

FAMILY AND INDIVIDUAL THERAPY

Comparisons and contrasts

Psychoanalytical and family therapies are contrasted: psychotherapeutic change involves a change of frame. The new frame in family therapy is the system; for analytical therapy it is the unconscious, but there are striking formal similarities between them. To achieve this change, there are two basic modes of therapy, reflective and directive. An essential ingredient in therapy is an uncoupling of action from effect, which occurs in play; psychotherapy can be seen as a special type of play. In family therapy, the therapist may use playful paradox: 'therapeutic double binds'. Transference, the vehicle of psychoanalytical therapy, is a metaphorical relationship that is also essentially playful—serious but not real. Some guidelines for considering the relative indications and contraindications of family and individual psychotherapy are offered.

It is one of the paradoxes of psychotherapy that, although most practitioners are fierce champions of their own particular approach or school, there is no firm evidence that any one method is more effective overall than any other. It seems, rather, that psychotherapy is a caucus race in which, as Luborsky and Singer (1975) have put it, quoting Frank quoting Carroll, 'everyone has won, and all must have prizes'; this alerts us to four important themes. Firstly, the notion of winning or losing has to be radically revised in the face of psychotherapeutic values – the substitution of 'ordinary human misery' for neurosis recommended by Freud (1916) is a long way from 'winning' in the Olympic sense. Secondly, it emphasises the importance of 'unconditional positive regard' ('all must have prizes') as an essential element in any psychotherapeutic endeavour. Thirdly, it points to the centrality of paradox in psychotherapy – a theme which will be developed in this chapter. Finally, it should not be forgotten that it was the Dodo which gave out the prizes at the Caucus Race; it is still uncertain whether publicly funded psychotherapy will, like the Dodo, become extinct, as some of its critics apparently wish (Shepherd, 1984; Medawar, 1984), or whether (as seems more likely) it will, like hysteria, outlive its obituarists.

The aim of this paper is to compare two very different modes of psychotherapy – individual analytical and family therapy. Although I see them as separate and autonomous disciplines, each with its own interests and therapeutic power, my aim here is to identify areas of overlap and similarity. A central objective is to find a theory of change that applies to both. A secondary aim is to find a framework within which to consider their indications and contraindications.

Some discussion of definitions is necessary. The terms 'individual' and 'family' therapy refer simultaneously to a practical arrangement and to a theoretical approach. By individual *psychotherapy* I mean primarily dynamic or analytically orientated therapy – derived from psychoanalysis, with a central focus on the unconscious as the arena of therapy and transference as the vehicle of change. *Family therapy* is harder to define. Madanes and Haley (1977) have differentiated at least seven approaches, ranging from behavioural to psycho-dynamic, through 'systemic' and 'strategic' techniques that are more specific to family therapy. It is perhaps best seen as an overall approach in which the family itself is the object of interest, a movement away from the atomic individual to molecular patterns of interaction in the family as a whole.

The family is a 'system', a term borrowed from cybernetics, and one that is hard to define in a way that is both useful and succinct. Hall and Fagan (1956) define a system as a 'set of objects together with the relationships between the objects and their attributes'. This, as it stands, may not seem very illuminating, but its emphasis on relationships and its focus on 'objects' (i.e. family members) as a set, rather than as individuals, are the key issues for family therapy. The great advantage of seeing the family as a 'system' is that a number of known properties and functions of systems – boundaries, sub-systems, hierarchy, openness or closedness, homeostasis and non-summativity (i.e. the sum being greater than the parts) – can then be applied to family patterns and pathology. It is worth noting that almost anything, including an individual or the 'unconscious mind', could be seen as a system. Finally, 'paradox' is defined by the OED as a 'seemingly absurd but perhaps well-founded statement'. This chapter could be seen as an exploration of absurdity and its foundations in relationship to two forms of therapy.

Change

Despite a considerable literature, it is still not known how psychotherapy brings about change. Although it is likely that the helpful elements in any therapy are much less specific than its practitioners like to believe, both analytical and family therapists have tried to isolate the 'mutative' elements in their work, and I shall now consider these.

Within family therapy, the most influential force has undoubtedly been Gregory Bateson and his followers – the Palo Alto group (Bateson, 1972; Watzlawick *et al.*, 1967). In their view, the aim of psychological methods of treatment is a change of frame or context within which the symptom is viewed. They follow Epictetus: 'Men are disturbed not by things, but by the view which they take of them' (Barker, 1983). This approach is inherently paradoxical. It suggests that, if you say to someone that reality cannot be altered, but your way of looking at it can, change will follow. Although the Batesonian view of change is cognitive rather than affective, this fits well with Freud's archaeological metaphor (1916); in this, he compared psychoanalysis to the disinterring of buried remains, which in the unconscious appear huge and terrifying but, seen in the light of day, shrink down to mere remnants of a past era.

Simply saying to a patient or family that they should look at their problems in a different light is unlikely to produce change. Both psychoanalysis and family therapy postulate built-in mechanisms which maintain the status quo: resistance or homeostasis. The techniques of therapy are designed to overcome these mechanisms, which Watzlawick called 'therapeutic double binds' – the patient is put in a situation in which they cannot *not* change. The most extreme example of this is the technique of 'prescribing the symptom', in which the patient is instructed to maintain his/her symptom – depression or anorexic behavior, for instance – often with the accompanying explanation that, by doing so, he will bring benefit through his own suffering and self-sacrifice to other members of the family (Palazolli *et al.*, 1978). According to the theory, this will lead to change whatever happens. The patient either follows the instruction, in which case he will have (a) shown that he has some control over his symptom and (b) implicitly accepted the authority of the therapist rather than that of the illness, *or* will disobey the instruction, and so will have (a) demonstrated some presumably desirable autonomy and (b) been relieved of the symptoms which led him to seek help.

An important element in the double bind hypothesis is the condition that the subject is 'held' in the situation, or, as Bateson (1972) put it, 'cannot leave the field'. Jackson and Haley (1963) have tried to apply the therapeutic double bind theory to psychoanalysis; they see therapy as a situation where the patient is 'held' and subjected to the 'be spontaneous paradox'. An example of this would be the patient who in his first psychoanalytical session, when told of Freud's 'basic rule' (i.e. say everything that comes into your mind, however embarrassing or irrelevant), replied, 'If I could do that, I would not need to be here in the first place.' When the patient *is* able to achieve the basic rule, he would therefore no longer need therapy (cf. Holmes, 2013). As Hans Sachs said (Watzlawick *et al.*, 1967), 'Therapy comes to an end when the patient realises that it could go on for ever.' This approach can be extended by seeing the analyst as a kind of Zen master (Watts, 1961) who sets his patient impossible tasks, such as 'find the sound of one hand clapping', which lead eventually to cure, or enlightenment, when the patient realises that there is no 'answer' and that he can be responsible for his own life, not needing to depend on a parental analyst or guru.

Although such anti-analytical analysis is witty and not without a grain of truth, this approach does not really take us to the heart of analytical therapy. Here, Strachey's classical formulation (1934) of the 'mutative interpretation' still holds sway after half a century (Sandler *et al.*, 1973; Malan, 1979); he saw the key change-producing interpretation as one that brings together the present relationship with the therapist, the patient's external 'problem' or situation, and the early childhood relationship, usually with the parents. The analyst's imaginative capacity to link together these three apparently heterogeneous elements into one coherent pattern is the core of his work. The analyst has simultaneously to enable a living, affectively charged relationship with the patient to develop and to be detached enough to interpret it.

There are two steps involved in this process. Firstly, the symptom – the 'external' problem – has to be seen in a new context; this is the context of the unconscious – the childhood conflict of which the patient is unaware, which nevertheless invisibly shapes his destiny. Secondly, this unconscious context is made manifest in the transference, which conjures up the past in a metaphorical and so controllable way. Transference makes the reality of unconscious determination an inescapable fact for the patient.

This more profound view of how change comes about in analytical therapy is still compatible with the Watzlawick model. Analytical change does involve a 'change of frame'; the patient learns in therapy to differentiate past and present, fantasy and reality, unconscious and conscious, body and thought, and to render unto each that which is appropriate to each. Change comes about through paradox in that it involves a 'real' relationship with a therapist that is laden with the unconscious 'fictions' or transference. To these, psychoanalysis adds two further elements: the need for an active transferential therapeutic experience, if change is to take place – intellectual insight alone not being enough (neither necessary nor sufficient); and the view that the central arena of change is in the unconscious – in those parts of himself of which the patient is mostly unaware and where primary processes predominate. These two elements are also to be found, albeit translated into systems language, in family therapy.

Family therapists would agree with the analytical emphasis on the importance of a living therapeutic experience, which Minuchin (1974) has called 'enactment'. The family does not merely describe their problem – they demonstrate it, as the family interactions unfold themselves before the therapist. A warring couple will row in the session, if necessary, before their differences can be resolved. A seductive and husband-undermining woman will exchange glances of exasperation with her son every time her husband speaks. In these living minutiae can be found, holographically, a microcosm of the total family pattern of relationships.

The concept of the unconscious is the hallmark of analytical therapy and one that family therapists, especially those with behaviourist leanings, have done their best to expunge. There are, however, important parallels between the concepts of the 'system' and the unconscious, both in the part they play in the theoretical structure of the two therapies and in their formal properties (Holmes, 1983).

Both system and unconscious are of a higher 'logical type' than the symptom, i.e. each provides a wider context within which the apparently incomprehensible symptom makes sense. An unconscious fear of paternal disapproval ('castration anxiety') might be seen analytically to account for repeated self-sabotage ('fear of success') in adult life, while 'a systemic need' for 'distance regulation' (Byng-Hall, 1980) which simultaneously keeps parents apart and holds them together, may explain disturbed behaviour in a child.

In both, system and unconscious provide an explanatory concept to which the illness is referred; each represents a reservoir of past experiences and present influence which mould the patient and of which he is unaware. Power is seen to reside not in the individual, but in the impersonal force of the system or the unconscious: the sick individual is trapped in illness by forces over which he has no control. Both theories hypothesise that a direct attempt at influencing the unconscious or system may be futile. Cure will involve a rearrangement of the relationship so that individual and unconscious or system are working harmoniously. As Freud saw it, the unconscious is a horse which the conscious rider has to control sometimes by giving it its head.

The paradoxical prescriptions of the Milan group, in which an anorexic or psychotic child is told to continue to sacrifice himself in order, say, to remind the family of a dead grandfather who is in danger of being forgotten (Palazzoli *et al.*, 1978), also contain the idea that change is more likely to occur by recognising the strength of the opposing forces than by direct confrontation. By referring symptoms to the impersonal 'not-I' of system or unconscious, both family and individual therapy eliminate the guilt which so often accompanies psychiatric disturbance, or, rather, they redirect it from the destructive self-referential guilt of neurosis to a reparative guilt, at having inauthentically avoided one's biological destiny and human responsibility.

The impersonality of system and unconscious allows the co-existence of opposites; as Freud put it, the unconscious knows no negatives – in it love and hate can co-exist. The system, too, contains apparent incompatibles. Silverstein and Papp (Papp, 1976) have developed a technique of therapy in which finely poised alternative interpretations are offered by each therapist, leaving the family free to choose which they accept. Just as analytical therapy opens up to the patient the range of forces within him of which he had been unaware and against which he is defended, so this technique reveals to the family members a wider spectrum of possibilities and roles than had seemed possible in their dysfunction. Both system and unconscious widen the range of choices, but neither therapy will choose for the patient; widened choice means more autonomy – an escape from the traps (Ryle, 1990) with which the patient and family presented themselves.

Bateson's attempt to 'go one meta-' over psychoanalysis by translating analytical procedures into therapeutic double binds can be accepted as possibly valid; the notion of the system also owes much to and is in many ways similar to that of the unconscious – the system might even be seen as an 'inside-out' unconscious.

Direction and reflection: clinical examples

Although there are some clear similarities between the formal theoretical properties of the unconscious and the system, as therapies they appear very different. Family therapy techniques are designed to act on the system in a directive way, while psychoanalysis appears rather to reflect on the unconscious. This polarity in treatment approaches is well established and has been described many times, e.g. as a dichotomy between 'directive' and 'exploratory' theory (Shapiro, 1981) or between 'doing to' and 'being with' the patient (Wolff, 1972). It may also be related to Piaget's (1954) accommodation/assimilation dichotomy, which he sees as fundamental to all developmental processes. Action, like accommodation, involves visible modelling and moulding between environment and organism; reflection, like assimilation, has to do with an invisible change of internal structures. Both are required for change. The interplay between the two therapeutic modes may be illustrated by the following clinical example.

> A divorced woman with three small children asked her GP for a psychiatric appointment for her boyfriend. This 'A asks for an appointment on B's behalf' constitutes an indication for conjoint rather than individual therapy, and they were therefore offered a joint appointment, at least in the first instance. Their problem as they depicted it was that they were fond of each other, got on well in almost every respect, and had been on the point of marriage several times, but, whenever the wedding day approached, the putative husband became beset with doubts and depression and insisted that they call it off; they had cancelled the wedding three times. What was surprising to them was that, in every other area of his life, he was strong and decisive.

An initial intervention was in the interpretive, reflective mood. It was suggested that his depression had to do not with his intended marriage, but with the death of his mother, which had occurred two years previously and which had been followed, in a very short time, by his father's remarriage to a young widow, who herself, like his fiancée, had three sons still at home. His difficulty in deciding whether or not to marry, it was suggested, reflected his grief at his mother's death, his unconscious guilt at wishing to find a substitute for his dead mother in his present girlfriend (whose eldest son had the same name as his own), and his Oedipal rivalry with his too-rapidly-remarrying father.

These comments were linked with and derived from tiny transferential elements of rivalry with the therapist, including openly expressed scepticism about the value of therapy, to which he had been dragged somewhat reluctantly by his girlfriend. This linked too with his evident pleasure but ambivalence about his outstanding academic gifts, his difficulty in deciding on a stable career, and his recurrent disappointment in tutors and bosses whom he sought as gods but whose feet he found were clay-infested.

The impact of these comments was hard to determine. The doubts continued and the pressure on the therapist to suggest some course of action other than reflection intensified. At this point, a different tack was tried, linking his doubts with the girlfriend's problems. It was suggested that his difficulties must be important in some way to their relationship: she had had a very difficult time, with a broken marriage and bringing up three children on her own, and it was important for her to feel decisive and competent and not to doubt her own capacity to make a stable relationship with a man. By 'carrying' all the indecision and depression, it was suggested, he was helping her to feel strong, and continuing to do so was probably as an expression of his love for her.

Rapid change followed. He changed his job for a better one, they married – to their apparent mutual satisfaction – and decided they no longer needed therapy. There was, however, an interesting sequel. Some 18 months later, they again made contact and asked for help. They said that their marriage was basically strong; they had had a baby – now four months old, but the wife – who had originally asked for help – had now become badly depressed, and this was leading to escalating rows between them, which they both found very upsetting. She complained that he had become just like his father, expecting her to be a subservient wife and to suppress her autonomy. He complained of her irrational angry outbursts.

On this occasion, the therapy centred on the wife – who had originally asked for help for her husband. The rebellious depressed part of her that had been suppressed in a rigid religious upbringing as an (unwanted) late last child finally surfaced within this marriage, which gave her the security to express her needs but lacked the flexibility to meet them. It was decided to refer her for individual therapy, but, once again, active directive intervention was needed to defuse the escalating rows and to help the couple to find common ground where they could be together without the demands of the children. When they presented originally, the wife had appeared the stronger, and the therapist had sided with the husband by suggesting to him that his depression was his way of helping his wife; the wife was now 'down'.

In an attempt directively to reverse this, it was suggested that she had an 'unfair advantage' over her husband, whose first marriage and first experience of parenthood it was. She must expect him to find it difficult to adjust and make it her task to help him to live in a family and to survive.

This is an example of how family therapy techniques can deal often rapidly and effectively with crises in relationships, but how underlying and longstanding difficulties may remain untouched. The initial period of therapy might have been seen as success, had the self-chosen 'follow-up' not happened. The distinction between active and reflective techniques illustrated here suggests that family therapy does not necessarily promote the understanding, and hence change, of internal mental structures that is required to sustain long-term benefit. Watzlawick *et al.* (1967) called these two models 'first-order' and 'second-order' change. The first might be likened to Freud's concept of transference neurosis, where the patient loses his symptoms in the early phase of therapy, only to replace them with a pathological dependence on the therapist which, if threatened, will lead to the re-emergence of the illness.

I have implied that family therapy can be equated with action, crisis and first-order change; analytical therapy with reflection, second-order change and long-term development. Although there may be some rather obvious truth in this, the distinction is far from simple. The directives of paradoxical therapy often prohibit change, with the aim of promoting it. The paradoxical message often contains quasi-analytical understanding of the problem (the case described above could easily be seen in terms of mutual projective identification), but phrased in action language. Similarly, the reflections of analytical therapy are implicitly designed to promote change; the structural arrangements of therapy – a commitment to regular and prolonged treatment – constitutes active direction of the patient's life. Khan (1983) gives some interesting examples of the structural arrangements that he insists on before working analytically with his group of privileged but disturbed young people, e.g. making regular attendance at school a precondition of undertaking analytical therapy and giving the parent the task of enforcing this.

In general, one can say that the active and reflective elements are present in both (probably all) psychotherapeutic techniques, but that the proportion and sequence with which they are applied varies with different therapies. Brief examples illustrate this.

The first shows how active techniques are often an essential preliminary to reflection. In family therapy it is inappropriate to try to explore family dynamics while a disturbed teenager is tearing the house apart: some degree of parental control has to be established first.

> In a joint referral, a depressed mother and a delinquent 15-year-old girl were presented. The family's main complaint was about this girl, who was often out all night, got into violent rows with her mother and fights with her father, used the telephone all day long, and played loud music in her bedroom while her parents were trying to rest. A paradoxical suggestion that her behaviour was an attempt to help her mother by showing her that *she* was not going to be depressed and was determined to have a good time produced just enough reduction in chaos for it to be established that both parents had been so confused in their adolescence – the mother by strict, puritanical elderly parents, the father by a liberal laissez-faire regime – that both felt too guilty to impose discipline on their children or to allow themselves some enjoyment.

A fundamental tenet of analytical therapy is the translation of feelings and actions into words: understanding has to substitute for action. This, as Freud saw it, was the great trade-off required by civilization – instinctual satisfaction (action) is renounced, to be replaced by thought. The child defers satisfaction, but gains an inner world of imagination, plan, structure; the word is the prize the child acquires in this struggle for development. In the Kleinian view, 'the depressive position' characterises this heroic renunciation that admits us to humanity; in exchange for a split and persecutory world of instinctive and immediate gratification, we may achieve wholeness and concern. In one sense, neurosis may be seen as a reversal or protest against this process. In therapy, the patient has to be led away from action to reflection, but, ultimately, the need for action returns. Psychoanalysis assumes that a change in internal structure will lead to effective action, just as directive therapies assume that a change in behaviour will produce internal (and so lasting) change. A second example illustrates this.

> After two years of weekly analytical psychotherapy, a 35-year-old man – who had presented with a cardiac neurosis apparently precipitated by a severe ill-ness in his mother – became engaged. As the wedding day approached, he became more and more preoccupied by his inability to tell his fiancée that he was in therapy, having concealed this fact from everyone – almost from himself. The action of entering therapy and the need to tell his fiancée were structural facts which lacked internal representation. Both were linked with a fear of being thought abnormal and with his intense jealousy of her previous boyfriends. This led to a retaliatory concealment of his secret relationship with the therapist. All this connected with his intense jealousy of his one-year-older sister and guilt about his collusive and father-excluding secret attachment to his mother. Only when he understood these connections was he able to act on them by telling his fiancée that he was in therapy.

Paradoxically, directive approaches are by no means confined to family therapy but are also to be found, often unobtrusively, within the analytical literature. Here is an example from the classical psychoanalytic canon.

Freud's Dora (1905) was an adolescent who found great difficulty in leaving home. This was partly because of her great love for her father and for her father's mistress's husband, Herr K. Freud 'cured' her after only three months of therapy when he suggested that she should marry Herr K, who would have to divorce his wife to do so, thus leaving her father free to marry Frau K; in Freud's words, 'this would be the best solution for all the parties concerned'. This paradoxical direc-tion seemed to have done the trick. Within a year, Dora had left home and was married to a suitable young man. The fact that this directive phase of therapy – this 'fragment' – was not followed by a reflective one accounts for the sad fact that, at 'follow up' 20 years later (Deutsch, 1957), Dora was as neurotic as before and as deeply and unplayfully involved with her teenage son as she had been with her father (Holmes, 1983).

Play

Both family therapy – in so far as it is not exclusively behavioural – and individual analytical therapy approach symptoms indirectly. Both assume that, as therapy proceeds, symptoms will disappear from prominence, to be replaced by uncon-scious or systemic issues. When this does not happen, it is usually a sign that the treatment is not going well.

In both forms, the client (patient or family) approaches the therapist expect-ing a solution to his/its problem, but what they are offered instead is a new problem – that of therapy. In individual therapy it is the therapist who becomes the object of interest, rather than the symptom; in family therapy it is the family itself. It is only when the patient begins to take an interest in the therapist – to wonder why they are always seen at such-and-such an o'clock, what the thera-pist's other patients are like, whether he/she is married, to wish they could meet for a drink, etc. – that mutative therapy in the Strachean sense can really begin. In family therapy the process is reversed, but the effect is the same. It is when the family forgets about the therapist and begins to interact among themselves, when the children begin to play and the parents to argue, rather than woodenly sitting and waiting for questions from the therapist, that the symptom slips away and the therapist can begin to reintroduce himself as an agent of change. This replacement of the problem by the 'non-problem', which in group therapy gradually takes over as a patient becomes assimilated, more interested in the life of the group itself and less in his own particular difficulties, has been described by Garland (1982). To take an analogy from the 'gate' theory of pain, the heat of the group, of family life, of the transference, like 'cupping', by raising the threshold for psychic pain, reduces it.

But how do we understand this new process that takes over from the symptom, this interest in the therapist who is not a 'real' person, in the group that is not a 'real' group, this family life that is so intense and yet (unlike the symptom which cries out to be removed) has no clear object? The common thread which runs through them all, I would argue, is that of *play*.

There is a deep seam in British psychoanalysis that centres on the notion of imagination and creativity: its exponents include Sharpe (1937), Milner (1971), Winnicott (1972), Khan (1983), Rycroft (1968), Wolff (1972) and Pedder (1979). The creative imagination is inherently playful: it must be in touch with the primary process but not be overwhelmed by it. Winnicott defined the essence of psychoanalytical therapy as learning to play, referring to play in its widest sense, including 'cultural' forms such as the arts and sport. Play is inherently paradoxical – both deeply serious and at the same time un-'real'; a still life is a picture of a bowl of fruit; its calorific value is nil. Play involves what Humphrey (1983) calls 'rhyme', in which 'cat' rhymes with 'mat', but not with 'cat'; it can be related to metaphor, finding likeness in difference. As Pedder (1979) has pointed out, transference is etymologically equivalent to metaphor; one is Latin, the other is Greek, but they mean the same: 'carrying across'. In therapy, the patient experiences metaphorically with the therapist the relationships, feelings and fantasies derived from the past and dominating the present; played with, they lose their power (Holmes, 1985).

If play is seen as a paradoxical conjunction of 'serious–unserious', we can ask how this state or mode is signalled. How does play stay play, remain outside the realm of the real? The essential mechanism is the uncoupling of action from consequence (Segraves, 1982). In a pre-match interview, a tennis player threatens to 'murder' his opponent: at the end of the game, they shake hands (just). Romeo is passionately 'in love' with Juliet, but they do not 'make' love on the stage (it is precisely this lack of uncoupling that separates pornography from art). The rules of analytical therapy, the regularity of time and place, the neutral stance of the therapist create just such an uncoupling. How many therapists have had to face the bitter complaints of their patients that they do not 'really' care for them, that they are just doing a job? Winnicott (1972) stated that the end of the session is the analyst's expression of 'hate in the counter-transference'; it is also his way of saying that he does not 'really' hate the patient – it is just that the game is over for today. When this understanding of the metaphorical nature of therapy breaks down, as in a psychotic transference, on the one hand, or in alexithymia (Lesser & Lesser, 1983), on the other, therapy cannot proceed.

Where do we just learn to play? It is of course in the family, at our mother's knee. The functions of play remain a subject for research and debate, but there is no doubt that, as well as being a rehearsal for 'real' tasks, play contributes to making humans into 'natural psychologists' (Humphrey, 1983). It is through play that we achieve the knowledge of our own and others' feelings that is essential for survival of a social species. In individual therapy, both therapist and patient are participants in play, which may resemble the intense involvement of a rebellious adolescent with a parent or the sometimes gentle and sometimes violent play of a baby at the breast. Winnicott (1972) describes the self-absorbed play of the small child in the presence of a watchful but non-intrusive mother as a prototype of one mood state that may be achieved in analysis and which may then generalise to the capacity to form intimate non-dependent relationships. The understanding which the patient seeks in analytical psychotherapy is more akin to this state – one in which the patient feels secure and attended to enough to begin through phantasy or 'thought-play' to understand himself – than it is dependent on any intellectual formulations or diagnosis.

The aim of the family therapist too is to rekindle the family's already existing capacity to play, not just in the sense of 'playing' cards, Monopoly, etc., but in the sense of teasing, joking, chatting, fighting, sulking, singing, hating, living, making up, without being overwhelmed by any of them, that is the essence of family life. In individual therapy, the therapist is an active participant; with a family, he is more like a referee who gets the game going and who throws the ball back into play when it goes out of touch. Here, too, uncoupling is central: the therapist tries to break up the repetitive and well-worn patterns of argument that lead nowhere (the 'gramophone record' that most families play at the start of therapy) and to generate playful interaction that, like speech itself, is an open system, an infinite source of variety and change woven from simple and repeated elements. Paradoxical techniques such as 'prescribing the symptom' and Kelly's fixed role therapy (Kelly, 1955) are uncoupling devices, designed to signify and generate play.

Indications and contraindications

Analytical and family therapies are both non-specific or broad-spectrum treatments, which include a mixture of different techniques and strategies. It is not possible to isolate a single active principle in them which would lead to cure, however much practitioners (and critics) would wish this were so. The consequence is, as several reviews have shown (Skynner, 1976; Martin, 1977; Clarkin *et al.*, 1979), that there are few clear-cut indications which would lead to choosing a particular therapy, only trends and tendencies.

This article would suggest that the two main issues affecting choice of treatment are *change* and *context*. Change in family therapy involves helping the family to find healthy patterns from within an existing repertoire, which will then lead through the family's own growth to new structures. In individual therapy, the therapist, rather than being a referee, is often a regression-inducing participant; new patterns will be generated within the treatment itself. It follows that family therapy is indicated either when the family is in a state of crisis or transition, which generates its own change, or when family members are changing rapidly themselves, as with the very young or the very old. Individual therapy, on the other hand, is indicated when there is no great biological drive towards change (i.e. adults) and when the pathology of the patient is too great for spontaneous improvement, but not so great that no change is possible (e.g. psychosis, severe personality disorder).

The second main factor determining choice of therapy is the *context* of the referral. As mentioned, when one member of a family asks for help on another's behalf, an initial family interview is usually desirable. When an individual patient is regularly accompanied by a spouse, or parent, or child who waits patiently outside while the official patient has their session, joint therapy is often indicated ('waiting-room syndrome'). Where there is multiple pathology in the family, joint interviews should be considered. 'Secondary gain' from illness often involves collusion between the family and the patient who has adopted a sick role, and, in this situation, family therapy can sometimes 'unstick' a chronically intractable case. Family therapy also often has something to offer where the more stringent requirements of individual analytical therapy would exclude the patient. Considerations of IQ, age, psychological-mindedness and psychosis are less important in family therapy than in individual therapy, but patients with severe paranoid anxiety do badly in any group situation, including family sessions. Motivation, commitment to change, and a positive view of therapy are important preconditions of any successful therapy, probably even more so in family than in individual therapy.

Conclusion

There are many points of contact and overlap between the two disciplines; no clear-cut guidelines indicate one or other therapy in any given diagnosis, and each case has to be considered on its merits. Psychotherapists should not despair of this, however, since therapy is always concerned with the individual case. We constantly confront the false alternatives ('dilemmas'; Ryle, 1990) with which patients torment themselves: 'Either I am unmarried (which I do not want to be) and strong, or married and weak (which I do not want to be).' The art of treatment is to unhook patients from this dilemma and help them to see that weaknesses may be strengths, and vice versa. The same is true for therapy itself. It is not a question of either family therapy *or* individual therapy. For example, in adolescence, family therapy can be immensely helpful in making a teenager feel less stigmatised and trapped and free him to leave home and make his own life. Equally, individual therapy may provide – may be the only way of providing – the intimacy and privacy that a disturbed young person needs to face fears of madness, perversity and death that prevent him from embarking on adult life. Therapists can offer no certainties in the face of the unpredictability of illness and neurosis: 'Phlegmatic rationality starts and shakes its head at those unaccountable prepossessions [passions] but they exist as undeniably as the wind and the waves, determining here a wreck and there a triumphant voyage' (Eliot, 1876).

Family therapy may be a beacon, psychoanalysis a sea chart. The wise sailor needs both.

CHAPTER 12

PSYCHOANALYSIS AND CBT
Confluence or watershed?

Prelude

Let's start well away from the consulting room, in what is rather quaintly known as the 'real world'. The venue is a local sub-post office, in the middle of a notoriously rough housing estate. Ahead of me in the queue are a very young-looking father with a baby in a push-chair and a couple in their early 40s, scantily clad, hair dyed respectively blond (male) and shocking pink (female), both with an opposite-sex moniker tattooed on their necks, presumably each of the other.

'Cheer up darling, it may never 'appen; got the 'ump or something?', shouts the man to a rather glum-looking shop-girl across the aisle. 'Nothing to be cheerful about', comes the reply. At this rebuff, his female partner comments, sotto voce: 'She's *breathing*, ain't she? That's all the 'appiness you need.' She turns to the push-chair baby: 'What lovely long hair; mine were all bald as coots. Oooh, but I do prefer pink ones to blue ones. Far less trouble.' 'No they ain't', retorts her man, 'you don't 'ave to say to them in a few years' time – no you *can't* sleep with 'im!'

This woman seems to be an enlightened being. She knows that for contentment one need look no further than an in-breath, offering the insights of mindfulness-based CBT to the depressed shop-worker, the 'patient' in this example of folk therapy. Meanwhile there is an inescapable sexual ambiance generated by the Oedipal confluence of man, woman and baby – the baby's infantile sexuality projected forward into her adolescence, the physicality and mock-aggressive banter of the couple suggesting somehow that bed is not far from their minds.

While none of the characters in this mini-drama would seem ideal candidates for therapy, it would be hard to deconstruct it without the help of *both* Beck and Freud. The girl needs immediate help with her misery. Focusing on the positive, while detaching herself from bad feelings through breathing meditation, may well be the first aid she requires. But, ultimately, there will likely be 'characterological' sexual/Oedipal ramifications to her unhappiness – she hasn't got a boyfriend and wants one; she's got one but wants a different one; she is pregnant and wishes she wasn't, or isn't and wishes she was.

Theoretical non-incompatibility

My aim here is to 'negate the negation' which typifies how CBT and psychoanalysis view one another. Both are adept at 'Othering', straw-man debating points, special pleading, polemics and tendentiousness (see, for example, Samuels & Veale 2009).

Psychoanalysts tend to dismiss CBT as a superficial, quick-fix, 'fast food' therapy which, while it may temporarily remove symptoms, is often followed by relapse, leaving fundamental dysfunctional character structures unchanged. The unconscious and its manifestations in the transference – the key province of psychoanalytic work – is ignored, glossed over, denied, or seen as irrelevant.

Equally, from a CBT perspective, the following is typical:

> The scandal is that GPs can't access CBT so they continue to send patients for outmoded treatments that don't work. When a severely health-anxious patient is told to 'lie on a couch and tell me about your relationship with your mother', he doesn't see the relevance and he drops out.
>
> (Salkovskis, quoted in Brearley, 2007, p. 20)

Implicit in this slur is the following: psychoanalysis a) is trapped in a fossilised past, b) is ineffective, c) lacks a collaborative culture, d) has high drop-out rates, and e) is generally absurd and contemptible; f) patients are made to do things that don't make sense to them, and g) practitioners are slightly mad and mother-preoccupied.

Conversely, psychoanalysts characterise CBT practitioners as therapeutic terriers, oblivious to personal and temporal boundaries, insensitive to client disappointment and hostility, obsessed with questionable psychiatric diagnoses, form-filling, homework and handouts at the expense of spontaneity and emotional expression, and blind to the interpersonal difficulties of their clients, especially those that arise in the therapeutic relationship itself.

Despite all this, a good argument can be made for a degree of theoretical compatibility between the two approaches (cf. Power, 2002). As Kuyken *et al.* (2005, p. 114) put it, depression is characterised by 'maladaptive beliefs about the self, the external world and the future, shaped through formative developmental experiences'. Common ground with psychoanalysis here includes: a) targeting mental phenomena of which the client is at presentation unaware; b) focusing on the combination of affect, wish and belief that typifies a people's fundamental view of themselves and others and the relationship between them; c) the avoidance of psychic pain by defence mechanisms; and d) the anachronistic persistence of such defences into adult life.

Through diary-keeping and pedagogic instruction, CBT helps its clients identify the 'automatic thoughts' which underpin depressive affect – 'I am useless', 'Nobody would want to be friends with someone like me', 'I'll never get better.' Until they are elicited in this way, these thoughts remain latent, out of conscious awareness. Psychoanalysis uses different means to a similar end: dream analysis, free association and transference-analysis. The distinction between preconscious and unconscious thoughts can be used to mark a radical divide between the two modalities but in clinical practice is often of little significance. Similarly, CBT's 'maladaptiveness' of depressive thinking is consistent with psychoanalytic defence analysis, in which patterns of self-protection appropriate to childhood persist into adult life to the subject's disadvantage.

CBT picks out typical predetermined patterns of inappropriate thinking in depression: overgeneralisation, catastrophising, black-and-white thinking, etc. Each of these is potentially translatable into psychoanalytic meta-psychology. Overgeneralisation illustrates Matte-Blancoian (1975) symmetrisation, the conflation of differences typical of the unconscious thought processes. Catastrophising arises when a single setback is taken as a signal of general disarray. It can be seen as a failure of Bionic 'K' – the lack of processing of beta into alpha elements due to the absence of an internalised 'thinking breast' (Bion, 1967). CBT protocols and exercises aim to instil this skill in the depression sufferer. Similarly, black-and-white thinking exemplifies pre-depressive-position defensive splitting of the world into good and bad, in order to protect the former from the aggressive aspects of the latter.

From an etiological perspective, The quote from Kuyken *et al.* shows that CBT readily acknowledges the childhood origins of depressive psychological difficulties at a theoretical level even if, in practice, less emphasis is placed on the past than on correcting current maladaptive tendencies. Contemporary psychoanalysis is concerned more with the 'present transference' (Sandler, 1976) than with reconstructions of a putative past. Linehan *et al.*'s (1994) Dialectical Behaviour Therapy model of Borderline Personality Disorder sees 'invalidation' in childhood as the key to pathology in adult life. Psychoanalysis may have a more detailed and nuanced theoretical account of infancy and childhood, and work with the ways in which people subject to invalidation, trauma or neglect may at an unconscious level contribute to their own victimhood, but it would be hard to find points of major theoretical disagreement here.

CBT arose in part from a dissatisfaction with certain aspects of psychoanalysis, the dominant paradigm in US psychiatry and psychology in the 1950s and 1960s: the cost and length of time needed to complete an analysis, lack of diagnostic precision, absence of scientific evaluation, and overvaluation of the unconscious as opposed to the conscious mind. However, the other main strand in the emergence of CBT flowed from the 'cognitive revolution' in which theoretical psychology began to acknowledge the limitations of stimulus-response psychology and to recognise an inner world characterised by mental models and maps (Westen, 2005).

In a typical acronymic fashion, CBT focuses on these in terms of 'EARS' – Expectations, Assumptions, Rules and Schemata. Young's (1990) 'schema-focused therapy' develops the idea of Early Maladaptive Schemata (EMS), i.e. unconditional beliefs about the self, and the self in relation to others, that form the core of a person's identity. These representations are a precipitate of early experience and the growing child's ways of coping.

One difference between the two disciplines is CBT's focus on the subject's relation to himself, while contemporary psychoanalysis, especially in its interpersonal, relational and intersubjective variants, homes in on the self-in-relation-to-others. However, Safran and Muran (2000) move CBT's intrapsychic tack in an interpersonal direction, building on schema-focused approaches by suggesting that EMSs influence behaviour in such a manner that a person's environment is shaped to respond in ways that confirm core schemata. Typical borderline sufferers may have EMS suggesting they are worthless and bound to be rejected by those with whom they try to establish emotional contact. Their unpredictable behaviour in intimate relationships then provokes and confirms the very rejectingness that lies at the core of this self-belief.

EMS seems to resonate easily with, and is no doubt in part derived from, the notion of the internal world as conceptualised by the Object Relations school, a fundamental constellation of self-in-relation-to-significant-others, instantiated in infancy and childhood and often persisting into adult life, with maladaptive consequences. There are of course important differences in emphasis. Psychoanalysis tends to emphasise the sexual and ethical (in the sense of splitting of 'good' and 'bad' aspects of the self and other) aspects of core beliefs and the representational world, rather than staying with the beliefs and assumptions themselves. But schema-focused and object-relational formulations map one to the other without too much awkwardness.

There is an ever shifting dialectic between experience and the language and narrative structures used to represent it. The stories people tell about themselves are 'representations of representations' in that they are attempts to encapsulate the mental structures which underlie them. The latter are 'unconscious', either in the descriptive sense of being out of awareness until activated through therapeutic dialogue or in the formal psychoanalytic sense of being repressed or split off in order to avoid the mental pain they embody. In either case, a developmental perspective suggests that these self-narratives derive from representations of actual relational events (cf. Stern, 1985; Representation of Interactions that have been Generalised, RIGs). The 'dialectic' refers to the way in which one's view of oneself determines experience, both literally (if one is expecting to be abused, one is more likely to 'choose' a potentially abusive partner) and in the narrative sense that the sense one makes of those experiences will be accommodated to fit pre-existing meaning structures ('the fact that men exploit me proves how useless I am').

Schema-focused approaches concentrate on the *consequences* of this dialectic, psychoanalysis on its *antecedents*. The CBT therapist tries to elicit the dysfunctional guiding principles/propositions by which a person lives – 'uselessness', passivity, unwantedness, etc. – and then to help her or him find ways to generate experiences which disconfirm them, including by implication the therapeutic relationship itself, which honours the intrinsic value of a human life and of a person's right to attention and respect. The main drive would be towards examining the client's current situation and relational constellations and trying, rather directly, to change them.

A psychoanalytic approach would focus more on the abusive events themselves, and their possible affective meanings for a child beset with external trauma and inescapable developmental priorities of establishing a gender identity, a sense of efficacy and ways of dealing with 'normal' Oedipal envy and rivalry. The mutative agenda here entails attending to ('mentalising'; Holmes, 2010) these thematic repetitions/manifestations in the transference. Both CBT and psychoanalysis adhere to Freud's dictum that 'effigies cannot be destroyed in absentia', but in CBT's case the transcendence of these false gods takes place outside the consulting room, through 'experiments', while psychoanalytically they are brought to life and then reworked in the therapeutic relationship.

'Mechanism of action'

CBT's theory of action rests on two planks: a) cognitive change, replacing dysfunctional assumptions with more appropriate and realistic ones, and b) exposure, in imagination and/or in vivo, to phobically avoided thoughts and affects. Translated into psychoanalytic terminology, the former corresponds to Freud's dictum 'where id is, there ego shall be', or the acquisition of mentalising skills, or 'alpha function', via interpersonal exploration in therapy sessions (cf. Holmes, 2010), the latter with the benign presence of the therapist providing a secure enough base for the patient to acknowledge and face disavowed feelings.

These ideas are at present no more than speculations. When it comes to testing them in the laboratory of psychotherapy research, the results tend to be confusing and contradictory. A core CBT mantra holds that changes in cognition result in changes in mood in depression. However, comparing outcomes in people with depression receiving CBT or pharmacotherapy, Imber *et al.* (1990) found that, in both groups, cognitive change followed rather than initiated mood changes. It is entirely possible that 'non-specific factors' in CBT – therapist attention, the attachment relationship, restoration of hope and attribution of meaning, whatever that meaning may be – are what produces change, not the supposedly 'active ingredient' of cognitive restructuring.

Similarly, great stress is placed on the role of accurate transference interpretations as a mutative element in psychoanalysis. Yet a much quoted study found that, the more the interpretations, the worse the outcome of psychoanalytic psychotherapy (Piper *et al.*, 1999). Recently, researchers looking at the role of interpretation versus support in psychoanalysis found in one instance that transference interpretations made things worse for people with low Quality of Object Relations (QOR) and better for the less disturbed (Piper *et al.*, 1999), while another found they were associated with sustained better outcomes in low QOR clients (Hoglend *et al.*, 2008). Capturing the subtlety of therapeutic interaction, both 'horizontally' in the minutiae of a session and 'longitudinally' in the overall strategy of a therapy, remains a huge research challenge (cf. Kächele *et al.*, 2009).

To make a rather grandiose comparison, psychotherapy currently finds itself in a place comparable to Darwinian evolutionary theory in the 1870s. Evolution by natural selection was an established fact but, pre-Mendel, pre-Watson and Crick, its mechanism of action remained obscure. Similarly, we know that psychotherapy 'works', but how change comes about is still unclear. Subtle dynamic models, encompassing both unconscious and conscious ingredients in the therapeutic relationship, are needed to tease out the mutative elements in psychotherapy. Disinterestedness, a genuine spirit of scientific enquiry, openness to 'soft' as well as hard data, not to mention generous doses of research funding, are preconditions for advancing the field, all of which are currently in short supply.

Technical non-compatibility

Despite the lack of serious theoretical dissonance between the two disciplines, when it comes to practice, CBT and psychoanalysis could hardly be more divergent, although, as we shall see, recent developments mean that even this must be somewhat qualified.

One striking difference is the ratio between meta-psychology and technique. CBT is concerned mainly with clinical practice; it is relatively unconcerned about developing itself as a general theory of the mind. By contrast, there is a distinct theory–practice gap in psychoanalysis. As Fonagy (2006, p. 26) elegantly puts it, 'clinical technique is not entailed in psychoanalytic theory.' The edifice of psychoanalytic theory is vast and diverse. Detailed accounts of what to do and when in psychoanalytic sessions are, with notable exceptions (e.g. Gabbard, 2004), relatively rare (but see Lemma, Roth & Pilling, 2008).

Whatever the theoretical overlaps, CBT is keen to differentiate itself from psychoanalysis as a practice. It claims to be transparent, 'problem-focused', 'collaborative' and 'scientific'. It relies on 'experiments', imparting 'portable skills', setting homework tasks, time-limitedness, and close evaluation of outcomes. However, although the proverbial prurient fly on the wall in the consulting room of a psychoanalyst and CBT practitioner would undoubtedly notice differences, these might not be as marked as either side would claim.

The opening and closing moves of sessions would likely be divergent, the psychoanalyst waiting for clients to 'bring' thoughts and feelings into the session, while the CBT therapist might ask what sort of week they had had. The implicit 'job' of the psychoanalytic client is to attend to his or her inner life, to freely associate and to bring dreams for consideration in sessions. The more directive CBT therapist, in collaboration with the client, typically sets an agenda for their hour together, unlike the psychoanalyst, who is alert to spontaneously emerging themes.

The middle sections of both sessions might be less dissimilar, with the therapist listening to clients' account of some episode in their week and/or its connections with past difficulties. Meaning-seeking interventions might also be comparable. Psychoanalysts undoubtedly make 'cognitive' comments, for example about the ways in which people's negative views of themselves become self-fulfilling prophesies, paying particular attention to how this plays itself out in the transference. Equally, CBT therapists allow freewheeling periods in sessions characterised by listening and speculation about the client's affective states.

There is a tension in any therapy between spontaneity and formulation. Meaning-making is central to any therapeutic activity (Holmes, 2012). Therapists need a guiding formulation which will help the client understand his difficulties. But too rigid adherence to a formulation inhibits the emergence of the uniqueness of an individual's experience. CBT therapists tend to work to normothetic, rather general formulations about the origins of depression, while psychoanalysts, schooled in 'Keats's 'negative capability' (i.e. tolerance of uncertainty), probe for the idiographic specificity of a person's life trajectory. Good therapists in either camp probably manage to strike a balance between these two poles.

As sessions draw to a close, differences surface once more. CBT therapists see inter-session work as an essential counterpoint to therapy itself, devising homework tasks, 'experiments' in which the client tests more positive assumptions about themselves, and 'bibliotherapy' in the form of handouts and reading assignments.

Psychoanalysts feel under no pressure to produce a well-rounded ending: 'Let's come back to that next week', or simply 'It's time to stop now', might be their rubric. It is hoped that the mutative aspects of therapy, including but not exclusively reliant upon, accurate interpretation, have penetrated defences into the unconscious life of the client, this in turn leading to a more positive view of the self, to acceptance of pain and loss, to empowerment and efficacy, and, armed with new-found skills of mentalising (Holmes, 2010), to interpersonal relationships more deftly handled. Psychoanalysis takes the inherently paradoxical nature of the unconscious and its workings into account: the more one tries directly to change things, the more resistance this may elicit; change may occur when one least expects it, in moments of mutual discovery, brought forth by the intimacy of one mind trying to understand another. CBT tends towards a more common-sense attempt to find 'solutions' to 'problems'.

Apart from the 'non-specific factors' of an attachment relationship and meaning-making in both therapies, recent developments suggest another area of partial convergence. Mindfulness-Based CBT (MBCBT; see Kuyken *et al.*, 2005) was devised in the light of the finding that, despite the short-lived helpfulness of conventional CBT, both chronicity and relapse are common in severe depression. In MBCBT, clients are encouraged, with the help of 'mindfulness' methods derived from Buddhism, to detach themselves from their depressive thoughts, to achieve affect regulation through breathing and quiet concentration, and to see negative ideations not as real but as 'just thoughts'. In a parallel development, conventional psychoanalysis has been shown to be relatively ineffective in severe Borderline

Personality Disorder (BPD) (Fonagy & Bateman, 2006). Bateman and Fonagy's (2004) modified psychoanalysis, Mentalisation-Based Therapy (MBT), addresses the difficulty which such clients have in differentiating their thoughts about the world from the world as it is. This is especially so when people are highly aroused (as people with BPD tend easily to become when stressed); their psychoanalytically informed 'partial hospitalisation' therapy package treatment includes exercises not unlike those used in MBCBT.

This illustrates theoretical overlap, at a much more therapy-near level. MBT, psychoanalytically derived, uses here-and-now transferential events in relation to the therapist and fellow group members as exemplars in which new learning takes place; skill acquisition arises in the course of 'living-learning'. CBT, less opportunistic and more protocol driven, teaches its clients to follow a meditation routine. Nevertheless, the connections are clear and probably merit further collaborative work.

Evidence of evidence

The success of CBT as the first-choice therapy for a wide range of disorders rests on its having from its inception in the mid-1970s successfully assimilated into talking therapies the blinded randomised controlled trial, the standard medical yardstick for effective treatments. Psychoanalysis has belatedly picked up the challenge and is beginning to show that it too can compete on equal terms in the world of evidence-based therapies (e.g. Leichsenring & Raybung, 2008).

It is beyond the scope of this chapter, and the competence of its author, to summarise and evaluate 30 years of complex and often contradictory psychotherapy research findings. Indeed, arguably the field still awaits an individual with the magisterial authority and Olympian detachment needed to do so. I shall instead briefly summarise the claims made on CBT's behalf as the definitive psychological therapy for most psychiatric disorders, and then present some of the arguments used by psychoanalysts in rebuttal of these claims and in support of their own position.

A good starting point is the recent 'meta-meta-analysis' offered in their 2006 article by Chapman and his colleagues (Butler *et al.*, 2006). This review summarises the current literature on treatment outcomes of CBT for a wide range of psychiatric disorders. Based on '16 methodologically rigorous meta-analyses', they found large effect sizes for CBT in unipolar depression, generalized anxiety disorder, panic disorder with or without agoraphobia, social phobia, post-traumatic stress disorder, and childhood depressive and anxiety disorders. Effect sizes for marital distress, anger, childhood somatic disorders and chronic pain were in the moderate range. CBT was somewhat superior to anti-depressants in the treatment of adult depression and showed, they claim, large but uncontrolled effect sizes in bulimia nervosa and schizophrenia.

This sort of data is routinely cited when advancing the merits of CBT, whether clinically or when applying for training and treatment funds. It has forced psychodynamically minded clinicians to rethink their position and find ways to defend their own shrinking corner.

There is in fact now a number of randomised controlled trials convincingly demonstrating psychoanalytic psychotherapy's effectiveness in a wide range of conditions. These include mild to moderate depression (Shapiro *et al.*, 1994), personality disorders (Bateman & Fonagy, 2004, 2008; Abbass *et al.*, 2008), panic disorder (Milrod *et al.*, 2007), somatisation disorders (Guthrie *et al.*, 1991) and eating disorders (Dare *et al.*, 2001). In addition, cost–benefit studies (Gabbard *et al.*, 1997) show that psychoanalytic psychotherapy, despite being resource intensive compared with pharmacotherapy and CBT, given 'cost off-setting' – less time spent in or visiting hospital, fewer medications consumed, reduced time spent on benefits, greater capacity for paid employment and there-fore more tax revenue – more than pays for itself.

However, the evidence for psychoanalytic psychotherapy is thus far generally less impressive than for its rival – compared with CBT, smaller numbers of trials, based on fewer patients, less replicated. Psychoanalysts tend to respond to this (Gabbard, 2005) in various ways. First, psychoanalytic psychotherapy is inher-ently less easy to research than other forms of treatment. Psychoanalytic therapies tend to be long term, so generating adequate research funding is problematic. In addition, the aims of psychoanalytic psychotherapy go beyond symptom relief to structural changes in personality, a deeper project, which is inherently more complex, time-consuming and expensive to study (Milton, 2001).

The argument runs that, given sufficient time and resources, psychoanalytic psy-chotherapy can and will be shown to be as effective as CBT, if not more so, and that its unique indications are gradually emerging: absence of evidence does not equate to evidence of absence (Holmes, 2001). Leichsenring and Raybung's (2008) meta-analysis of Long-Term (defined as more than one year) Psychoanalytic Psychotherapy, LTPP, supports this. Compared with short-term psychoanalytic psychotherapy (in which relapse post-therapy is common in all modalities of therapy (Parry *et al.*, 2005)), LTPP patients showed effect sizes of around 1.8 (a very respectable figure, higher than the average anti-depressant) for target problems, overall effectiveness and personality functioning. Although only around ten studies met their stringent criteria, they estimate that more than 350 studies showing contrary findings would be needed for their conclusions to have arisen by chance alone. An example included in their analysis is the Bateman and Fonagy (2004, 2008) Borderline Personality Disorder Project, an intensive programme which shows impressive reductions in suicidality, use of medical services and psychiatric consultation rates up to five years post-therapy. These findings are especially important given both the possibility that standard therapies (including short-term psychoanalytic therapy) with this diagnos-tic group may actually make patients worse and the failure of cognitive approaches to show maintenance of gains once therapy comes to an end (Levy, 2008).

Another defence of psychoanalytic psychotherapy revives the famous 'dodo bird verdict' of equal outcomes irrespective of therapy modality. Head-to-head studies show few major differences in outcome for psychoanalytic psychotherapy compared with CBT, although those differences that do arise tend marginally to favour CBT. The argument here is that, when it comes to 'parcelling out' the contributions of various factors affecting outcome, the role of 'common factors', such as the therapeutic alliance and remoralisation and the severity of the client's condition itself, far outweigh the technical contributions of specific therapies (Wampold, 2001). This aspect is played down by CBT enthusiasts, who are wont to cite the 15 comparisons in which CBT out-performed other modalities and to omit to mention the 298 studies which failed to show any significant differences (Mollon, 2009).

Further, there is a case to be made that the real-world clinical impact of CBT is far less dramatically effective that those responsible for health-care funding (usually non-clinicians) have been led to believe. Outcome indicators in research studies do not always equate to clinically significant improvement. In clinical practice many, if not most, cases treated by psychotherapists show complexity and co-morbidity, where the results for all forms of therapy, including CBT, tend to be less impressive. Also, as mentioned, long-term follow-up suggests that relapse is the norm for short-term therapies, which is where most of the outcome evidence favouring CBT is clustered.

The disingenuousness underpinning in CBT's pitch to funders and managers of mental health services has recently been exposed in a rigorous meta-analysis looking at the impact of CBT on major mental illnesses (Lynch *et al.*, 2009). They start from the premise that allegiance effects are widespread confounders in psychotherapy research. Researchers are reluctant to publish the results of studies that fail to support the particular therapeutic modality they espouse. Indeed, this could be adduced as an argument for a psychoanalytic perspective acknowledging the role of unconscious bias – these presumably being manifestations of unconscious wishes rather than deliberate deception – although this stricture applies to psychoanalytic researchers no less than to their CBT counterparts.

Lynch *et al.*'s (2009) meta-analysis looked only at studies which a) took allegiance into account and b) provided robust controls such as a weekly 'support group' without CBT content, since, given the huge impact of placebo effects, especially in psychotherapy, 'no therapy/treatment as usual' is no longer acceptable for comparison. Confining themselves to studies of CBT that met these stringent criteria, they found that, in the major mental illnesses with which most psychiatric services are concerned, i.e. schizophrenia and bipolar disorder, *CBT has no demonstrable effect beyond what occurs with non-CBT controls, while its impact in depression was relatively minor*. It seems that the emperor is, at best, very scantily clad!

A final argument, ironically closest to the heart of psychoanalytic psychotherapy yet perhaps least likely to cut ice in the public arena, is that the project of outcome evaluation is fundamentally misguided and contrary to the spirit of psychoanalysis, which is concerned with idiographic individual life stories, not normothetic, instrumentalist 'best buys'. This applies particularly to 'full' psychoanalysis (e.g. five times a week for five years), which has never been, and perhaps never will be, subject to an RCT, although various methodological modifications which, on the whole, tend to be strongly favourable can be used to evaluate its outcome (see Sandell *et al.*, 2000). While it might appear at first sight to be an untenable 'backwoods' defence, there are growing hints of a wider dissatisfaction with over-technologised and compartmentalised health care and an emerging interest in qualitative methodology and narrative-based medicine (e.g. Avdi, 2008), with which psychoanalysts following this tack might usefully ally themselves.

The politics of therapy

The CBT/psychoanalysis debate, especially on the CBT side, tends to present itself as a disinterested 'scientific' dispute about the effectiveness of various forms of therapy. But, while the scientific method may be neutral, the uses to which science is put arise in a particular historical context. Behind the CBT/psychoanalysis conflict loom sociological and political realities: the need to contain health-care costs and to search for cheaper forms of therapy; an assault on the hegemony of the professions and a move towards demonstrable competencies rather than professional titles; instrumentalism and pragmatism and the 'end of ideology'; the search for quick, simple, 'solution-focused' answers in the face of increasing complexity; the rise of clinical psychology (allied with CBT) and the decline of psychiatry (associated with psychoanalysis); and the need to limit the costs of training therapists.

In all of these arenas, the zeitgeist seems to favour CBT. This in turn is reflected in the UK government's National Centre for Clinical Excellence (NICE) guidelines for psychotherapies in major mental disorders, which almost exclusively advocate CBT (NICE, 2009). Cries of anguish from psychoanalysis go unheard; there is a real danger of it becoming an endangered species, especially in the public sector. 'Dodo bird'-type arguments carry little weight, for if outcomes between different therapies are equivalent, why not invest in those that are cheapest and require least intensive training?

In psychoanalysis' favour there is the argument that, 'on a rising tide, all ships float'. In other words, psychoanalysis need have little to fear from the rise and rise of CBT, since at least psychological therapies, as opposed to pharmacotherapy, are gaining their rightful place in the treatment of mental illness, and in the long run its niche will emerge. While acknowledging that this argument has overtones of a sop designed to dampen envy, psychoanalysis does need seriously to consider what its niche might be.

In my view, psychoanalysis' contemporary role is fourfold. First, buttressed by attachment theory, it has an indispensable contribution to make to the science of intimate relations, whether parental, spousal or therapeutic (Fonagy *et al.*, 2002; Holmes, 2010). Second, it is likely that psychoanalytic treatment will find its place among the psychotherapies as a first-line treatment for people with long-term complex illnesses and personality disorders. Third, derivative and modified forms of psychoanalysis, such as Balint groups, will increasingly be needed to underpin short-term approaches, especially in supporting front-line mental health staff. Finally, as a cultural presence, psychoanalysis need have no fear of extinction, albeit one confined mainly to 'high culture'. Like opera, nuclear physics and avant-garde architecture, psychoanalysis is an essential ingredient in the intellectual and aesthetic mix of modernity.

To return, finally, to the scenario with which we started: the CBT project of providing functional help for the mental miseries of the poor exemplifies a social democratic scheme that has driven the politics of the Western world for over a century, and is to be welcomed as such. But the limits of that project are beginning to be acknowledged. Despite progressive government policies, most Western democracies remain riven with social inequity and widely discrepant health outcomes between rich and poor (Wilkinson, 2006). There is a need for a more nuanced, reflexive approach, taking into account unconscious as well as conscious factors, one that encompasses the 'helper' as well as the 'helped', and the interactions between them. In my view, psychoanalysis has a unique contribution to make to that new beginning. But then, to paraphrase the immortal words of Mandy Rice-Davies, not a million miles from my post office protagonists, thanks to the allegiance effect, 'I would claim that, wouldn't I?'

CHAPTER 13

INTEGRATION IN PSYCHOANALYTIC PSYCHOTHERAPY

An attachment meta-perspective

In Isaiah Berlin's (1953) famous trope, writers can be divided into one of two categories based on Archilocus' dichotomy: 'The fox knows many things, whereas the hedgehog knows one big thing.' Using this Procrustean rule, psychoanalysts might be classified roughly as follows – *hedgehogs*: Freud, Klein, Bion, Kohut; *foxes*: Jung, Anna Freud, Winnicott, Balint. Among contemporaries – *hedgehogs*: Britton, Caper, Fonagy, Steiner; *foxes*: Bollas, Lear, Ogden, Parsons. Readers will doubtless disagree and are invited to play the game (which Berlin claimed he did not intend to be taken seriously – or was this a disingenuous defence?) with their friends.

Foxes are by nature integrationist. Definitions of integration in psychotherapy (Holmes & Bateman 2002) may refer to theoretical integration (e.g. finding comparable theoretical ideas despite differing nomenclature); integration at the level of clinical practice (e.g. combining homework tasks with transference interpretation); or administrative integration (offering a range of therapies in the same clinic). Psychoanalytically, integration may be intra-psychoanalytic, referring to reconciliations between divergent psychoanalytic ideologies – Kleinian, Lacanian, relational, self-psychological, etc. – or extra-psychoanalytic, e.g. integrating psychoanalytic with non-psychoanalytic approaches such as supportive work and CBT.

The starting point of this paper is the view that 'psychoanalytic theory does not *entail* psychoanalytic practice' (Fonagy, 2006, p. 67). What happens in the consulting room is only partially related to the avowed theoretical perspective of the practitioner. What follows is an attempt to use attachment ideas and research as a meta-position from which to view psychoanalytic psychotherapy practice (Holmes, 2010). I argue that practitioners are intuitively – unconsciously in the descriptive sense – integrationist to the extent that they follow attachment principles, irrespective of their therapeutic allegiance. The aim of the paper is to delineate those principles, organising the discussion around the therapy's three principal components (Castonguay & Beutler, 2006): the therapeutic relationship, meaning-making and change promotion. (En passant, I suggest that this *intuitive integration* is seen most commonly at the extremes of the therapy life cycle, in naive therapists or in mature clinicians. Senior students and recent postgraduates are perhaps those most likely to stick to a strict non-integrationist agenda).

The therapeutic relationship

Attachment styles and therapeutic engagement

Attachment theory suggests intimate relationships have specific interactional dynamics, prototypically between children and parents and spouses, and sometimes among siblings and military or sporting 'buddies'. Threat or illness trigger attachment behaviours, which involve seeking proximity to a figure able to assuage distress – in the case of children, one who is older and wiser. Once soothed and safe, and only then, the sufferer is able to explore his or her world, inner or outer, in the context of 'companionable interaction' (Heard & Lake, 1997) with a co-participant. An integrative perspective on therapy suggests that the attachment dynamic is likely to apply also to the therapist–client relationship.

In this model, exploration and threat-triggered attachment behaviour are mutually incompatible. In infants and young children this is manifest in observable behaviours – pulling 'in' to the secure base figure when threatened, turning 'out' into the world of play and exploration when secure. Inhibitions and compromises of this pattern are the mark of insecurely attached children. In adults these shifts are usually more subtle, although most will have had the experience while in the public arena of 'holding on to'/'holding in' pain, whether physical or emotional, until the secure presence of a loved one makes 'letting go' possible, usually with physical accompaniments such as holding, hugging and tearfulness.

The basic interpersonal architecture of therapy is a) a person in distress, seeking a safe haven, in search of a secure base, b) a care-giver with the capacity to offer security, soothing, and exploratory companionship, and c) the resulting relationship, with its own unique qualities. This process applies to the initiation of therapy itself, to the start of sessions, and to moments of emotional arousal as they occur within each session. Since a central therapeutic aim is eliciting and identifying buried feelings (Malan & Della Selva, 2006), there will, in the course of a session, be an iteration between affect arousal, activation of attachment behaviours and their assuagement; companionable exploration of the triggering feelings; further affective arousal; and so on.

This process is inevitably coloured by past experience, especially expectations about how a care-giver will respond to expressed distress. This can be construed as transference in that the client brings to the relationship largely unconscious schemata, or internal working models, based on, but not identical with, previous experiences of care-seeking.

Classifying attachment styles in adults, Shaver and Mikulincer (2008) see insecure attachment as a spectrum ranging from deactivation (corresponding to avoidance in children) of attachment needs, at one pole, to hyperactivation (corresponding to ambivalent attachment), at the other. This hyperactivation/deactivation dichotomy captures the relational expectations clients typically bring into the consulting room. Some seem 'switched-off', describing their difficulties in clichéd, minimalist ways, resistant to therapists' probes for feelings. Others overwhelm the therapist and themselves with emotion, seemingly confusing present and past, leaving little space for the therapist to stem the tide of emotion or assuage distress so that difficulties can be reflectively considered.

Real-life therapists are far from passive observers, neutral elicitors of 'material', or objective commentators on their clients' difficulties. A proportion of them will have insecure attachment styles, usually towards the hyperactivating pole (Diamond et al., 2003). Therapist and patient actively engage in an attachment/exploration cycle, in which the actuality of what the therapist offers, and the client seeks, is counterpoised with long-established expectations, potentially threatening that very process of productive engagement.

Mallinckrodt and co-workers (Mallinckrodt et al., 2005) illustrate how skilful therapists accommodate to and gradually modify the presenting stance of the client vis-à-vis attachment. They suggest that successful therapy requires initial 'concordance' (cf. Racker, 1968) on the part of the therapist. This means partial acceptance by the therapist of the role allocated by the patient's unconscious expectations and procedures. This might entail allowing for a degree of intellectualising with deactivating clients, waiting patiently for the client to begin to allow feelings to surface – for example, in relation to breaks: 'I used to take gaps in my stride, just telling myself that you were a hard-working professional and were entitled to holidays; now I really resent your going away, and wonder who you are going away with.' Conversely, with hyperactivating clients, a degree of boundary flexibility and gratification might be allowable, accepting intersession letters and text messages and occasionally offering extra sessions. Later the therapist will move to a 'complementary' (as opposed to 'concordant'), more challenging, role, thereby disconfirming maladaptive client expectations and opening the way for psychological reorganisation.

From an attachment perspective, the therapeutic relationship can be seen as the resultant of two opposing sets of forces. On the one hand, the analyst attempts within the limited framework of therapy to provide a secure attachment experience – to identify and assuage attachment needs and to facilitate exploration; on the other, the patient approaches the relationship with prior expectations of sub-optimal care-giving, and, unconsciously assuming an unloving and/or untrustworthy or narcissistically self-gratifying care-giver, aims mainly for a measure of security. The attachment viewpoint suggests that the therapeutic relationship is shaped both by the dynamic of its actuality and by the distorting effects of transference. Secure therapists *redress* their client's attachment insecurities, while insecure ones more likely reinforce them. As therapy proceeds, the soothing presence of the analyst enables the client to expose themselves to, tolerate and learn from increasing levels of anxiety.

Emotional connectedness

What makes a potential secure base 'secure'? How does an infant 'know' to whom to turn when attachment behaviours are activated? How does an attachment hierarchy, normally with mother at the apex, followed by other kin such as aunts, older siblings, father, grandparents, and non-kin 'alloparents' (Hrdy, 1999) such as child-minders, become established? For adults, at what point does friendship and companionship become 'love', and what is the relationship between this and the establishment of a secure base? (Attempting to tap into this vector, I routinely ask clients at assessment, 'Who would you contact first if there were an emergency or crisis in your life?') Relatedly, when does a therapist move from being a helpful professional to the role of an indispensable attachment figure, and how does this connect with the establishment of an 'analytic process'? Attachment research suggests at least partial answers to some of these questions.

Konrad Lorenz (1959), Bowlby's mentor and colleague, was famous for his 'imprinting' experiments in which goslings would follow, and take as their mother, any largish moving object to which they were exposed in the first few hours of life – whether this was the actual mother, Lorenz himself, or even a cardboard box! Imprinting-type temporal 'windows' do not seem to apply to the more fluid relational system of primates, and especially humans. Ongoing intimate proximity and availability, together with the 'knowing' – the holding in mind through absence and interruption that is integral to parental (and spousal) love – are some of the essential ingredients of a secure base. The mother–infant literature suggests that, among other characteristics, a secure base parent also offers responsiveness and 'mastery' (Slade, 2005); reliability and consistency; 'mind-mindedness' (Meins,

1999); and the ability to repair disruptions of parent–infant emotional connectedness (Tronick, 1998). Each of these is a thread that also runs through the fabric of successful therapeutic relationships.

Overall, *care-seeker/care-giver emotional connectedness* is the key feature of secure base (Farber & Metzger, 2008). The restriction, exaggeration or uncoupling of such connectedness is what leads to the three varieties of insecure attachment. No less than in secure relationships, in insecure attachments the attachment figure is present in the mind of the care-seeker as a sought target for attachment behaviours, but there is a discrepancy between what is desired and what is available. Transference analysis in therapy attempts to place the minutiae of this disjunction under the therapeutic microscope.

Contingency and marking

Are there analogues of therapeutic intimacy in developmental studies of parent–child interaction? Gergely and Watson's (see Gergeley, 2007) landmark paper focuses on affective sequencing between parents and infants. They identify 'contingency' and 'marking', in the context of intense mutual gaze, as the basis of mirroring sequences in which, to use Winnicott's (1971, p. 51) phrase, the 'mother's face is the mirror in which the child first begins to find himself'.

'Contingency' describes the way in which the care-giver waits (her response is 'contingent upon') for the infant to initiate affective expression. Her response is then 'marked' by an exaggerated simulacrum of the infant's facial and verbal affective expression. For example, the child might be slightly down-at-mouth; the mother might then, while maintaining intense eye contact with her child, twist her face into a caricature of abject misery, saying, in high-pitched 'motherese', 'Oh, we *are* feeling miserable today, aren't we?' She thereby offers the child a visual/auditory representation of his own internal affective state. This sets in motion the child's capacity to 'see' and 'own' his feelings.

Contingency gives the child the message that he is an actor, a person who can initiate and make a difference to the interpersonal world in which he finds himself, and introduces him to the dialogic nature of human meanings. Marking links representation (initially in the mother's face, then re-represented in his own mind) to the child's own actions and internal feelings, while 'tagging' that these are his, not the mother's, feelings. This proto-linguistic envelope has a soothing, affect-regulating quality.

These interactive sequences thus involve a) *affect expression* by the child; b) *empathic resonance* on the part of the mother, able to put herself into the shoes of the child; c) *affect regulation* in that the parent tends to up-regulate or down-regulate depending on what emotion is communicated (stimulating a bored child, soothing a distressed one); resultant d) mutual pleasure and playfulness or, to use Stern's (1985) phrase, the evocation of 'vitality affects', *enlivenment*; leading to e) *exploratory play*/companionable interaction (Heard & Lake, 1997).

Goal-corrected empathic attunement

Similar sequences characterise in-session therapist–client interactions. McCluskey (2005) has shown that initial attunement, a mirroring *affect-identifying* response on the part of the therapist, in itself is insufficient to make up a satisfactory therapeutic interaction. Further steps are needed in order to release exploration and companionable interaction. Step two is affect-regulatory, as the therapist 'takes' the communicated feeling and, through facial expression, tone of voice and emphasis, modifies or 'regulates' it: softly expressed sad feelings are amplified, perhaps with a more aggressive edge added; manic excitement is soothed, vagueness of tone sharpened. Mirroring here becomes dialogic.

These moves are comparable to the 'marking' of the Gergely and Watson schema. The therapist might say: 'You did *what*?!'; 'That sounds *painful*'; '*Ouch!!*'; 'It sounds as though you might be feeling pretty sad *right now*'; 'I wonder if there isn't a lot of *rage* underneath all this.' It is interesting to compare this empirical account with Grotstein's (2007, p. 29) account of his analysis with Bion:

> virtually every one of the words in my associations was taken up, used, and rephrased so that I was receiving from him in a somewhat altered and deepened version what I had uttered. It was like hearing myself in an echo chamber or sound mirror in which I was being amplified while being edited ... what the classical analyst would point to as a resistance he would point to as a focus of great anxiety ....

The therapist is a 'sound mirror', representing the analysand's self to himself. Further, 'resistance' is reframed as anxiety which has to be soothed if the analysis is to progress. Thus two very different theoretical and evidential standpoints arrive at similar technical conclusions. The common theme is affect regulation and mirroring as the pathway to self-understanding.

Translating this into consulting room practice, the therapist communicates to the patient that he has heard and felt her feelings, regulates their intensity, and implicitly or explicitly adds something, e.g. the sadness that underlies mania, the anger that can be an unacknowledged feature of depression. The security associated with being understood leads to enlivenment on the part of the patient. This in turn opens the way for companionable exploration of the content or meaning of the topic under discussion. McCluskey (2005) dubs this sequence *Goal Corrected Empathic Attunement* (GCEA), in which there is a continuous process of mutual adjustment or 'goal-correction' between client and therapist as they attempt, emotionally and thematically, to entrain the client's affective states and imagine the contexts which engender them. Mentalising (Holmes, 2010) can be thought of as an umbrella term covering all aspects of this process.

Rupture and repair

Such sequencing is of course a council of perfection. Like parents and spouses, and indeed anyone whose goal is intimate understanding of another person, therapists regularly 'get it wrong'. Tuckett *et al.*'s category (2008, p. 29) of therapist actions defined as 'sudden and glaring reactions not easy to relate to the analyst's normal method' can be seen as ruptures, comparable to the normal and expectable ruptures in parent–infant connectedness, which in well-functioning parent–infant couples are 'repaired' as the parent responds to the child's signals of distress.

The GCEA framework tells us that being understood reduces anxiety, liberates vitality affects, and initiates exploration. Conversely, being *mis*understood is anxiety-augmenting and aversive, triggering withdrawal and avoidance and/or defensiveness and anger. But, just as security-providing mothers are able to repair lapses in attunement with their infants, so the capacity to repair therapeutic 'ruptures', a concept developed by Safran and Muran (2000), is associated with good outcomes in therapy.

Using the 'still face' paradigm, attachment researchers have looked at attachment styles in relation to the capacity of mother–infant dyads to resume affective contact following a brief one-minute affective withdrawal on the part of the mother in which she is asked to 'freeze' her expression (Crandell, Patrick & Hopson, 2003). Securely attached children are least disrupted by this procedure. Children with organised insecurity resort to self-soothing via looking at their own faces in the mirror when the link with mother is broken, but can generally resume contact once the break is terminated. Disorganised children are least likely to get back on track with their mothers on resumption and most likely to resort to self-soothing, and fail to link up again with the security of the mother's gaze even when it becomes once more available.

Extrapolating from these findings to adult psychotherapy, therapists need to be highly sensitive to client reactions to 'freezing' or discontinuities of contact both within sessions and in relation to the normal interruptions of holidays and illness. Even though psychoanalytic psychotherapists are trained to focus on manifestations of 'negative transference', the evidence suggests that clients hold back negative feelings from their analysts no less than in other modalities of therapy (Safran & Muran, 2000). An attachment perspective suggests a) that in any intimate relationship quotidian misunderstandings are the norm; b) the implications of these depend in part on prior expectations and attachment styles of both participants; and c) the therapeutic issue is not so much to eliminate misunderstandings as to focus on the feelings associated with them and find ways to talk about them.

'Transferential' expectations are brought into play in relation to the regular mistakes, weaknesses and idiosyncrasies applicable to therapies and therapists. Therapist 'enactments' (e.g. starting a session late, drowsiness, inattention or intrusiveness, etc.) need to be non-defensively acknowledged. Such ruptures are understood as 'induced', often outside the awareness of both therapist and client, in the unconscious matrix inherent in an attachment relationship. Reflexively thinking about them by therapist and client together strengthens the therapeutic bond and is itself a change-promoting manoeuvre, enhancing clients' capacity for self-awareness and negotiating skills in intimate relationships.

'Paternal' aspects of the attachment/therapeutic relationship

A key early finding in attachment research was that attachment classification in the Strange Situation was a relational not a temperamental feature, since at one year children could be secure with mother and insecure with father, or vice versa, although by 30 months the maternal pattern tends to dominate (Ainsworth *et al.*, 1978). Nevertheless, the role of fathers in attachment has been relatively neglected, in the case of disorganised attachment because, sadly, most of the children studied come from mother-only families (Lyons-Ruth & Jacobvitz, 2008). The Grossmanns' longitudinal studies (Grossmann, Grossmann & Waters, 2005) are an exception, showing that paternal contributions in childhood to eventual security in early adulthood is as important as that of the mother, and that their combined parental impact is greater than the sum of each alone.

The Grossmanns delineate the 'paternal' role as somewhat different from the 'maternal' one. (The sexist implications of this dichotomy are acknowledged, perhaps better reframed as 'security-providing' and 'empowering' parental functions.) When asked to perform a brick-building or sporting task (e.g. teaching a child to swim), security-providing fathers offer their offspring a 'you can do it' message, creating a zone of protection within which sensory-motor development can proceed. In the Strange Situation, as compared with mothers, fathers tend to use short bursts of intense distraction and activity as comforting manoeuvres, in contrast to the more gentle crescendo and diminuendo of hugging and soothing characterising female care-givers.

Comparing parent–child relationships in disorganised and secure children, measures of maternal sensitivity are insufficient to capture security-providing functions. A dimension of 'mastery' also contributes to the variance, communicating not just intimate protectiveness but also the presence of a competent adult in charge of the play space (Slade, 2005). The importance of space – physical and metaphorical – links with the Vygotskyian notion of the 'zone of proximal development', where the child is directed to tasks that are neither too easy nor too hard (Leiman, 1995), and the 'defensible space' surrounding the child whose security it is the parent's responsibility to guarantee. Similarly, therapists provide therapeutic space (which is also a 'space of time') mindful of Freud's (1914) injunction that interpretations should be aimed at patients' emergent thoughts, being neither too 'deep' nor too superficial.

Effective psychotherapy is *both* soothing and empowering. In the Western world, 'naming' is construed as a 'paternal'/masculine function. The famous Lacanian pun – 'le no(m) du père' (the name of the father; the *no* of the father) encapsulates the 'negative' paternal Oedipal prohibition which severs the infant's phantasy of merging with the mother, but also the 'positive' liberating, linguistic function which enables one to stand outside, think about, and manipulate, experience and, ultimately, understand one's self (expressed in the patronymic). In order to alleviate client anxiety, the therapist needs not just to be empathic but also to communicate 'mastery' (with its 'paternal' resonance) – a sense that she knows what she is doing, is in control of the therapy and its boundaries (without being controlling), and is relaxed enough to mentalise her own feelings. Mastery and empathy are not mutually exclusive but denote a good 'primal marriage' of sensitivity and power from which the client can begin to tackle his difficulties.

The 'fundamental rule'

A feature of secure relationships, whether parent–infant or spousal, is open communication ('I can say anything to my mum/husband and know she/he will listen without judging me'). Freud's 'fundamental rule' (inviting the patient to say anything that comes into her/his mind, however irrelevant or embarrassing) could be seen as an attempt to establish a similar culture within the consulting room. Much of the work of psychoanalytic psychotherapy revolves around identifying and removing barriers to unfettered communication. 'Free association' typically requires a contingent interactive culture in which the therapist awaits and follows the client's lead. The flow of communication becomes possible once an atmosphere of security is established, often following the identification of, and challenge to, the myriad ways in which clients habitually evade emotional intimacy in the service of security.

Bollas (2011) bemoans the attrition of free association in current psychoanalytic practice, which he sees as having been driven out by an excessive preoccupation with transference interpretation. For him a mark of good analysis is one that liberates the flow of free association. But there is no inherent opposition between transference interpretation and free association. Indeed, Freud viewed transference interpretations as necessary only when the flow of free associations was interrupted. Interpretations can be seen as means of identifying ways in which the patient feels insecure in the presence of the analyst. An interpretation, which acknowledges and helps understand a painful affect – if transferential in relation to the therapist – facilitates exploration once greater security/intimacy is re-established.

Meaning

Meaning-making is intrinsic to all therapies. An explanatory framework brings order to the intrinsically inchoate experience of illness, whether physical or mental (Holmes & Bateman, 2002). A 'formulation' is anxiety-reducing in itself and provides a scaffolding for the mutual exploration that follows once attachment anxiety has been assuaged. A symptom or troublesome experience is 'reframed' via an explanatory system, which helps make sense of the sufferer's mental (or physical) pain. The use of the word 'sense' here acknowledges that meaning transcends mere cognition and ultimately derives from bodily experiences.

Language

New meanings emerge in the cut and thrust of psychoanalytic work in part through the analyst's close attention to language. Freud saw the inherent ambiguity of language as an entrée to the unconscious, viewing words as 'switches' or junction points between conscious and unconscious thoughts, or, to use a contemporary metaphor, nodal points in neural networks.

In Tuckett *et al.*'s (2008) attempt to categorise psychoanalytic interventions, one group of comments is described as 'unsaturated' or 'polysemic'. 'Unsaturation' is Bion's (1978) chemical metaphor. An unsaturated solution is one that can always accept more without precipitation; an unsaturated compound is one capable of further reactions. Polysemism means 'many meanings'; so it and unsaturation refer to the possibility of multiple (or arguably infinite) meanings. As the literary critic Eagleton (2007, p. 22) puts it: 'Language is always what there is more of.' Therapist and patient co-create a space from which to look at feelings, behaviours and speech-acts from all possible perspectives and angles – concrete, metaphorical, sexual, adult, child-like, coercive, intimidated, anxiety-influenced, and so on. The analyst is ever alert to the polyphony of the words and phrases used by the client, ready to explore the many meanings thereby revealed and concealed.

In the consulting room, sensitivity to the ebb and flow of attachment and exploration is the hallmark of the skilful therapist. As discussed, GCEA entails 'secure base' responses to client distress. This is in part a matter of timing and tone of voice, but accurate verbal identification of feelings – i.e. the emergence of shared meanings – is in itself soothing.

As in any intimate relationship – spousal, parent–child, sibling, close friendship – highly specific meanings derived from the minutiae of a person's life are co-created by therapist and client. Elaborating this personal vernacular or 'ideolect' (Lear, 1993, 2009) is a crucial aspect of psychotherapeutic work. In Bollas's (2007) terminology, the 'receptive unconscious' of the analyst is tuned into the 'expressive unconscious' of the client; the task of the analyst's conscious ego, like that of the good-enough mother in Winnicott's (1971) model of the child playing 'alone in the presence of the mother', is to guard the therapeutic space in a non-intrusive way.

The meaning-making function of therapy picks out significance from this unending flux and free play of the imagination, or stream of consciousness. Once verbally 'fixed', meanings can be considered, by therapist and patient together, from all possible angles: tested, refined, held onto, modified, or discarded as appropriate.

Main is credited with attachment theory's decisive 'move to the level of representation' (Main, 1991) – i.e. the instantiation in the mind of attachment relationships. Clearly 'representation' is neither exclusively nor necessarily verbal. 'Teleological' thinking, characteristic of pre-verbal, 'pre-mentalising' toddlers (Holmes, 2010), is both representational and meaningful in the sense that the infant begins to develop a mental map of the interpersonal world based on 'if this, then that' logic. However the capacity to represent the Self and Others and their relationship *verbally* is a vital developmental step, enabling children to negotiate the interpersonal world which will be the matrix of all future existence once the physical 'matrix' (i.e. mother) is relinquished. Language underpins a Self which becomes both a centre of experience and an object in the world which can be described and discussed and 'worked on' through the vicissitudes of everyday life – and, when necessary, in psychotherapy.

Narrative styles and the meaning of meaning

The Adult Attachment Interview suggests that *how* we talk about ourselves and our lives, as much as *what* we talk about, reveals the architecture of the inner world. Like the 'fluid attentional gaze' (Main, 1995) of the secure infant who seamlessly negotiates transitions between secure base-seeking, social referencing and exploratory play, Main characterises secure narratives as 'fluid autonomous' – neither over- nor under-elaborated, and able to balance affect and cognition in ways appropriate to the topic discussed.

In the context of therapy, secure narrative styles are 'meaningful' in the sense that they facilitate an open-ended 'language game' (Wittgenstein, 1958) between therapist and client. 'Meaning' is inherent in the interactive mutuality of a language game. Clearly it is possible to have a private language, as for example in psychosis, but it is only when it can be shared that it becomes meaningful in the sense used here. Therapy can be seen as continually helping the client to move from private to shared meanings. Insecure attachment styles lead to therapeutic conversations that are under- or over-saturated with meaning (dismissive or enmeshed, respectively) or with breaks in meaning (incoherent), depending whether they represent deactivating, hyperactivating or unresolved attachments.

A key part of therapeutic work is not so much about making 'correct' interpretations as moving the client towards the exploration of mutual meanings, based on a more secure narrative style. 'Can you elaborate on that?'; 'What exactly did you mean then?'; 'I can't quite visualise what you are talking about here; can you help?'; 'What did that feel like to you?'; 'I'm getting a bit confused here, can you slow down a bit'; 'There seems to be something missing in what you're saying; I wonder if there is some part of the story we haven't quite heard about?' The therapist is probing in this kind of dialogue for specificity, visual imagery and metaphor which enable her to conjure up, in her mind's eye and ear, aspects of the patient's experience. This then becomes a shared object, or 'third' (Ogden, 1989; Benjamin, 2004), which can be 'companionably explored' (Heard & Lake, 1997), often a metaphor to be played with and extended.

There is evidence to support the idea that successful therapy is associated with the replacement of insecure by more secure narrative styles (Avdi & Georgaca, 2007), towards the acquisition of what I have called 'autobiographical competence' (Holmes, 2001). Main's schema contrasts the fluidity of secure styles with the fixity, prolixity or incoherence of the insecure. Psychic health is characterised by some psychoanalytic writers in terms of a harmonious and creative collaboration between unconscious and conscious parts of the mind (Rycroft, 1985). Secure narrative styles are open-ended, polysemic systems, 'infinite' (in Matte-Blanco's (1975) sense of the unconscious as an 'infinite set'), always subject to further 'vision and revision' (Eliot, 1986), in contrast to the fixed, overwhelming or inchoate narratives of insecure attachment.

Finding the right meaning

As therapists we are continually struggling to find the 'real', 'right' or 'true' meaning of our client's communications, verbal and non-verbal. The client will in turn respond by telling us whether a particular comment on the part of the analyst, or an idea they have generated themselves, 'feels right'. In his neurophysiological critique of Cartesian dualism, Damacio (1994) suggests that mind and body work in tandem to let us know when our cognitive and intellectual faculties are on track. Implicit in Cavell's (2006) notion of 'triangulation' is the idea that a child cross-checks the veracity and validity of their perceptions of the outside world with those of the care-giver, and so begins to build up a picture of the real world distinct from his or her perception of it. The Winnicottian ideas of mirroring, contingency/marking and empathic attunement suggest that we learn about our inner world in a comparable way, using the *care-giver's understanding* to develop our own *self-knowledge*. In psychotherapy sessions the analyst makes guesses or suggestions about how clients may be feeling; clients then compare this proffered empathic understanding with what their introspection tells them. Exploring whether there is a near match or a misalignment (empathy is never an exact match, more a 'rhyme' leading to further informed guesses), therapy helps the client gradually better to know him- or herself.

Attachment and empathy, apparently abstract concepts, are ultimately psychophysical phenomena. Proximity is sought – tactile (hugging, sitting on a lap), auditory (via a telephone) or visual (a picture, which may be in the 'mind's eye'). This lowers arousal – slowed heart rate, less sweating, oxytocin release (Zeki, 2009). A mentalising conversation (e.g. a therapy session) may also be seen in those terms. The physical posture and tone of voice of the client reveals his or her emotional state. The therapist imaginatively or even actually (via contingently marking and so altering their own physical posture) mirrors this state, which, in turn, via 'mirror neurones', triggers a version of the client's emotional state in the therapist's receptive apparatus (Hobson, 2002). This can then be introspected, identified, verbalised. Thus, change is set in train.

Finding the 'right' meaning emerges from a three-stage process. First, in a state of 'reverie' (Ogden, 1989), the therapist 'tunes into' her own affective and corporeal sensory-affective world, i.e. her 'counter-transference'. Describing such sensations in words constitutes stage two, an attempt at verbal description, transforming 'preconceptions' into 'conceptions' (Bion, 1970). Stage three, the full expression of meaning-making, is the therapist's attempt to weave a) her own affective reactions, b) knowledge about the client's history, and c) relevant understanding of developmental/psychoanalytic theory into a pattern that captures the internal world of the client in the context of the interpersonal situation generated in the *in vitro* atmosphere of the session.

Herein lies the argument for psychoanalytic pluralism. The therapist's affective response to the client is involuntary and, if the therapist is working well, ineluctable.

Her task then is to find an appropriate theoretical metaphor or 'fit' with this counter-transferential feeling. She might want to work with defences, with loss, with splitting, with the simultaneous need for and fear of attachment, with the fragile narcissistic self, with rage, and so on. The amalgam of counter-transferential response and theoretical formulation forms the prevailing 'focus' (Malan & Della Selva, 2006) of the session. The more theoretical perspectives are available to the therapist, the more sophisticated this response is likely to be. Lear (2009) argues that seemingly incompatible theoretical ideas can be reconciled as long as they are directed to the overall goal of therapy, i.e. emotional freedom. In the end, all roads, not just dream-analysis, lead to Rome. Which is chosen depends on where one is starting from (clinical context – NHS/private sector, etc.), the time available for the journey ('route one' or scenic route), how heavily one's companion is baggage-laden (client's clinical state), the means of transport at one's disposal (therapist's background and training) and a degree of whim (the ephemeral counter-transferential moment).

To summarise, attachment theory's contribution to meaning-making underpins a meta-theoretical perspective in which it is not so much specific interpretations that count as the restoration or fostering of the *capacity to find/make shared meanings*, irrespective of their content. Lyons-Ruth and the Boston Change Process Study Group (2001) have similarly focused on the mutative aspects of 'non-interpretive mechanisms' in psychoanalytic work. Therapist and client come together in a meaningful shared 'present moment' (Stern, 2004). Meaning in itself is not mutative; it is the *mutuality* of meaning-*making* that matters – which brings us to the third leg of the psychotherapy tripod: promoting change.

Promoting change

Psychoanalysis is inherently ironic (cf. Lear, 1993) in that it avoids explicit efforts to produce change, yet its implicit aims are no less 'mutative' than those of any other therapy. This paradox follows logically from psychoanalysis' theoretical base. People get into psychological trouble because of conflict between the conscious and the unconscious mind. Direct appeals on the part of therapy to the sufferer's consciousness will therefore merely activate resistance of the unconscious to change in the status quo and be counter-productive. The unconscious must be approach by stealth and taken unawares. Difficulties based on paradox require paradoxical means if they are to be overcome.

Exposure

An integrative approach to psychoanalytic work sees the key to psychic change as based on exposure to previously avoided/warded off mental pain and trauma. In the safety of the consulting room, past pain is revived and relived in the transference. Focusing on this in safety enables sufferers to experience, process, name and gain perspective on unexpressed feelings that bedevil their relationship to themselves and their intimates. In that it is based on trauma, avoidance and exposure, this formulation is consistent with cognitive-behavioural theory, even if the methods – spontaneous free association and transference interpretation as opposed to pen-and-paper self-observation and directed homework exposure tasks – are radically different.

In a series of studies, Mikulincer and colleagues (reviewed Mikulincer & Shaver, 2008; Mikulincer *et al.*, 2009) show how the experience of security, even if subliminal, enables insecurely attached people to confront rather than defensively deactivate or hyperactivate mental pain. In one study, participants who had completed a questionnaire tapping into attachment styles were asked to write a description of an incident in which a close partner had hurt their feelings. They were then exposed to security-enhancing subliminal 'primes' (words such as 'love', 'secure', 'affection') or neutral ones ('lamp', 'building', etc.). Next they were asked to reconsider the hurtful event and to describe how they would feel if it were to occur again. In the neutral priming condition, deactivators reported less, and hyperactivators more, pain than in the initial task. This would be expected if, with the passage of time, pre-existing defences were reinforced. However in those exposed to the positive prime, both anxiety and avoidance were greatly reduced, and the insecurely attached subjects' responses were indistinguishable from those of the securely attached. As (Mikulincer *et al.*, 2009, p. 318) put it: 'protective armour can at least temporarily [be] softened by an infusion of felt security ... even a small security boost can allow an avoidant person to be more open to inner pain ... which can then be addressed clinically.'

Transposing this into the consulting room, the benign presence of the therapist offers a validating, encouraging environment, helping clients to face, bear, process, live with, master, transcend and incorporate pain and trauma. It matters little whether the latter is seen as externally inflicted or arises from within from the intrinsically rage and envy-wracked psyche. Kleinian psychoanalysis is sometime caricatured as focusing on negative emotions such as aggression and envy, relegating more benign attachment-influenced approaches as manic defences or obfuscations. In skilful hands there is, however, no real incompatibility. Positive priming, via the implicit validating presence of the analyst, is a precondition for meaningful exposure to negative emotions. Conversely, support without challenge can be collusive rather than mutative.

Mentalising

According to Gustafson (1986) (drawing on Bateson (1972), who based his ideas on Bertrand Russell's 'theory of logical types'), psychic change invariably entails taking a perspective at a *meta-level, or 'higher logical type'*, from the problematic behaviours or experience which has led the sufferer to seek help. 'Mentalising' – 'thinking about thinking' or 'mind-mindedness' (Meins, 1999) – clearly fulfils the Gutafson criterion. Moving from action and impulse to reflecting on one one's own and others' mental states is crucial to therapeutic action in psychoanalytic psychotherapy, and perhaps the psychotherapies generally (Allen, 2013b).

Bleiberg (2006) suggests that mentalising is an essential social skill for group living. Being able to mentalise or to read the intentions of the Other became a vital 'friend-or-foe' appraisal as small groups of hominids learned to collaborate and to cope with competition. However, once the Other is identified as unthreatening, mentalising is inhibited. With the appraiser's guard down, psychic energy is available for other uses. Extreme instances of this are seen in intimate relationships between infants and their mothers and romantic partners. Brain patterns in both are similar, with inhibition of the neuroanatomical pathways subsuming mentalisation (Zeki, 2009). This releases psychic energy from the appraisal task, and perhaps explains the necessary idealisation inherent in such relationships ('my baby/lover/mum is the best baby/lover/mum in the whole world') in which negative features are ignored or discounted.

A similar sequence may apply in psychotherapy, as the client begins to imbue the therapist and therapeutic situation with secure base properties and to relax into a comfortable state of held intimacy. However, while encouraging the development of trust, the therapist will simultaneously insist that clients examine their feelings about the therapist and the therapeutic relationship – aiming to help them acquire, activate and extend mentalising skills. A psychotherapy session is *recursive* in the sense that it loops back on itself in ways that normal relationships tend not to, except perhaps when repair (which can be thought of as an everyday form of 'therapy') is needed. To take a commonplace example, there is often a tussle between therapist and client – especially if a deactivating one – about reactions to breaks. The client may insist that it is perfectly alright for the therapist to have a holiday, ('Everyone needs time off, especially in your sort of work'), while the therapist relentlessly probes for signs of disappointment, rejection and anger, sometimes much to the client's irritation. The client is made to mentalise avoided affect in the service of therapeutic change.

The 'benign bind'

Seen this way, psychoanalysis puts the client in a 'benign bind'. In Bateson's (1972) classic formulation of the double bind, the potentially psychotic adolescent is given an approach/avoidance message from his 'schizophrenogenic' parent while at the same time being unable to 'leave the field', this triggering a psychotic response as the only possible escape from an intolerable crux. While this etiological model has been conclusively disproved, it lives on in Main's approach/avoidance model for disorganised attachment (Main, 1995). A positive feedback loop is initiated in which a child feels threatened by the very person (i.e. the parent) to whom he would naturally turn for succour. The more attachment behaviours are activated, the more he seeks out a secure base but, as he approaches the 'secure base'/source of threat, the more threatened he feels, and so on. The bizarre self-soothing manifestations of disorganised attachment such as furling into oneself, rocking and head-banging – and later, perhaps, deliberate self-harm, risky sexual behaviours, drug and alcohol abuse, etc. – can be seen as attempts to 'solve' or escape from this impossible dilemma (cf. Holmes, 2001).

But because it leads inevitably to change of *some* sort, a 'double bind' can also foster positive developments. Therapy puts the client in a paradoxical 'change/no change', 'inhibit mentalising/mentalise' bind, forcing the emergence of new structures and extending their range of interpersonal skills and resources. Clients have no choice but to think about feelings and identity in ways that would normally be dealt with by repression, avoidance, acting out or projection.

A psychoanalytic formulation consistent with this comes from Lear's (1993) extension of Strachey's classic 'mutative interpretation' hypothesis (Strachey, 1934). Lear sees transformational transference as a three-stage process whereby the therapist first enters the client's pre-existing internal world, with its unique assumptions and preconceptions and linguistic manifestations or 'ideolect' – the shared associations and meanings that develop in the course or a therapy. Once 'in', secondly, the therapist begins to disconfirm transferential expectations, neither colluding with the client's preconceptions nor allowing herself to be discounted as alien, irrelevant and expellable. The client is now in a bind. His internal world has been 'colonised' by therapy; but the therapist neither conforms to transferential expectations *nor* accepts 'de-colonialising' expulsion. This is often most manifest around therapeutic 'ruptures' – an idealised therapist is seen as failing or a denigrated one as loving. Moments of discrepancy, disappointment or confusion arising out of the therapeutic relationship, if they can be expressed and fully experienced and then thought about and discussed, now become productive points for psychic growth (Safran & Muran,2000). Thus, thirdly, the patient is forced to revise his expectations, assumptions and schemata about intimate relationships. In so doing, as his perceptions of himself, the therapist, and their relationship become 'de-transference-ised', he becomes more realistic in his appraisals and more skilful in managing them.

Conclusions

The main arguments of this chapter are that a) the psychotherapy process may be best understood by theoretical perspectives – in this case attachment theory – orthogonal to those espoused by its practitioners; and b) once such an 'external' perspective is adopted, apparent differences between differing psychoanalytic philosophies become less salient.

Research findings from non-psychoanalytic therapy illustrate the point. Castonguay and colleagues (Castonguay *et al.*, 1996; Hayes *et al.*, 1996) studied transcripts of CBT treatments for depression. Surprisingly, they found that good outcomes were predicted by processes unrelated to CBT theory: good working alliance; 'experiencing' (i.e. affective expression in sessions); and exploration of interpersonal difficulties. Rigid adherence to CBT protocols was associated with *worse* outcomes. It seems that psychodynamic processes underpin CBT success as much as they do psychoanalytic good outcomes. This should not, however, lead to complacency on the part of psychoanalysts. It may well be that psychoanalytic therapists, like their CBT colleagues, are similarly blind to what it is they do that makes their patients better. Attending to the pull and push of the attachment dynamic and freeing oneself from dogma (including , of course, dogmatic views on attachment) may lead to better therapy, productive research questions, and an integrative perspective – both within and without psychoanalysis – that transcends both petty rivalries and superficial compromise.

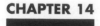

CHAPTER 14

SUPEREGO

An attachment perspective

Introduction

According to Freud, minds are like cities: prototypically Rome, in which ancient structures persist, overlaid with the accretions of modern civilisation (Freud, 1930). The same might be said of psychoanalytic meta-theory, in which old and new ideas jostle, co-existing sometimes peacefully, sometimes less so (Blass, 2010). Psychoanalysts tend to deal with this in different ways: remaining steadfastly loyal to time-honoured concepts; allowing them to pass gracefully into oblivion; replacing them with contemporary additions to theory; rejuvenating old models.

The aims of this paper are a) to review the superego from an attachment perspective; b) to revisit the idea of the 'benign superego', somewhat overshadowed in recent formulations; c) to reconsider Strachey's notion of the part played by the superego – both analysand's and analyst's – in therapeutic action; and d) to look at transgression and its role in analytic work. Throughout, it will be argued that the superego is 'heir' not just to the Oedipal relationship, but to attachment constellations of infancy and early childhood.

Historical background

Current superego thinking can be traced back to the 'controversial discussions' between Melanie Klein and Anna Freud and their followers in the 1930s and 1940s. They disagreed both about the superego's role in the psyche and about the timing of its development. Freud's theories about depression (Freud, 1917) paved the way for the structural model (Freud, 1921) forming the germ of the object-relational account of the psyche. The superego, as 'shadow of the object', represented an identification with, and internalisation of, parental/paternal authority. But, a decade later, Klein argued that the superego predates the prohibitive Oedipal father. The child does not just feel 'bad' because he/she wants to collapse the family triangle into a self-centered dyad, but because of oral-sadistic feelings towards the nurturing breast – biting the inconstant hand that feeds. The superego's origins, as she saw it, lie in the 'archaic' pre-Oedipal period, when 'the earliest feelings of guilt ... derive from the oral sadistic desires to devour the mother' (Klein, 1948, p. 388).

Klein's tripartite model of the archaic superego in its modern form now runs as follows: a) devouring, destructive, rageful desire b) projected externally into the 'bad breast', c) reintrojected as an archaic guilt-meting 'superego nucleus'. Britton (2006) describes this incorporation, externalisation, reintrojection process as 'recycling'.

Kernberg's account is similar: 'Earliest superego structure derives from internalisation of fantastically hostile, highly unrealistic object-images reflecting expelled, projected, and reintrojected bad self-object representations' (Kernberg, 1984, pp. 70–71). The Kleinian superego embodies the inevitable aggression that accompanies love, turned towards the self. Bad feelings are evacuated; the external world becomes threatening and persecutory; the badness is then reintrojected; the threat now lies inescapably within, albeit in a walled-off superego nucleus. If its influence can be mitigated by good experiences of holding and 'detoxification' (Bion, 1967), and/ or bringing together bad and good internal representations based on concern and depression, all will be well; if not, the consequence is psychic ill-health. The violent, self-destructive, autonomous 'archaic' superego is held to underlie pathological phenomena such as the 'negative therapeutic reaction', deliberate self-harm, suicide, and self-defeating addictive behaviours (Kernberg, 2009).

For Anna Freud, the family is an interactive matrix in which individuation continues throughout the developmental period. Parents (and child analysts as surrogates) occupy the controlling, judging, criticising – but also praising, valuing and encouraging – functions later to be internalised as the superego. Thus Anna Freud emphasised the *benign* aspects of the superego in parallel with its strictures. The 'positive superego' had been implicit in Freud's notion of the ego ideal, but this fell away in his later formulations and even more so once the Kleinian viewpoint began to take root. Nevertheless, Freud had, albeit somewhat *en passant*, paved the way for the 'friendly superego' in his brief late paper on humour (Freud, 1927; Christie, 2009; Lemma, 2009). Here the superego is a comforting, friendly, older, wiser entity, a good parent who 'speaks ... kindly words of comfort to the intimidated ego' (Freud, 1927, p. 166).

The technical implications of this theoretical divergence meant that Klein repudiated Anna Freud's model (1998), in which the superego, the orchestrator of guilt, conscience and social responsibility, is not fully formed until late latency/early adolescence. Klein was highly critical of what she saw as Anna Freud's inappropriate and unnecessary advocacy of a species of supportive paedagogy: 'She [Anna Freud] omitted to explain the *deeper* causes of the sense of guilt ... if Anna Freud had submitted the instinctual impulses to a more thorough analysis, there would have been no necessity to *teach* the child how to control them' (Klein, 1948, p. 176; emphasis added).

Nevertheless, Anna Freud's successors continued to develop the idea of a benign superego. Attempting to operationalise psychoanalytic concepts for child psychotherapy research, Sandler asserts: 'parental introjects serve not only to criticize and punish but also to encourage and support' (Sandler & Rosenblatt, 1962, p. 141). Shafer emphasises the idea of internalised relationships in his picture of the 'loving and beloved' aspects of the superego, underpinning 'pride, fortitude, humour, and the effective transmission of cultural ideals' (Shafer, 1960, p. 187).

Let us track these two contrasting trends within superego theorising – the 'archaic/sadistic' and the benign picture – in the context of attachment theory and research findings in the hope of their at least partial resolution.

Attachment theory and the superego

Attachment theory's distinctive contribution to contemporary psychoanalytic discourse (cf. Bowlby, 1988; Slade, 2008; Fonagy, Gergely & Target 2008) includes a) an account of *divergent developmental tracks*, starting in infancy, characterised by secure, insecure-avoidant, insecure-ambivalent and insecure-disorganised epige-netic pathways; b) an exposition of a *security-driven dynamic* in which the object is a source of safety in parallel with libidinal satisfaction; c) *vicissitudes of the security system* in which, with sub-optimal care-giving, full expression of security needs are inhibited, distorted or dissociated; d) the resulting *disruption of narra-tive capacity* and restrictions on conscious exploration and awareness, including sexual and aggressive feelings; e) *replication of the security dynamic in the trans-ference*, in which the analyst is experienced by the analysand in terms of the primary attachment relationship; but f), through her sensitivity, responsiveness, reliability and boundedness, the analyst helps the client move *from a position of insecure attachment to one of 'earned security'*.

Before continuing with the theoretical discussion, some clinical material is con-sidered. The aim is to illustrate, first, the role of the superego as part of the system's unconscious and conscious; second, the superego's moral precepts as defensive strategies, both helpful insofar as they ensure security, and unhelpful in that they inhibit full expression of emotional need; and, third, how the sex and security dynamic interweave one with another.

Case example 1: security and sex in the superego constellation

Alison came into once weekly, sitting-up psychoanalytic psychotherapy not ostensibly for herself, but because her son Tom, aged 14, was 'going off the rails'. Her older child, his sister, aged 17, was everything a parent could wish for: helpful, studious, intelligent, charming and popular. Tom, by contrast, had always been 'difficult', prone to tantrums as a baby, reluctant to go to school, and now holing up in his room play-ing internet computer games, falling behind in his grades, and possibly, Alison thought, taking drugs. If only he could be like his older sister! Just getting Tom to school every morning was an hour-long ordeal; he did no homework, and no amount of cajoling or draconian measures seemed to work. He was becoming pale, thin and withdrawn, and she feared for his future and his life. He had been referred to various counsellors and doctors but had refused to cooperate. She was now seeking help in her own right, hoping that she could be shown how best to rescue her son and put him on the path leading, as it should, to school, university and a good job.

Alison's own childhood history was one of not-so-benign neglect. 'My mother's priorities were: number one herself, number two her horse, number three the dogs. We came in a poor fourth.' An early memory was of being locked out of the house by her mother after breakfast in charge of her younger sibs and not allowed back until lunchtime. Meanwhile her mother was out hunting and hobnobbing with her friends. At 12 Alison was sent to boarding school while her parents worked abroad. She saw them once a year, spent holidays with her grandparents, and was expected to make her way to the airport and back on her own. Somewhat shy, she discovered academic prowess and put all her energies into her school-work. Arriving at university at 18 to study mathematics, she had a heady and unsettling sense that she could do whatever she wanted. After leaving university she worked in the financial sector and soon became a successful stockbroker. Sporty as well as clever, she loved skiing. In her late 20s, after the breakup of a relationship, she toyed with the idea of 'giving it all up' and becoming, as she put it, 'a ski bum', but was discouraged by her father, who could not tolerate the idea of a clever daughter 'throwing herself away'. Emotionally self-sufficient, she was rather surprised when, in her early 30s, she met an older man, a lawyer, who, in her words, 'insisted' that they get married.

The marriage was basically happy, especially when they had lived abroad for two years, far from his controlling family. When she became pregnant with her first child they returned home and settled into a comfortable life of middle-class suburbia. She continued to work part-time, but the principal focus of her life was her children. The intrusions of her in-laws were the main marital irritant – she particularly resented the fact that her husband's mother had apparently vetoed through her husband their choice of name for her son. He had remained innominate for eight weeks, and Tom was semi-randomly chosen at the last moment on the way to the registrar of births. Now she felt that her husband was disengaged, didn't see what danger his son was in, and was leaving everything, including coming to therapy, to her.

At first Alison was nonplussed by her therapist's apparent refusal to give her directions about how best to handle Tom, focusing instead on *her* feelings of frustration, exasperation and panic about the situation. 'Why don't you tell me what to do? I am at my wit's end, and you just sit there' – this was likened to having been sent out into the garden to fend for herself and having to control a group of unruly younger sibling/feelings. Were the therapist to tell her what she should do (if that were indeed possible), would he not be just another mother-in-law trying to control her – inserting the wrong name-of-the-father into her family?! Everything seemed at odds, he suggested: the conflicting parts of herself (her love for Tom and her fury at his unresponsiveness); herself and her husband; and between herself and her therapist – (his seeming passivity and failure to give advice).

We were in the territory of 'benign bind' (Holmes, 2010) – she accepted the therapist's professional integrity, but chafed at his failure to conform to her representation of what a therapist/parent's role should be. How could 'letting be' (Lear, 2009) and giving her and Tom and his father a chance to work things out for themselves possibly be helpful? What was she to do? Therapy was no real help, yet, now she was embarked on it, she could not quite bring herself to walk away.

Alison could see that her attempts to fit Tom into her achievement-oriented mould were not working. Something new *was* needed. Perhaps letting him make his own decisions about school and computer time and career did not necessarily correspond to the negligence she accused herself of. Perhaps laissez faire (he refused to let her test him on his French verbs!) did not have to be construed as neglect and was not necessarily a repetition of her mother's self-preoccupied emotional and physical absence. Maybe, too, the therapist suggested, there was a rebellious, 'drop-out' part of herself that had been swept aside when her father insisted that she choose the stock-market in preference to the ski-slopes. Perhaps a similar autonomy was emerging in Tom, his passive rebelliousness chiming with a part of herself she had for too long pushed down into the realms of the unconscious. She began to see that Tom was a being in his own right, making his own choices, not an extension of her; and that the behaviour she found intolerable in him was not so far removed from a thwarted part of herself.

The struggle against her need to be in control was not easy. Alison found it almost impossible not to try to run Tom's life for him – not to get him up in the morning, ask him if he had done his homework, check whether he had contacted any friends, insist on a detailed itinerary on the rare occasions when he did go out. Her tongue, ever ready to issue 'helpful' directives and reproaches, had constantly to be bitten. She saw that it would be better to hand over a lot of the parenting to her husband, but could she be sure he would do things the 'right' – i.e. her – way? She wanted to pursue her own interests – work, seeing friends – but found it hard to square that with the feeling that she was neglecting her duties as a mother. Without her omnipresence Tom might fade away – how could she possibly enjoy herself with that at the back of her mind? There was an insistent, demanding, critical part of herself over which she had little jurisdiction, urging her to 'do something' rather than just 'sit there'. But as time went on and she learned to hold back, the struggle began to seem worthwhile. Things improved: Tom was getting himself to school; his reports acknowledged that he was at least trying; he was beginning to go out and see friends. She could imagine a time when he would lead his own life, even find a career, albeit a non-academic one that she might not approve of, and that she and her husband could one day enjoy themselves again as they used to.

Discussion

How does the concept of the superego help thinking about this case? Alison was clearly a person divided against herself: part kept persisting with ineffective mothering strategies; another recognized that this was not helpful. Part of her desperately wanted to make everything right for Tom; another felt furiously and impotently angry with him. Aware of how counter-productive this was, she was nevertheless unable to stop her controlling and critical ways with Tom. There did indeed seem to be an 'agency' within her, of which she was at best only partially conscious, beyond her control, dictating her behaviour in unhelpful ways. The essence of this could be encapsulated in a series of implicit rules for living: 'Be self-sufficient'; 'Study hard to the limits of your ability'; 'Don't be a neglectful mother as your's was'; 'Suppress subversive desires'; 'Don't tolerate laziness or backsliding.'

These precepts fit with the superego model in that her sense of 'right and wrong', and how a child *should* be brought up, was shaped and dictated to by forces 'within' her yet, seemingly, over which she had little control. These implicit guiding rules represented her own defensive strategies as a child, unconsciously transmitted to her own children, successfully in the case of her daughter, but not so with Tom. They had served her fairly well and enabled her to survive her own distant and rebuffing parenting. In her developmental history Alison had traded exploration and libidinal satisfaction for security and self-sufficiency. Intimacy and reciprocity were jettisoned for the sake of financial and social independence. These superego-ish strictures of which she was only partially aware, and which she could subject to critical scrutiny only with extreme difficult, seemed to have a life of their own, beyond the reach of her conscious ego.

Alison's superego 'rules' ensured her freedom from dependence on unreliable attachment figures and underpinned the rewards of worldly success. On the other, their rigidity and inhibition of affect compromised her ability to respond to Tom's unique personality and 'difference'. Her superego was an amalgam of identifications ('Like my mother, I must impose order regardless of its impact'), dis-identifications ('A first priority is not to be neglectful like my mother'), and functioning defences ('Hard work and study will get you independence and freedom from anxiety and depression').

In the structure of her superego, the search for security and the vicissitudes of her sexuality were intertwined. If being a 'ski-bum' was a surrogate for sexual freedom, her father's intervention ensured that she remained on the 'straight and narrow' of her career path. Her superego was also anti-libidinal in that the 'marriage' in the family was more between Alison and her children – echoing that between her husband and his mother – than the parental couple themselves, just as her narcissistic mother was primarily in Alison's eyes 'married' to her horses! Despair, rage and desolation about all this were feelings to be avoided at all costs. Tom's possible misery about the lack of a close parental couple in the family was undiscussable.

Psychoanalytic therapy seemed to help in a number of different ways. It offered an environment based on acceptance rather than control, suggesting that non-directiveness does not necessarily equate to abandonment. This could be seen as the gradual installation of the Sandler/Shaffer-like 'benign superego' in Alison's psyche. It stayed with her while she wrestled with her anger at the therapist's refusal to 'help' or tell her what to do, thereby providing a 'benign bind' (see below) as a catalyst for change (Lear, 1993). Therapy began to provide a language, clichéd perhaps, but self-generated rather than imposed, for looking at and revising her own habitual thought processes – 'letting go', 'doing my own thing', 'staying with it', verbal expressions of a less constraining, more self-sensitive superego.

It is being suggested here that the superego as the fount of a person's moral universe is shaped as much by the attachment dynamic as by an Oedipal or pre-Oedipal one; and that change in therapy can be catalysed by the juxtaposition of 'archaic' aggression (Alison's disappointment in her mother, son, husband and – transferentially – therapist) with the benignity of the therapeutic environment. Let us now turn to some empirical findings from the attachment literature to buttress this viewpoint, before considering its limitations and need for extension.

The relational superego

A semi-popular book by a Kleinian psychoanalyst starts with the striking – but reifying – statement 'Everyone has a superego' (Roth, 2001, p. 3). Clearly everyone does not 'have' a superego in the sense that they have a liver or a vertebral column. Superego, ego and id are not so much entities, agencies or regions as interacting functions – waves, rather than static particles, creating psychic ripples as they engage with one another. Dichotomies of action and observation, attack and submission, criticism and self-hatred, desire and frustration animate the 'action language' (Shafer, 1960) of the inner world. This dynamic view is consistent with the psychoanalytic conceptualisation of the superego as a defensive structure (Gray, 1994). Any particular superego constellation is a resultant of the balance of forces within the self, of the possible and the permissible.

Attachment theory similarly reformulates Anna Freud's theory of defences in dynamic relational terms (Mikulincer *et al.*, 2009). As development proceeds, the growing child negotiates an ever shifting balance of exploration and security. Thanks to the sensitivity and mastery of the responsive parent, when faced with temporary abandonment, secure children can tolerate and express feelings of fear and rage without jeopardising their secure base. Curiosity and exploration need not be inhibited, because comfort and companionship can be relied upon to be there when required (Heard & Lake, 1997). Bolstered by parental support, the secure child is confident that her hopes and wishes will be fulfilled, or, if not, disappointment is tolerable as a mere temporary setback. The relationship between the internalised parent and the self and its desires is essentially benign; defensiveness, with concomitant unconsciousness and lack of narrative competence, is minimal. There is an internal containing, regulating, facilitating presence, distinct from the autonomous ego, yet located within the self. This internal secure base, like the benign superego, or Freud's humorous parent, oversees the ego in all its vicissitudes.

In the 'organised' forms of insecure attachment greater defensiveness comes into play. The relationship between the self and the internalised parent is a necessary compromise. The child wishes to explore and to experience feelings – including feelings of closeness – but to do so runs the risk of rebuff and disapproval. In the hypoactivating/avoidant pattern, awareness of feelings is suppressed for safety's sake. The superego, as it were, says: 'Don't *feel* your feelings of fear and rage and desire; damp them down, even if in doing so you are diminishing the richness of your inner world and may miss affective the signals you need to guide you towards good choices in life.'

The hyp*e*ractivating/ambivalent pattern of defence similarly trades off exploration for security. Here the price paid for security is regression. The superego's message runs: 'Succumb to your flooding emotions, indulge them, stay regressed and uncontained – that way someone will take notice, even if it means your autonomy and self-efficacy are compromised.'

In disorganised attachment, the superego is dangerously disengaged from the self and its desires, unable to support or help the fragile ego. Either it stands apart, mimicking the behaviour of the frightened withdrawn parent (Lyons-Ruth & Jacobvitz, 2008); or it intrudes, attacks and blames the self, heartlessly disregarding its needs or feelings. Either way, the self is depleted, forced to try to become its own parent. In this radical state of dissociation, the self cannot 'hear' injunctions for self-preservation and is likely to ignore warnings to avoid risky or self-defeating behaviours. In the absence of a guiding internalised parent, it is on its own, doing its best to achieve a modicum of security and satisfaction, even if this entails self-soothing via deliberate self-harm or drug abuse. In these pathological states the relational superego is either absent or abusive; sub-sections of the self are forced to make do without an integrating, coherence-producing, meaning-making, consciousness-raising, over-viewing part of the self.

These early relational experiences with parents lay the foundation for moral behaviour. Avoidant children tend to be bullies; hyperactivating children to be clingy and helpless; disorganised children to resort to role reversal in their relationship with their mothers (Lyons-Ruth & Jacobvitz, 2008). Relational models are internalised which include precepts about how things 'should' be. The morality of the ego ideal reflects the handling which preceded it. Secure children are natural mentalisers (Slade, 2008) – they can see others as sentient beings and treat them accordingly, while insecure children may set up narcissistically derived ego ideals – doomed to disappointment when confronted with reality – as defences against feelings of abandonment, isolation or intrusion.

The attachment typology outlined above is consistent with Bowlby's (1980) view that normal and pathological development should be seen as distinct, self-maintaining pathways. Secure children experience cascading 'broaden and build' experiences as they ascend the developmental ladder. Insecure children, by contrast, may enter self-perpetuating vicious circles of relational disturbance. This epigenetic perspective is robustly supported by longitudinal prospective studies looking at children classified in the first year of life and followed through into young adulthood (Grossmann, Grossmann & Waters, 2005).

Prohibition and the superego

From this viewpoint, rather than being an universal developmental stage, the 'archaic' pre-Oedipal superego model may apply particularly to developmental *pathology*, especially the disorganised attachment patterns underlying Borderline

Personality Disorder. The clinical phenomena usually explained by the archaic superego model include the negative therapeutic reaction and various forms of self-defeating behaviours. For such people, healthy strategies of self-protectiveness and seeking out good rather than bad experiences seem to be in abeyance. The sufferer appears driven by hate, including self-hatred, rather than love. Attachment thinking suggests that the dynamic here is not so much the internalisation of a hated inconstant object as the overwhelming need to have some sort of security, even if this means clinging to a 'bad' object. Better a bad object than none at all: as Fairbairn (1954, p. 27) puts it: 'it is better to be a sinner in a world ruled by God than to live in a world ruled by the Devil.'

From an attachment perspective, avoiding bad experiences is far more important than achieving good ones. In man's evolutionary past, it was better not to be eaten than to go hungry; better to avoid poison than to indulge one's appetite. Bitter fruit chewed spells death; eschewed, one lives to love another day. While our taste buds are sensitive to one part of sugar per 200 parts food, they can detect one part of bitterness per 2 million parts food (Ito *et al.*, quoted in Music, 2009). Thus we are 10,000 times better at detecting danger than enjoying pleasure. To stay safe, we need to be good at representing, and then avoiding or negotiating, bad experiences. The mother who says 'No' as her toddler approaches an electric socket is pitting 'external' superego power against the capacity of the environment to cause harm. The primitive infant mind may similarly view love as more fragile than hatred, walling off aggression towards the loved object, and ultimately turning against the self. The superego plays an essential role in maintaining safety, even if this means prohibiting, or at least postponing, pleasure. In disorganised and borderline states this process goes awry.

In sum, the superego is 'heir' not just 'to the Oedipus complex' but also to the attachment relationship which an infant needs in order to survive into adult reproductive life. The benign superego in this model is the internalisation of the protective parent. Rather than being a 'pure culture of death instinct', the superego has the job of keeping death at bay. It is only in severe pathological states that the superego perversely turns against itself and becomes the very source of danger and disorder which its primary role is to counteract.

The subliminal superego

Bowlby summarised his view on the superego as follows: '[There are] ... rules for appraising action, thought and feeling that together are usually referred to as constituting the super-ego ... applied automatically and outside consciousness ... hard to change either because they are ingrained or because of defensive exclusion' (Bowlby, 1971, p. 54). The psychoanalytic notion of 'working through' acknowledges the power of 'ingrainedness' and the time needed to unlearn defensive habits and to acquire new, more appropriate and adaptive ways of dealing with intra- and interpersonal experience. Recent attachment-informed research, however, suggests that both ingrainedness and defensive exclusion can be over-ridden by subliminal messages from the immediate environment.

In a series of studies, Mikulincer, Shaver and colleagues (reviewed Mikulincer & Shaver, 2008; Mikulincer *et al.*, 2009) have shown that dispositional attachment styles influence responses to affect-laden tasks, but that these can be altered by appropriate environmental 'priming'.

Their findings apply across a range of situations. In a visual exploration study, subjects were asked to rate their liking for and interest in a Chinese ideograph. In a textual study, subjects were exposed to a traumatic story in which a child was killed in an automobile accident, and the levels of compassionate responses towards the parents were rated. Studies looking at intimate relationships asked subjects to consider a relationship problem that had occurred in the previous week, and then to think about how such difficulties might be resolved. In each of these situations, secure individuals (previously rated) showed more 'positive' and exploratory responses than their insecure counterparts. The experiments were then repeated, but subjects were now 'primed' with either positive or neutral stimuli, either subliminal (words such 'love' and 'support' being flashed onto a screen so briefly that the subjects did not consciously register them) or supraliminal (asking the subjects to think about a loving or supportive relationship, or showing them a picture of a mother cradling a baby). The general outcome was that *insecure subjects, when primed with positive but not neutral stimuli, then behaved and thought in ways that were indistinguishable from those of their secure counterparts.*

These studies could be seen as tapping directly into an individual's superego function or moral dispositions, measuring compassion, concern for the other, and prejudice. They suggest that individuals' moral perspectives are influenced *both* by their attachment history *and* by the prevailing ambiance, and that the latter's impact does not depend on conscious awareness. Compared with secure subjects, insecure people are less likely to be compassionate and concerned and more likely to be negatively judgmental and to adopt self-serving ethnocentric perspectives; but these tendencies can be over-ridden by intercurrent positive attachment messages from the environment. As we shall see, these findings lend empirical support to stage 1 of the Strachey–Lear model of therapeutic action.

The maturation of the superego

The discussion so far suggests a number of modifications of classical superego theory. First, the internalised parent or parent–child relationship as represented by the superego is concerned not just with sexuality or with primitive feelings of hatred but also with maintaining safety. Sex and security are linked in that a secure child will feel free to explore sexual feelings, whereas an insecure one will either be inhibited or confuse sexuality with the need for security. Second, a mechanism whereby internalisation of parental function occurs is suggested by the Mikulincer experiments. Parents create a subliminal atmosphere which, to a varying extent, elicits 'good' behaviours and discourages 'bad' ones. The security and degree of neglect or aggression implicit in this atmosphere will determine the character of a person's superego. Third, this environmental perspective suggests there is a maturational process within the superego from a 'primitive' archaic black-and-white, talion-law viewpoint into a more nuanced, 'new testament' morality, more forgiving, more able to see both sides of an argument (cf. King, 2003). This could, crudely, be seen as a developmental progression from the Kleinian to the Anna Freudian superego. Benign transgression, which is the essence of adult sexuality, is predicated on a sense of safety which enables the mature individual to see that 'rules are there to be broken'.

Clinical implications

What is the relevance of this to the quotidian work of the psychoanalyst and analytic psychotherapist? Can thinking about the superego lead to a deepening of our understanding of 'therapeutic action' (Gabbard & Westen, 2003)? Here I shall follow Lear's (1993, 2003) updating of the classical Strachean view (Strachey, 1934) of 'mutative moments' in psychoanalytic therapy, before concluding with a consideration of the analyst's professional superego.

Strachey's (1934) classic paper started from the then prevailing view that neurosis was the result of superego-mediated repression and inhibition. The principal aim of therapy therefore was to help modify the harsh strictures of the superego. As 'heir to the Oedipus complex', the superego represented an anachronistic presence within the self, controlling the ego and prohibiting Oedipal desires and rivalries. The role of the analyst was in effect to say to the adult ego: 'It's alright to experience strong feelings of desire and aggression: the old prohibitions no longer apply.' Strachey's insight was to see that simply *saying* that would not necessarily produce change: the superego would continue to defend itself and its right to control the ego. Since the superego is formed through idealisation, identification and internalisation, Strachey argued that, if it could, via positive transference, be persuaded to absorb into itself a portion of the analyst's more lenient superego, able to tolerate a necessary degree of transgression, it would then in turn adopt a more benign attitude towards the self as a whole. Tracking the tension between the newly internalized benign superego and transferential expectations of censure were the main focus of 'mutative interpretations'.

Strachey used Freud's theory of hypnosis to support his argument. The hypnotherapist gains sway over the subject's mind by infiltrating a portion of the superego; 'falling in love', the beloved assumes the position of the ego ideal; and in groups the leader similarly colonises followers' superegos. In the Strachey model, the hypnotic power of the analyst is put to therapeutic use. Temporary submission to the analyst's influence rearranges the balance of psychic forces. Anna Freud's idea of the therapist as a pedagogue was implicit in this – the nonjudgmental, accepting attitude of the analyst teaches the patient to be more loving and lenient towards himself.

The Mikulincer findings provide a possible mechanism for Strachey's idea that psychic change entails analysands internalising therapists' 'benign superego'. The analyst, unbeknown to the patient or even herself, transmits a benign 'prime' – acceptance, attention, focus, security, reliability – thereby enabling the patient to become less hard on himself, more able to examine and accept his id-derived desires and rages.

But would that analytic work were so simple! While the above model might explain 'flight into health' and the benefits of supportive therapy, it fails to take into account resistance and the sheer difficulty of achieving psychic change. For example, Taylor (2009) describes a psychoanalytic therapy research project with treatment-resistant depression sufferers: after an initial period of improvement seemingly related to patients being listened to and taken seriously, the old depressive patterns invariably reassert themselves.

This takes us to Lear's reworking of Strachey's 'mutative interpretation' (Lear, 1993). His three-stage model starts from the accommodation of the analyst to the linguistic and intrapsychic world of the analysand as the former begins to enter into and share the analysand's 'ideolect'. Here the analyst's benign superego *is* absorbed into the client's world (this could be construed as the 'supportive' stage). Next, as Strachey suggested, there is a *discrepancy* between client's transferential expectations – negative or positive – and analyst's response. The analyst neither colludes nor rejects, nor allows herself to be expelled, while consistently resisting pressure to conform to the dictates of the client's fantasy. At this disjunction or 'rupture' point (cf. Safran & Muran, 2000) the client is forced to mentalise (cf.

Fonagy *et al.*, 2002) – to subject her 'automatic' responses to scrutiny and articulation, while remaining held within the analytic field. This opens up a 'mutative moment': the unlearning–relearning process of psychic reorganisation that is the essence of therapeutic change.

In this third stage, analyst and analysand together examine in slow motion or 'action replay' moments that have spontaneously arisen between them. Mentalising is subsumed under the self-scrutinising aspect of the superego, one of the three components originally proposed by Freud – the capacity to look at oneself and one's thoughts as though from the outside. For Lear (2003), this capacity is essentially 'ironic' in the sense that an interpretation is not simply a plain statement of analytic 'truth' (to which the analyst but not the analysand is privy) but incorporates the capacity to subject that 'truth' to ironic scrutiny. The 'benign superego' is not merely a Strachean, less harsh, 'good parent' vector, but one at a level of 'higher psychical organisation' (cf. Bateson, 1972) endowed with the capacity to communicate and transfer that 'higher level' of self-understanding to the analysand.

In Britton's (2006) Klein–Bion model, this is an 'Oedipal heir' function, deriving from the child's capacity to 'allow' his parents to be together, and to be able to think about their togetherness without being overwhelmed with envy and intrusiveness. This is then metaphorically transposed to the act of thought itself – freedom of thought follows from acceptance of, as opposed to attacks on, linking. But Britton's formula 'where superego was, there ego shall be' (Britton, 2006, p. 132) does not acknowledge that self-scrutiny/mentalising is a psychological function distinct from the executive role of the ego. It is a case not so much of superseding the superego as replacing sequestration and rigidity with creative communication between different psychic functions. Civil war is replaced by democratic discussion and harmonious tolerance of difference. This includes the capacity to take full 'depressive position' responsibility for one's negativity – hatred, envy and destructiveness – rather than 'blaming' one's superego as the inner representative of less-than-perfect parents. Attachment suggests this is likely to be achieved only under conditions of security. Maturation is a matter not just of tempering hatred with love but also of mastering the anxiety that inhibits exploration, including exploratory self-understanding.

Case example 2: the three-stage mutative model

Fran, a single woman in her mid-40s, suffered from Borderline Personality Disorder. She presented with alcoholism, depression and a wish to find a stable relationship (she had had numerous traumatic sexual experiences) and a coherent direction in life. Due to her mother's mental illness, she had been brought up in multiple foster homes in the early part of her childhood. When her mother was finally able to look after her, she was sexually abused by her step-father.

Four years into twice-weekly couch-based psychoanalytic psychotherapy, her life pattern had stabilised, she had successfully completed a university course, she was far less depressed and she was able to be more sociable and out-going. However, her drinking remained problematic and she continued to feel lonely and isolated. She managed to stay sober for the day before her therapy sessions, but usually drank afterwards and for the next night or two, until she again became abstinent for the time leading up to her next appointment.

During an extended analytic break she attended a three-week Buddhist retreat. On her return she happily reported that she had been abstinent since going to the retreat, and recounted an epiphanic moment that had arisen during a meditation session there. She had suddenly had a powerful vision of herself pouring, as she put it, 'poison [i.e. alcohol] down my throat'. She then thought: 'That's not something that I would ever do to someone I love.' She had returned home determined to be more nurturing and loving of herself, and so far had been alcohol abstinent. The therapist suggested that she was perhaps unfavourably comparing what he had to offer – two 50-minute sessions punctuating an otherwise bleak existence – with the all-encompassing love which she had experienced at the retreat. This led her tearfully to acknowledge the horror of coming back from sessions to her lonely apartment and how drinking controlled this desperation.

She returned next week saying that she had once more been drinking. The therapist pointed out how difficult it was for her to 'bring' her drinking self to the sessions, in which, generally, she was sober, serious and collaborative. What would it be like, he speculated, if the drunken part of herself were to come into view?

Responding perhaps unconsciously to the unwitting sexual undertones of the word 'come', she replied, 'Oh, I'd probably "come on" to you.'

The therapist said: 'Hmmm: that would mean that whatever I did it would be wrong. If I responded, I would be like your abusive step-father and the other men in your life; if I held back I would be like your absent unresponsive mother. It is as though your sexuality is forever condemned to loneliness or abuse; its only hope is to be lulled to oblivion with alcohol.'

She said: 'Actually, perhaps this is not really about my so-called sexuality; maybe I just want to feel safe and accepted and validated – up to now the only way I know to get anything even approximating to that is through drunken sex.'

Discussion

Fran's experience at the retreat suggests that the subliminal positive messages implicit in a group religious experience produced beneficial effects. In the embracing atmosphere of the retreat she developed compassionate feelings towards herself, just as, in Strachey's model, the analyst's 'benign superego' lodges in the patient's psyche. Psychoanalytic sessions similarly benefit clients even when the therapist relentlessly focuses on the negative (cf. Music, 2009), because the subliminal message is one of warmth, reliability and non-judgmental validation. But the impact of the retreat was short-lived. Similarly, the subliminal positive messages of therapy produce benefit only for the duration of the treatment, or perhaps for the session itself. To go beyond supportive psychotherapy, the mutative 'value-added' of psychoanalytic work requires a further ingredient.

Fran's borderline 'archaic superego' orchestrated her self-destructive drinking and negative sexuality: hate towards the 'bad' depressed mother/breast turned against herself. From an attachment perspective it represented the disorganised attachment of her infancy and childhood. Her overwhelming anxiety was, to an extent, contained in a split-off 'bad me'; clinging to drink provided a source of pseudo-security. The lack of an internalised protective benign parental superego meant that she failed to protect herself from danger, in part through failure to read warning signs, in part in a perverse attack on the absent secure base.

The subliminal support of therapy sessions and of the retreat offered the security that her childhood had lacked but failed fully to engage with this self-destructive aspect. The archaic superego remained sequestered. When, in the context of a benign superego, Fran could express her transferential neediness openly towards the therapist, the disjunction between her expectations and his response provided the therapeutic leverage that had been lacking. By neither reciprocating nor rejecting Fran's advances, he forced her to think about and put into words what she *really* wanted – a safe place – a Secure Base – to which she could turn when feeling lonely and sad, rather than resorting to drink. This mentalising 'meta-self' was the first step towards the instatement of a 'better self' in place of the self-destructive superego.

Transgression and the therapeutic superego

A paradox of the superego is that, as heir to the Oedipus complex, it prohibits 'illicit' sexuality, and yet a well-functioning superego must lower its restrictions when the time is right so that mature sexuality can flourish, with its necessary admixture of assertiveness and healthy aggression. The structural link between the 'heir to the Oedipus complex' and 'heir to the attachment relationship' is that it is under conditions of security that such lowering of transgressive boundaries becomes possible.

Strachey pointed to a similar paradox for the analyst. Change in therapy flows from the mitigating effect of the therapist's benign 'good parent' superego vis-à-vis the patient's transferential expectations of seduction or rejection. But, he argues, giving transference interpretations is no easy task:

> there is a … lurking *difficulty* in actual *giving of the interpretation*, for there seems to be a constant temptation for the analyst to do something else instead. … the giving of a *mutative interpretation is a crucial act for the analyst* … he is *exposing himself to great danger* in doing so …. at the moment of interpretation the analyst is … deliberately evoking a quantity of the patient's id-energy while it is … aimed directly at himself. Such a moment must above all others put to test his relations with his own unconscious impulses.
>
> (Strachey, 1934, p. 140; author's emphasis)

An attachment perspective on the superego can help elucidate this 'great danger'. If part of the superego's job is to police the boundaries of social relations, transference interpretations are difficult because they are *inherently transgressive*. That is, they flout the strictures of the 'normal' superego. A psychoanalytic conversation, especially when interpretive, disobeys the rules of 'civilised' non-intimate social intercourse: don't make personal remarks; don't discuss sex, rivalry or aggression; don't refer directly to the relationship of the interlocutors; be helpful, polite and tactful; if any of these taboos are involuntarily broken, make a joke of it or apologise.

In everyday life, these topics are unsafe because they potentially expose the power relations between people. Where the relationship is inherently 'unequal', one party is in a position to exploit the other – physically, sexually, financially. Secure intimate relationships – between parents and children, spouses – and therapists – are built on the possibility (and hope) of mutual advantage and non-exploitation. Attachment theory holds that danger can be negotiated with the help of a trusted other or 'secure base' – i.e. someone who won't use the inherent inequality of the relationship for their own ends. Freud's 'fundamental rule' is a message to patients that it is OK to explore taboo territory, even if it means going against what their superego tells them. But therapists themselves also need to feel that what they are doing is acceptable to *their* superego. This is why prolonged training is needed to overcome the 'ingrainedness' of convention, and to instate a professional ethic that values truth above triteness and confrontation over collusion.

In Fran's case, all was fairly plain sailing, with the therapist facing the challenge of the patient's sexual comment in a way that was neither seductive nor evasive, leading to further opening up and enhanced awareness of the conformist and rebellious aspects of her personality, embodied in her drinking and non-drinking selves. However, as the final case illustrates, analysts will recognise that this smooth running cannot always be relied upon.

Case example 3: flouting the professional superego

Joel, a 45-year-old, had given up his beloved dairy farm when a heifer crushed him and injured his back. His insurance company threatened to withdraw his injury pension, and he was referred for psychoanalytic therapy by his GP, with whom he had a very close relationship, for help with depression, sense of persecution, feelings of hopelessness and suicidal ideas.

Joel, an only child born out of wedlock and stigmatised in his rural community, had never known his father. His mother had managed subsistence-level farming to support herself and her son. A difficult woman, she would retire to her room for days if offended. In his late teens Joel inherited the farm from his grandfather, making a great success of it until the accident and the fateful day when he had to sell his beloved 'girls' (i.e. cows). His 20-year-old son lived on the farm with him and his semi-estranged partner.

He was seen in once-weekly psychoanalytic psychotherapy, lying down. Sessions were relentlessly dominated by his story of the insurance company's wrongdoings. He presented himself as a passive victim of their persecution. Interpretations were made along the lines of the insurance company's attitude a) as a repeat of his feelings of being bullied by his peers at school and at home by his unpredictable mother, and b) as a surrogate for an unseen, unknown, abandoning father. Both fell rather flat.

The therapist felt increasingly oppressed, hopeless, impotent and irritated. In one session he found himself unleashing a vigorous 'non-analytic' challenge, encouraging Joel to stand up to the insurance company's onslaught, to see it for what it was – unfortunate but not a disaster – to find strength and to put things into perspective. He was dimly aware of how bullying and persecutory were his comments and the way he was delivering them, but persuaded himself that he was acting like the father the patient had never had, trying to put some 'backbone' into a collapsed child, rather than reinforcing Joel's sense of helplessness and victimisation. In the last minute of the session Joel said: 'So you are telling me I am a worthless waste of space.' Shocked, the therapist tried to backtrack, but time had run out, and as Joel departed he was left feeling worried and guilty and rang his keyworker to tell her what had happened, warning of Joel's suicidal potential.

Meanwhile, self-supervising, the therapist suddenly saw the insurance company incident, reinforced by his own onslaught, as a 're-traumatisation', both of the precipitating loss of his dairy herd and of the childhood sadness of Joel's absent father and depressed mother. His feelings switched instantly from annoyance to compassion. After arriving for the next session, Joel clumsily tried to hug the therapist as though to make amends, before lying on the couch and saying that he was feeling much better and had written letters taking the fight to the insurance company. In response to the therapist's acknowledgement of his unwarranted attack, and proffering the 're-traumatisation' interpretation, Joel spoke movingly about his cows, how attuned he had been to them, their condition and illnesses, and how important it was that his milk yields had been so high – unlike most farmers he milked three times a day rather than the usual twice, both for their comfort and for his pride. This in turn deepened the therapist's compassion, as he realised that Joel's relationship with his cows and their milk represented the nourishment, both literal and metaphorical, that had been so lacking in his childhood and his consequent despair at its traumatic loss. The accident, and now the insurance company's refusal, represented the ultimate 'no' on the part of the 'archaic superego', prohibiting mother–child intimacy and love. Following this incident, Joel became less 'concrete', more open to, and initiating of, metaphorical and playful conversation, and reported increased closeness with his son, who was beginning to undertake some of the farming jobs that had lain fallow during the years since the accident.

Discussion

The therapist's attack in this case constituted an enactment as opposed to an interpretation, the therapist semi-unwittingly – unconsciously – embodying aspects of the patient's split-off rage and disappointment at his ill-treatment. The irony was that, once mentalised – made conscious – this seemed to have more beneficial effects than the conventional interpretations previously offered. It exemplified perhaps Symington's (1983) idea of the analyst's occasional necessary 'act of freedom' in which she goes 'off piste' but in a way that communicates pre-interpretive spontaneity and engagement to the client.

In enactment there is a double danger: the therapist transgresses not just conventional mores but also the rules laid down by his professional superego. In his challenge to Joel, the therapist was caught up in a force field over which he had only minimal control – he just decided to 'go for it', knowing that what he was doing was in some way 'wrong', while at the same time needing to follow his instinct that this might somehow lead to an escape from the impasse. Confident that this was boundary-crossing, not boundary-breaking (cf. Gabbard, 1989), he trusted the setting to hold both himself and the patient. His 'attack' was transgressive in the way that barriers are breached in dreams or in theatre – i.e. within a context that clearly demarcates fantasy from reality. Therapists, although immersing themselves in role-responsive enactments – 'nature subdued to what it works in, like the dyer's hand' (Shakespeare, 1974) – can still be still guided by a wider trust, secure in the benignity of a mature superego (cf. Stern, 2010).

Conclusions and summary

A key part of the superego's role is to manage boundaries. The 'archaic', 'Kleinian' superego uses crude symmetrising categories of 'good' and 'bad'. The mature 'Anna Freudian' superego uses more differentiated, forgiving, subtle criteria in judging what is permissible and impermissible. The progression from these primitive to more mature states depends on an internalised parent–child relationship that maintains safety, which in turn allows for exploration, including sexual exploration.

Values are gradually acquired and internalised throughout life. The environmental ambiance transmits these values, which, under favourable circumstances, become instated in the maturing superego. Psychic change means negotiating the disjunction between new and old value-systems. In therapy this proceeds by thinking about the conflict between transferential expectations and the analyst's actual behaviours. Training as an analyst means unlearning conventional social mores and, within the confines of the consulting room, incorporating a new 'professional superego'. In the course of professional maturation, this too becomes gradually modified and sophisticated, so that occasional boundary crossings can be tolerated in the service of a greater good. For both analysand and therapist, a degree of existential commitment is needed in order to brave these transgressions. A secure attachment history instantiated in the superego makes such benign leaps in the dark more likely to succeed.

In sum, in the course of this paper a number of points have been put forward:

1   There is a tendency in psychoanalytic thinking to conflate normal and patho-logical developmental pathways. Many of the attributes classically ascribed to the punitive superego can be seen as manifestations of disorganised attachment.
2   As well as being 'heir to the Oedipus complex', the superego is 'heir to the attachment relationship' – secure, insecure, organised or disorganised.
3   The capacity to make moral judgments resonates with surrounding circum-stances, often subliminally.
4   The superego can be seen as a defensive structure, balancing desire and aggression against the need for security.
5   Strachey's 'mutative interpretations' entail a) accommodation to the client's unconscious 'ideolect'; b) transgressive moments in which the therapist nei-ther conforms to conventional mores nor fully enacts the substance of the client's inner world; c) mentalising the anxieties evoked in this sequence.
6   In mature psychological functioning the superego no longer wields absolute power within the psyche. Transgression is possible when deemed appropriate, and new sets of rules can be instated alongside or superseding those of the 'archaic superego'.
7   The capacity to mentalise – from the position of a meta-self/better self – represents a developmental step in the unfolding of the superego, going 'beyond good and evil' to objectivity, humour, acceptance and 'letting be' (Lear, 1993).

To return, finally, to the question implicit in the genesis of this paper: is the superego still an essential part of the psychoanalytic theoretical armamentarium? If seen as a quasi-physical locus within the mind, then the answer must be no: as Stern (2010, p. 3) neatly puts it: 'The era of psychic geography is dead.' But if we think of the superego as a regulating *function* ('system superego'; Barnett, 2007), con-cerned with observations, ideals and prohibitions, then, equally, Roth (2001, p. 3) was not far wrong in her claim that 'everyone has a superego'. Perhaps clinical change parallels theoretical development here. The movement from rigid structure to fluid functioning is synonymous with the movement from insecure to secure attachment patterns. I have tried to illustrate how this mutation might happen in the course of attachment-informed psychoanalytic treatment and, *pari passu*, in the evolution of our theories.

CHAPTER 15

RELATIONAL PSYCHOANALYSIS

Given its ambitions, psychoanalysis can be surprisingly parochial, intellectually and geographically. Relational psychoanalysis is a burgeoning psychoanalytic movement in the US but is relatively overlooked in the UK. Its founding father, Stephen Mitchell, whose untimely death was a major loss to psychoanalytic thinking, is known in Britain mainly for his co-authored book with Jay Greenberg *Object Relations in Psychoanalysis* (Greenberg & Mitchell, 1983), which could be seen as an attempt to understand and introduce an American public to the British Object Relations school. Sadly, this open-mindedness has not been reciprocated: his subsequent work and the journal he founded, *Psychoanalytic Dialogues*, finds few British contributors or readers.

The aim of this article is to introduce some key contemporary relational concepts through the work of one of its leading exponents, Donnel Stern – not to be confused with his namesake, Dan Stern (1985, 2004), on whose work Donnel draws, especially through the Boston Change Process Study Group (Stern *et al.*, 1998). Stern is best known for his concept of 'unformulated experience', which has resonances with Bollas's 'unthought known'. I shall trace the connections in the course of this chapter, which is based mainly on Donnel Stern's two books (Stern, 1997, 2010). Both are collections of previously published papers, in which he eloquently and passionately expounds relational psychoanalysis in an accessible yet never oversimplified way.

Gadamer

In addition to the psychoanalytic canon, a major influence on Stern's thinking is the work of the Heideggerian philosopher Hans-Georg Gadamer (2004 [1965]). This poses problems for the empiricist Anglo-Saxon mind, constitutionally resistant to the speculations and intellectual pirouetting of 'continental' philosophy. There follows a brief attempt to summarise Gadamer's ideas insofar as they are relevant to Stern's work. The everyday terms which Gadamer uses in a quasi-technical way are italicised.

For Gadamer, a Kantian hermeneuticist, there is no *a priori* position from which to grasp the truth – *understanding* is all. But this presents a seemingly inescapable existential dilemma. The full truth – the thing in itself – is never within reach. All that we have are our 'understandings', but these are inevitably tinged with '*prejudice*' – the historical and sociological preconceptions of the subject. From a psychoanalytic viewpoint, transference could be seen as a species of prejudice.

However, prejudice *can* be transformed into understanding through '*true conversation*' with another. This leads to a gradual process of '*unconcealment*' of implicit or latent truths, albeit they are intrinsically '*uncompleted*', in an endlessly unfolding process. This dialogic exploration of the nature of reality ultimately leads to a '*fusion of horizons*' in which the participants arrive at a shared viewpoint. There are clear links here with the later Wittgensteinian view of truth as a 'language game' in which there are no intrinsic truths but, rather, sets of shared meanings that emerge in the course of conversation.

Gadamer's dialogic, conversational approach fits well with the contemporary 'relational turn' in psychoanalysis. In Stern's model, the aim of a psychoanalytic conversation is to achieve a '*fusion of horizons*' in which the client feels, perhaps for the first time, 'understood' in the Gadamerian sense. This experience is often expressed by clients using vernacular expressions such as 'being on the same wavelength', 'getting the measure of me', 'understanding where I am coming from'. Here 'understanding' has not just to be seen as an intellectual process but includes procedural as well as episodic memory. It thus encompasses the non-verbal 'dance' – the playful reaching out to another that is the precondition for Gadameric horizon fusion. The hermeneutic circle is always provisional, so that a psychoanalytic conversation can be seen as an endless dialectic of confusion, fusion and defusion, followed by further attempts at understanding, and so on.

With these Gadameric underpinnings, Stern's key ideas fall into four interrelated themes: the nature of therapeutic conversation; dissociation; enactment; and the search for new meanings. These in turn represent a critique and restatement of the standard psychoanalytic concepts of free association, defence, impasse and interpretation.

The nature of therapeutic conversation

What goes on in psychoanalytic sessions remains, despite valiant research attempts (Kächele *et al.*, 2009), something of a mystery. Could the proverbial fly on the consulting room wall, especially that of a mature as opposed to a trainee clinician, reliably tell whether he or she was witnessing a Kleinian, Lacanian, self-psychological or relational therapy? For the most part, probably not, although there might be giveaway moments – Lacanian wordplay, Kleinian transference interpretations, self-psychological support, or relational self-disclosure.

Bollas (2007) describes two basic models of psychoanalytic dialogue: free association and transference interpretation, representing Freud's classical method and the prevailing neo-Kleinian paradigm. He passionately advocates a return to the former on the grounds that too much interpretation interferes with patients' freedom of thought, over-privileges the analyst, and inhibits the patients' autonomy, the fostering of which is one of the prime aims of treatment (cf. Holmes & Lindley, 1997). In Steiner's (2002) terms, classical technique is primarily patient-centred (i.e. free associative), modern approaches analyst-centred (i.e. interpretive). Neither model fully reflects therapy as a joint creation, a 'third' (Benjamin, 2004; Ogden, 1987), contributed to by each party but more than the sum of what each brings and unique to any particular analyst–patient dyad.

The Gadamerian perspective as expounded by Stern – he points out that Gadamer had no particular interest in psychoanalysis – offers a more interpersonal account of what actually happens in psychoanalytic sessions than either of these models. If psychoanalysis is in essence a conversation, 'Psychoanalysis is about what two people can say to each other if they agree not to have sex' (Bersani &

Phillips, 2008, p. 1). Two people are working together to try to understand what is going on in the mind of one of them. In this process of goal-corrected affective attunement (McCluskey, 2005) there is a cyclical feedback loop between therapist and patient as they circle ever closer to emotional truth. The work continues until a 'fusion of horizons' moment is reached, a moment of meeting, akin to the Boston Change Process Study Group's (2008) 'something more than interpretation'. At this point there is a moment of repose, before confusion, enactment and dissociation resume and the ever renewing project of understanding begins again.

Relationists are at pains to differentiate the models and metaphors which they claim encapsulate their approach from classical and neo-classical approaches. Relationship is all: the baby's mind exists from birth only as a mind-with-another(mother)-mind. The here-and-now, 'present transferential' aspects of the therapeutic relationship are the key. The focus of the work is the unconscious matrix which exists between therapist and patient; the task and talk of therapy are to attend to that unspoken tissue of feelings and connections and to draw relevant lessons from them. The therapist has a twofold job – as co-contributor to the matrix but also as someone whose expertise lies in the capacity to reflect on that process.

In practice most contemporary analysts of whatever stripe would see it as important to attend to the minutiae of the ebb and flow of the therapeutic relationship. But relationists argue that classical and neo-Kleinian theory fail fully to encompass practice, and that a more radically interpersonal model of clinical theory is needed to describe the realities of psychoanalytic work as it actually goes on in the consulting room (cf. Holmes, 2010).

Dissociation

In place of repression, Stern's primary picture of psychopathology is that of dissociation, first described, pre-Freud, by Janet in his account of hysteria, and conceived by him as a deficit rather than as a defence. Stern draws on Sullivan's (1954) notion of 'not-me' to characterise the dissociated/repudiated parts of the psyche leading to a diminished sense of self, helplessness, unmourned trauma and reduced capacity for intimacy. Stern sees 'not-me' as the unwitnessed, unmirrored aspects of the self, which exist in a latent unexperienced, 'unformulated' form and which contribute (see below) to enactments in which repudiated parts of the self become embodied in the thoughts, feelings and behaviour of the analyst.

Stern's version of dissociation is akin both to the Kleinian notion of projective identification and to the Fonagy–Target model of unmentalised experience and the alien self (Fonagy & Target, 2007). Clearly, dissociation and splitting are related, and the projection of split-off unacceptable parts of the self via projective identification into the analyst is not far removed from Stern's idea of enactment of 'not-me' in the Other. However, as a relationist, Stern's views differ from those of the Object Relations model in two ways. First, rather than viewing splitting/dissociation as an intrapsychic, 'normal' defence aimed at preserving the good object from the hatred and destructiveness of the monadic primitive mind, he sees it as arising in a relational context. His is a 'deficit' model, albeit arising not from 'degeneracy' – as Janet would have viewed it – but out of the relational matrix in which the developing child is embedded.

Thus, second, dissociation emanates from the 'group mind' – co-constructed relational world – of mother and baby. This links to the Fonagy–Target attachment-derived picture, in which parental mirroring and marking reflect back the child's experience, which is 're-presented' in the nascent mind as 'me', albeit sometimes 'conflictual me'. As development proceeds, this process is internalised as 'reflexive function' (whose absence represents the 'deficit' underlying psychopathology), enabling the subject to represent and therefore own the disparate aspects of the self, including troubling, unacceptable and potentially disruptive elements. Where, through neglect, trauma or parental illness, this process is deficient or disorganised, the child is potentially inhabited by an 'alien self', a 'not-me' nidus. This, beyond the reach of interpersonal and intrapsychic regulation, becomes a driver for self-destructiveness and perversity. Stern's recipe for overcoming the trauma of non-mirroring is that of the analyst as *witness*, the unblinking, non-judging *eye* that can restore narrative capacity and enable the victim to gain or regain a sense of 'I'. The analyst, rather than participating in the dissociative process, faces up to that which thus far has been unrepresented and unrepresentable in the patient's mind.

Stern is at pains to differentiate his concept of dissociation from these more familiar versions. The difference lies mainly at a philosophical–metapsychological rather than a clinical–practical level. For Stern, the mind is intrinsically 'distributed'. Just as for Winnicott there is no such thing as a baby – only a baby and a mother together – so for Stern there is no such thing as a mind – only a mind in relation to another mind. In Stern's 'constructivist' account, 'The interpersonal field is a primary influence on the contents of consciousness' (2010, p. 94). What we can or cannot think depends on who we are 'with', either in fact or in imagination, since, in the Gadamerian sense, all thought is a conversation with actual or imaginary others. Dissociation 'is not conceived in interpersonal theory as disavowed intrapsychic conflict. It is, rather, the subjectivity we never create, the experience we never have' (p. 95).

I suspect that a last-ditch defender of the psychoanalytic status quo might argue that this is no more than a restatement of the Bionic idea (Bion, 1970) of 'beta elements', waiting for a container, an alpha function, which would enable the 'unthought known' (Bollas, 1987) to be made mental flesh. Stern's riposte to that might be to say that the Bion model remains unidirectional, while he is trying to capture the reciprocity, the two-wayness, of unconscious communication. This is an ongoing and necessary debate. Whatever its outcome, Stern challenges us to follow the consequences of radical intersubjectivity and to see where they lead, theoretically and clinically.

Enactment

Features of ideal psychoanalytic technique and ethics include: substituting thought for action; remaining neutral; being reliable, consistent and self-abnegating; eschewing encouragement, seduction, support, criticism and moralising. But there is an inherent paradox here: most of us fall short of these ideals from time to time yet, when failings and mistakes are handled right, they are often highly productive. Winnicott was keenly aware of this dilemma and tried to theorise it via the concept of 'good-enoughness', pointing to the dangers of narcissistic perfectionism in both parenting and analysis. For him, minor parental faults and misattunements provide the child with an opportunity to sense his true self, own his legitimate aggression, and enhance his capacity to survive setbacks and disappointments.

Stern's relational focus helps resolve the paradox by viewing enactment as central to psychoanalytic work, an inevitable and indeed desirable feature of intimate engagement between two subjects. In psychopathology, as he sees it, intrapsychic conflict (between acceptable 'me' and the repudiated 'not-me') is located in the interpersonal space *between* the subject and his object – in this case the analyst:

> When the analyst participates in an enactment, it is because she dissociates; and when she dissociates she finds herself in circumstances that make her vulnerable in a way she can manage, for the time being, only by dissociating ... the patient cannot provoke such dissociation if the analyst is not vulnerable to it ... the negotiation of an enactment requires growth from the analyst in just the way it requires growth from the patient. The analyst's role is not defined by invulnerability ... but by a special (though inconsistent) willingness, and a practiced (though imperfect) capacity to accept and deal forthrightly with her vulnerability.
>
> (Stern, 2010, p. 98)

The key points in this beautiful and compressed passage are:

- Enactments in analysis entail mutual dissociation.
- The analyst's counter-transference has to be understood in both the classical and the contemporary sense – a manifestation of her own vulnerability *and* a resonance with the patient's conflict.
- The analyst is and must be vulnerable and be able to address her vulnerability.
- Enactment can be resolved if it can be 'negotiated' (a very Gadamerian concept).
- Change in psychoanalysis is not confined to the patient: it involves growth in the minds of both patient and analyst and cannot occur without this mutual widening of thought and experience.

In Stern's model, to the extent that this negotiation can happen, 'conflict' (getting in touch with 'not-me' elements of the self) will then begin to be located 'in' one or other or both of the subjects rather than 'between' them: 'The experience of internal conflict by either the analyst or the patient ... is the necessary and sufficient condition for the negotiation of an enactment' (2010, p. 93). This helps theorise the everyday experience of therapy in which the analyst might ask herself 'What's going on here?', 'Why did I feel like that when the client came in?', 'Why did I forget to mention that I would be away next week?', etc.: 'Mutual enactments are our only route of access to these parts of our patient's minds [i.e. their emotional pain]; as enactments end, the experience can finally be formulated' (p. 179). Stern's model here fits well with Safran's 'rupture/repair' model (Safran is another relationist; Safran & Muran, 2000), in which in which quotidian breaks in attunement can, if 'repaired' via a mentalising focus, lead to a strengthened therapeutic alliance, or, if not – especially if stimulating self-justifying and client-blaming interpretations on the part of the therapist – to the reverse, and ultimately to poor outcomes and drop-out.

One way of thinking about Stern's model of enactment is to see it as a mutual non-mentalising pact between patient and therapist. Each party 'helps' the other not to feel uncomfortable with – to turn a blind eye towards – this collusive state of affairs. Only when the analyst – *or* the patient – allows herself to *feel* the discomfort and sense of transgression can psychic change be initiated. Again, this can be seen as little more than a restatement of generally accepted views of impasse. But, once again, the traditional viewpoint is restated in dyadic interpersonal terms so that analyst and patient together create the dissociation, and either has the opportunity and moral courage to bring it to an end.

At a clinical level the 'devil is in the detail'. Only through minute examination of the to and fro of analytic work can the vicissitudes of dissociation, enactment and the elusiveness of the repudiated 'not-me' be captured. Consider one of Stern's case examples (2010, pp. 120–24). The patient was a vulnerable young man with a 'demanding and easily disappointed father'. Therapy was proceeding smoothly but uneventfully, with the patient always at pains to conform and cooperate with the treatment. However, on one occasion the patient was late for a session. Stern, hungry, goes off to have something to eat, and on his return the patient is in the waiting room, standing expectantly. The patient then uncharacteristically attacks Stern, saying that his coolness in the waiting room confirmed his suspicions that he despises him and tolerates him only because he is paid to do so. Stern finds himself responding somewhat defensively. He then begins to see that the patient's repudiated 'not-me' is finally beginning to manifest itself. He must at all costs not be in touch with his depressive feelings of being despised, not good-enough, unwanted – and his rage that this is the case. His last-ditch defence is to attribute these views to the analyst rather than owning them for himself. In relational terms, the patient's dissociated, vulnerable, low self-esteem 'not-me' had been, by unconscious mutual consent, relegated to the sidelines. Finally it erupted into the interpersonal space, with consequent discomfort for both analyst and patient. Stern then acknowledges to the patient that he may indeed have been less than friendly in his greeting in the waiting room. He owned his 'not-me' – a hungry, curmudgeonly self, at variance with his view of himself as an ever warm, friendly, healing analyst. This in turn enabled the patient to explore his disowned 'not-me' feelings – especially the possibility that he might indeed have been a burden to those who cared for him, and that his precipitating lateness was an indirect protest about this. Stern sees this sequence as illustrating the reality that, far from interpretation or intellectual intervention, 'Therapeutic action lies in becoming a different person, usually in a small way, in the here and now' (2010, p. 124). A key point is that both analyst and patient, despite differing starting points, became 'different persons' in the course of this sequence.

The emergence of latent meaning

Another of the enduring dilemmas which Stern tackles is the question of the origins of new meanings in psychoanalysis. In the not entirely outmoded classical model, the analyst, aseptic as a surgeon, 'the one who knows' (Žižek, 2006), is a whole-psyche scanner whose evenly suspended attention gave him privileged access to the patient's inner world. Based on the patient's dreams and free associations and his knowledge of the soul's anatomy – Oedipal, pre-Oedipal, paranoid–schizoid functioning, bizarre objects, etc. – he pronounces a diagnosis that is also mysteriously therapeutic.

Stern tries to steer a course between this caricatured version, in which the analyst is working deductively from predetermined theory, and an inductive anything-goes, 'post-modern' model in which meanings are all equally valid and capable of being entertained. He quotes Fingarette (1963) approvingly: 'Insight into an unconscious wish is like noticing a well-formed "ship" in the cloud instead of a poorly formed "rabbit". On the other hand, insight is not like discovering an animal which has been hiding in the bushes' (Stern, 2010, p. 184). As conceived by Stern, meaning-making in therapy is an interactive process, a 'true conversation' in the Gadamerian sense. As described in the previous section, through mutual enactments, latent meanings – 'unformulated experience' – become embodied and therefore potentially accessible to reflection. Stern sees the origins of meaning as an unfolding 'continuous emergent process' (p. 185) in which new meanings arise in the mind, 'New narratives arise unbidden in the analytic space' (p. 124). But his is not an anything-goes view of meaning-making. Meanings are invariably and inevitably constrained by 'culture'. There is never, in Nagel's phrase, 'a view from nowhere' (Nagel, 1986). Participants in meaning-making 'understandings' are inescapably shaped by their historical and cultural positions – both at the micro level of their family history and at the macro level of class, gender, race, etc.

The latent meanings which become manifest in the course of therapy are those that have been dissociated, 'exported' into the interpersonal no-man's land where, at the level of individual experience, they are 'non-conflictual', i.e. they work as defences, although of course they routinely produce interpersonal conflict. By mentalizing enactments in therapy, these dissociated aspects of the self are returned to their rightful locus – allowing the patient to take responsibility, to experience warded-off pain, to mourn appropriately, etc.

But – and here is the relational caveat – the therapeutic relationship takes place 'between two unconsciously intertwined subjectivities' (Stern, 2010, p. 171). The analyst, no less than the patient – however 'well analysed' – needs to examine his own dissociations and be aware of the ways in which his/her own vulnerabilities, fear of chaos, weaknesses, powerlessness, loneliness and suffering ('bad me') are projected onto the patient.

Conclusions

It is difficult from a UK viewpoint to gauge fully the significance and place of relational psychoanalysis within the psychoanalytic family. Apart from the key relational thinkers themselves – Sullivan (1954), Mitchell (2000), Aron (1996), Bromberg (2010), Benjamin (2004) – Stern's most frequently cited authors are Winnicott, Bion and the Boston Change Group (2008). There are obvious links between relational psychoanalysis and the independent stream of British psychoanalysis. Stern makes passing references to Loewald, Kohut, Symington and Ogden. Jung, Balint, Gabbard, Kernberg, Rycroft and Parsons are conspicuous by their absence. Fruitful interchange between these broadly compatible authors and relationalism seems in order. Clarifying what is genuinely innovative about relationalism is also an ongoing project. Echoing the well-worn phrase 'what's true is not new, and what's new isn't true', Carmeli and Blass (2010, p. 222) summarise their objections: 'Not only is traditional analysis more relational, but relational psychoanalysis is much more traditional than relational analysis would have it.' (Straw man-ism is a besetting sin on both sides.)

Much of the relational perspective is consistent with, and to some extent arises out of, attachment-informed psychoanalysis (cf. Holmes, 2010) – although, in saying this, I am perhaps guilty of the 'Oh, we know all that already' resistance to what is genuinely new in Stern's theorising. 'Fusion of horizons' is what mothers and infants do when attunement, sensitivity and therefore secure attachment holds sway. Insecurely attached children are forced to dissociate – (a) affect (avoidant attachment), (b) autonomy (ambivalent attachment) or (c) coherence (disorganised attachment) – when their care-givers are rejecting, distracted or themselves dissociated. The capacity to explore and entertain a range of meanings is a mark of narrative competence (Holmes, 2001), as revealed by the Adult Attachment Interview, and links with the capacity to establish and maintain secure romantic relationships in young adults. As Stern puts it: 'Imagination is our capacity to allow language to work within us as it will; dissociation is our inhibition of that capacity' (2010, p. 64).

From an attachment perspective, the most innovative of Stern's ideas is his conceptualisation of enactment as an avoidance of conflict and the need in therapy to move conflict into the intrapsychic realm, where it then becomes a lever for change. This links with the view of therapy as a 'benign bind' based on confrontation and challenge rather than collusion, in which, within overall conditions of security, the patient is helped, via mentalising (another attachment-derived concept), to use that security as a springboard for exploring insecurity (Holmes, 2010).

Stern's quartet of therapeutic conversation, dissociation, enactment and meaning-making made a compact and practice-near reef-knot which merits close attention. Several aspects are eminently manualisable and researchable. A text-based approach, looking at transcripts of relational therapy sessions, would reveal the extent to which theory does indeed guide practice. The relationalists' much vaunted – and much questioned – valuation of self-disclosure could similarly be examined. Does self-disclosure enhance the therapeutic alliance or muddy it? What, if any, is its relation to outcome? In CBT, self-disclosure is associated with good outcomes (Farber, 2006); but the same might not be true for analytic work.

Operationalised versions of relational therapy would also seem feasible. Setting 'fusion of horizons' as a goal for understanding makes clinical sense – if seen as the attempt between therapist and patient really to touch the depths of the sufferer's being. This is far removed from the goal of making clever interpretations. Working with 'me' and 'not-me' makes the concept of dissociation accessible to beginning therapists and clients alike, rather than the sometimes elusive notion of projective identification. A focus on enactments as the key to self-knowledge – arrived at by close examination of counter-transference – for both patients and therapists can and should be highlighted in training and supervision. Finally, emergent meaning depends on mentalising, and robust measures of mentalising function are beginning to be available (Fonagy *et al.*, 2002).

Relational psychoanalysis is perhaps best seen as part of a dialectic, an antiphone to establishment psychoanalysis – if there is still such a thing in an increasingly pluralised world. From a relatively uncommitted perspective, it remains unclear whether it is genuinely a new set of ideas and practices or primarily a political turn in which traditional ideas are restated in contemporary, and sometimes deliberately contrary, terminology – or both!

PART V

HEROES

Humans learn by imitation. Piaget's model of this process is based on the digestive metaphor of accommodation, absorption and assimilation. When we eat, we first accommodate the food to our bodies by ingestion – seemingly 'inside', it is still 'outside' in the digestive tract. We then absorb and assimilate the nutrients by making them our own. At this stage we truly 'are we are what we eat'. Similarly, children and students learn by first imitating their parents and teachers – trying on their mother or father's shoes for size. Then, gradually, what is imitated is transformed, by absorption and assimilation, until it becomes integral to the Self.

This section celebrates of some of the giants in whose footsteps I have trod, who have influenced my thinking and practice, and whose tradition I have tried to promulgate, preserve and rejuvenate: John Bowlby, father of attachment theory; Michael Balint, whose student groups first drew me to psychiatry; David Malan, Balint's protégé, whose studies of brief dynamic psychotherapy inspired me to see that science and psychotherapy were not incompatible; Anthony Storr, a friend and supporter, whose book *The Art of Psychotherapy* I have revised and updated; Jonathan Pedder, my role model and predecessor as chair of the Psychotherapy Faculty of the Royal College of Psychiatrists; and last, but very much not least, my analyst, Charles Rycroft.

HEROES

CHAPTER 16

BOWLBY'S 'TRILOGY'

According to Steele (2002), Bowlby's 'trilogy' – *Attachment*, *Separation* and *Loss* – had by 2010 been cited 12,000 times. By this measure at least, John Bowlby is the most influential psychoanalyst of all time. And yet, as he disclaimed in his introduction to *Attachment*: 'In 1956 when this work was begun I had no conception of what I was undertaking' (Bowlby, 1971, p. 11). This 'undertaking' turned out to be no less than a new psychological paradigm, with implications for child development, child and adult psychiatry, parent–infant research, child-rearing practice and psychoanalysis itself.

The phrase 'paradigm shift' is something of a journalistic cliché. Thomas Kuhn, its coiner, describes how 'the usual prelude to changes of this sort is ... the awareness of anomaly ... that does not fit existing ways of ordering phenomena' (Kuhn, 1977, p. xvii). Bowlby's initial aims were relatively modest. He wanted to observe and understand the responses of children separated from their mothers and their developmental sequelae. His Kuhnian anomaly was that neither of the prevailing theories – psychoanalysis and behaviorism – accounted adequately for the facts of the parent–infant tie. Both relied on an individualistic 'secondary drive' model in which parent–infant love was a by-product either of feeding or of mere propinquity.

Attachment lays out, in typical Bowlbian fashion, a detailed, logical, exhaustive account and demolition of these theories, clearing the way for his own novel model. Drawing on neo-Darwinistic ethology, which he had encountered through the work of Lorenz and his friend Robert Hinde, and control systems-theory, he proposed the attachment bond as a primary motivational force. Bowlby saw attachment as a product of humans' 'environment of evolutionary adaptation', in which protection from predation was essential, especially in view of our prolonged period of childhood dependency. The 'set goal' of attachment is physical proximity to a Secure Base when a child is threatened, stressed or ill. Only once attachment needs are assuaged can exploration and play resume.

Bowlby was primarily a clinician and a theorist. The co-creator of attachment theory was the Canadian psychologist and experimentalist Mary Ainsworth. Volume 2 of the trilogy, *Separation*, is largely devoted to the implications of her work, especially the Strange Situation, an experimental set-up in which individual differences in one-year-olds' responses to brief separations from parents can be reliably observed and classified. The familiar concepts of insecure and secure attachment, and the sub-types of insecure, insecure-avoidant, insecure-ambivalent and insecure-disorganised attachment, all flow from this work.

Findings from the Strange Situation continue to be a benchmark for attachment research – new paradigms bring with them new methodologies of observation and measurement. Ainsworth established two central attachment concepts: a) the differentiation of the attachment bond from temperament, thus establishing attachment as a truly relational phenomenon; and b) how maternal sensitivity and responsiveness in the first year of life was the key to security of attachment later. Long-term follow-up studies have shown how subsequent social competence is linked to early security of attachment, delineating the self-perpetuating nature of developmental pathways and supporting the psychoanalytic hypothesis of the determining influence of early relationships.

In *Separation*, Bowlby analysed anxiety disorders, especially agoraphobia, in terms of insecure attachment persisting into adult life. Anger is seen as a normal and adaptive response to separation, a negative reinforcement schedule aimed at maintaining proximity. The clinical manifestations of anger, including deliberate self-harm, and the rage of Borderline-sufferers can be seen as pathological attempts to restore a threatened attachment bond.

Loss was strongly influenced by two sets of experimental findings. First, Parkes's studies of bereavement and its stages: denial, protest, anger, apathy, despair and restitution – explicable if grief is seen in attachment terms as a response to irretrievable separation. Second, Brown and Harris's studies of loss and depression, where the balance between adverse events and the presence of a Secure Base to which the distressed person can turn determine whether depression or recovery is the outcome.

Bowlby's trilogy remains the secure foundation for half a century of 'normal science' (the post-paradigmatic phase). Ainsworth's student Mary Main identified disorganised attachment as a risk factor for severe psychopathology and devised the Adult Attachment Interview as a systematic measure of mental representations of attachment. Fonagy and colleagues have extended her model into the concept of 'mentalising' and its deficiency in psychopathology. The implications of this post-Bowlbian world make attachment theory one of the most fertile of developmental models.

Some paradigm shifts leave one dumbstruck – like Keats, 'Silent, upon a peak in Darien'. Others feel so familiar that one thinks 'Why had no one thought of that before?' The trilogy stirred up much opposition when first published, but today attachment is part of the air we breathe. None of this would have been possible without Bowlby's courage, persistence and synoptic vision. He bemoaned the divide between 'biological' and psychodynamic psychiatry, insisting that his ethological-developmental model was rooted in evolutionary biology. Today's epigenetics and attachment-informed developmental research suggest that divide is narrowing. Psychiatry may be on the brink of another paradigm shift, one that that Bowlby would have welcomed joyfully.

CHAPTER 17

MICHAEL BALINT

I was one of the smallish band of 'Balint boys' (and girls) who were lucky enough to be in his seminars at UCH for medical students, which ran in the mid-1960s, several of whom, like myself, ended up as psychiatrists. I remember that first electrifying seminar well. Balint instantly reminded me of my maternal grandfather, a powerful influence in my life: stocky, bull-necked, thin swept-back hair, obviously Jewish in an assimilated way, myopic, intriguingly deformed hands, bossy, yet an acute listener. In retrospect, the resemblance was probably pretty superficial, but Balint, like all charismatic people, had the ability to evoke strong transference reactions. One could not help projecting onto him significant aspects of figures from one's life: the father one wanted to please, the feared critic, the Goliath one would have to slay in order to find one's manhood, the encyclopaedic polymath one admired and envied, the attentive and protective lover. As for the last: an aquaintance who had been a patient of his always referred to him as 'my darling Balint'. She was still seeing him at the time of his premature death and, like many others, was not given time to resolve her positive transference.

Balint's skill with medical students was to persuade us that we – role-less lowly nothings in the medical hierarchy which then prevailed in hospital medicine, even in a liberal institution like UCH – were the 'experts' on our patients. Only we – not the consultants and other gods – had the time, he insisted, to sit and talk with our patients, to hear their fears, hopes and frailties. He taught us how to take a psychological 'history' – the *real* histories of people's lives, their attachments, losses, traumas, dreams and disappointments – that complemented and illuminated the medical histories we were being groomed to extract and regurgitate on ward rounds. This subversively seductive message was manna to Balint devotees. Not only did it make us feel special, its down-power view chimed with the zeitgeist – this was the 1960s after all.

Once we told our stories in the seminar, Balint's facilitative dogmatism opened up new vistas. Incredibly, he seemed to want to know what we *felt* about our patients, and he had the ability to get us to talk without embarrassment about our reactions in a group of peers! He had a master-narrative to help make sense of our patients' (not to mention our own) lives. The child is father of the man. We have to separate from our mothers; find, fight and love our fathers; discover our sexuality; identify and dis-identify with our heroes; and adjust to the realities of life without compromising our desires. Illness can be an escape route from these vicissitudes. Our patients were regressing to earlier stages as they stepped off, by choice or necessity (Balint, a diabetic and GP's son, knew all about illness), the developmental train.

Part of Balint's magic was his insider/outsider role. He had the transfixing charm typical of the Hungarian male. At the same time he was clearly drawn to and respectful of British values and the democratic traditions embodied in the NHS. He had perfect command of English (his third language, after Hungarian and German), yet used it in that creatively idiosyncratic way that only non-native master stylists (one thinks of Conrad or Nabokov) can. Phrases such as 'interpenetrating harmonious mixup' (mother–baby intimacy), 'the drug, Doctor' (positive transference and the placebo effect) and 'the basic fault' (the deep pain of disturbed and traumatised 'pre-Oedipal' patients) have a vividness and unforgettability that is uniquely Balintian. As an antidote, perhaps, to his exceptional verbal facility, Balint was also an advocate of the healing powers of silence in psychotherapy.

Another aspect to Balint's appeal was that, despite his psychoanalytic mystique, he remained very much a *doctor*. He combined an acute analytical and theoretical mind with down-to-earth pragmatism. *If it works, use it*, was intrinsic to his attitude. He is famous in the psychoanalytic world for 'the somersault' episode. A patient had complained on his couch for years of her fear of physical exertion: 'I've always wanted to do a somersault, but never had the courage', she bemoaned. 'Why not do one right now?' says Balint. Up she gets, twirls on his consulting room carpet, and never looks back. Or so the story goes.

This is often cited as an example of psychotherapeutic integrationism, combining psychoanalytic and behavioural techniques in one session. Balint earned opprobrium among some psychoanalysts for that sort of thing; it is exactly what makes him so appealing to GPs and psychotherapeutic eclectics like myself. It is also part of the legacy of his own analyst, Ferenczi, also Hungarian, who pioneered 'active techniques' and maintained that, in the end, it is the analyst's love that cures the patient.

The somersault paradigm also illustrates another Balintian insight: that psychic change rarely proceeds in a simple linear fashion. Balint's concept of 'the flash' captures these moments of spontaneous insight shared by doctor and patient: e.g. '*Oh my goodness*, I've suddenly realized that my tummy-ache is all about how furious I am with my step-dad and the things he did to me.' This quasi-paradoxical approach calls for courage and confidence on the part of the therapist. Balint used to encourage us as students to take risks – for example, in delving into our patients' sex lives – reminding us that the way to ski safely was, counter-intuitively, to lean into the slope rather than away from it.

One easily forgets what an innovator Balint was. He was one of the few psychoanalysts to take epidemiology seriously. He realised that psychoanalysis could never be available for 'the masses'. The Balint movement was a response to that insight: since most people consult their GP several times a year, equipping GPs with psychological-mindedness is a way both of touching those parts of the psyche that conventional medicine can't reach and of reaching populations for which the ivory couches of Hampstead are inaccessible.

Balint was also a world pioneer in psychotherapy process-outcome research. David Malan's Tavistock brief therapy studies were instigated under his tutelage. Here too he was trying to find ways to abbreviate psychoanalytic work, and thus to widen its applicability. The concept of 'focality' in therapy – that at any given moment in therapy the themes of a session centre around one pivotal psychic point – is another Balint coinage, today taken for granted. He was a relational psychoanalyst before its time. He insisted on a 'two-person' psychology to understand the analyst–patient relationship, abhorred analytic omniscience (despite not being immune to the lure of it himself), did not eschew limited and judicious personal revelation in therapy, and saw the therapeutic relationship as a more significant curative factor than any specific technique or interpretation.

What would Balint make of today's General Practice? With counsellors and CBT therapists embedded in most practices, and group experience firmly rooted in GP training, is the 'job done'? Are we all Balintians now? I think he might have demurred. Psychological mindedness is always hard won. The mind and its institutions have myriad ways of avoiding pain and failing to face the truth. Social fragmentation, neglect and trauma, and population mobility (Balint knew what it was like to be an immigrant) take their toll in ways that impact on the GP surgery. De-professionalisation, abdication of leadership, the retreat of whole-person medicine, and lack of continuity of care are endemic among doctors, breeding cynicism and self-servingness.

Redressing these tendencies and bringing out the full potential in medical workers is never easy, but the basic Balintian principles remain as true today as they were 40 years ago. In summary:

- a fundamental belief in the primacy and healing potential of relationship, including the doctor–patient relationship
- valuing the potential of groups within which to explore feelings and the power of many minds when they set to work on an 'impossible' problem
- the importance of moral courage and the ability to risk anxiety as one seizes the moment, including the therapeutic moment when it arises
- trusting the 'butterfly effect', the small change that makes a big difference, whether this be in brief therapy or the 'small but significant' change in personality that a Balint group can induce in its members
- acknowledging the ubiquity (including in the consulting room) of the demands of sex and aggression and, if unmitigated, of their possible destructive consequences
- valuing the constructive potential of secure attachment and creativity.

CHAPTER 18

DAVID MALAN AND BRIEF DYNAMIC THERAPY

On the whole, Brits don't do festschrifts. Maybe we are too suspicious of hierarchies, too allergic to idealisation, too democratic, too healthily sceptical, too polyphonic – or perhaps just too envious! And, so often, 'A prophet is not without honour, save in his own country, and among his own kin, and in his own house.' But if any UK psychoanalytic psychotherapy researcher deserves to be celebrated for a lifetime contribution, and any guru be more modest and un-envy-provoking, it would be David Malan.

It is more than 60 years since Malan first started his MD thesis on brief psychotherapy at the Tavistock – and he is still going strong (2014). One of his many attributes is that he has always been open to influence and change. There have been significant mutations since he first enunciated his seminal Brief Dynamic Psychotherapy (BDP) credo in *Individual psychotherapy and the science of psychodynamics* in the 1970s, especially those attributable to Davanloo and McCulloch.

What are the essential qualities which Malan has brought to the field? They can be summarised as openness and honesty, clarity of thought, the scientific spirit of enquiry, simplicity that does not sacrifice subtlety, and an active stance that does not preclude receptiveness.

One of the key features of his work from the start is the recognition that, if psychotherapy is to be properly studied, for purposes of both research and supervision, it must be in the public domain. The use of audio or videotape recording – with appropriate confidentiality safeguards – is integral to his work in a way that is notably absent from all other established therapies.

Nevertheless, this spirit of openness is beginning to be accepted within the psychodynamic research community. It is not that therapist's own written process recordings are deliberately dishonest, but rather that unconscious forces are ubiquitous. Therapists, no less than their clients, are shaped by narcissism, the Oedipal need to please, obsessional fears of failure, and the desire to bend reality to conform to a preconceived story or theory.

Malan's second great contribution, his clarity of expression and thought, sets him apart from many psychoanalytic writers. 'Malan's triangles' may not be entirely of his own making (they derive from Karl Menninger), but in his hands they become a rubric in which the therapist can reflect upon what she is doing and where she 'is' in relational space at any given moment.

This capacity to demystify and penetrate the aura of mystique which surrounds psychoanalytic work, yet not devaluing or vulgarising it, is one of Malan's extraordinary gifts. Therapists from a variety of backgrounds can understand his approach to BDP without feeling that they need to undergo a pronged period of priestly initiation before they can embark on psychoanalytic therapy. Malan's triangles are an invaluable *vade mecum* in introducing the principles and practice of dynamic therapy to trainee therapists. These are often experienced professionals from medicine or clinical psychology who need to 'unlearn' the tendency to 'help', advise and prescribe and begin to acquire a new set of skills, including receptiveness and 'active passivity'. Like many great ideas, the triangles are deceptively simple yet, however convoluted the clinical situation or sophisticated the analyst, it is always worth thinking about what is going on in Malan's-triangles terms.

Malan started his professional life as a scientist. From the outset he promoted the need for accurate, reproducible clinical descriptions and the prediction of desirable outcomes prior to embarking on therapy (i.e. 'intention-to-treat'), followed by unbiased evaluation post-treatment. This approach was, to its detriment and shame, viewed with intense suspicion by the analytic community in the 1950s, not least among Malan's colleagues at the Tavistock Clinic. Malan managed, far ahead of his time, to do justice to the subtlety of psychoanalytic assessment of character and dynamics, while at the same time to subject it to scientific scrutiny. Brief dynamic therapies are finally beginning to accumulate a respectable evidence base (Abbass, 2006), an impetus which can be traced directly back to Malan's influence.

Another of Malan's crucial contributions, manifesting his analytic heritage through Balint and Ferenczi, is that of the 'active therapist'. This is the 'masculine' psychoanalytic vector whose counterpart is the 'feminine' capacity for receptive encouragement of free association. The 'active therapist' reaches its apotheosis with Davanloo's quasi-surgical (i.e. using violent means for curative ends) assault on the patient's defences. This is based on the conviction that, once the walls come tumbling down, the patient will finally get in touch with warded-off affects in need of expression. As Dr Johnson famously said, nothing concentrates the mind more than the prospect of a hanging (the built-in termination for brief therapies) in the morning.

One of the most useful BDP formulations, deriving directly from Davanloo, is the distinction between strategic and tactical defences. The wider psychoanalytic community is familiar and comfortable with the range of strategic defence mechanisms, systematised originally by Anna Freud and explored empirically by Valliant. The innovative aspect of the idea of tactical defences arises out of a focus on the 'minute particulars' – a Keatsian phrase picked up by another brief therapy theorist, Robert Hobson (1985) – of patient–therapist interaction. The ways in which people avoid painful affect in the here and now – by gaze aversion, vague generalisations, changing the subject, adopting a physically defensive posture, and so on – are all grist to the psychodynamic mill. They provide the entry point for therapists' compassionate probes into the psychic pain they are designed to protect.

There is an obvious link between video recording and tactical defence analysis in that, in supervision, the therapist can observe defences in action and how she responds to them: by collusively going along with the avoidance; by over-enthusiastically trying to break them down in a species of 'friendly fire', which may serve merely to reinforce defensive manoeuvres; or by a sensitive sticking to the point, so that the patient feels both sufficiently held and challenged to be able finally to express and to let go long-suppressed painful emotions.

Relevant to tactical defence is the idea of the 'character hologram', a metaphor based on the idea that, like a hologram, every part of the client's existential being is contained in each fragment of interaction and behaviour. Thus the first session contains in embryo all of the subsequent treatment; focusing on a fragment of clinical interaction can not only illuminate the whole of a session but may typify the patient's problems more generally. Malan-influenced therapists strive holographically to make a Strachean (1934) 'complete interpretation' – one that brings together into a single focus the patient's current relationship outside therapy, the transferential constellation n the consulting room, and the childhood and family structures which underlie both – T, O and P.

An interesting facet of Malan's approach is the way in which he breathes fresh life into classical psychoanalytic formulations. The idea of the character hologram, for instance, loops back to Freud's observation that:

> He that has eyes to see and ears to hear may convince himself that no mortal can keep a secret. If his lips are silent, he chatters with his finger-tips; betrayal oozes out of him at every pore. And thus the task of making conscious the hidden recesses of the mind is one which it is quite possible to accomplish.
>
> (Freud, 1905, p. 94)

One difference that distinguishes BDP, and perhaps contemporary psychodynamic therapy generally, from Freud's 1905 formulation is that, in the latter, the therapist's task is primarily cognitive: to 'make conscious the hidden recesses of the mind'. BDP, with its Ferenczian antecedents, sees emotional avoidance – affect phobia – as the crucial target for interpretation and intervention. The movement from avoidance of painful affect to release of pent-up feelings, as the therapist both warmly holds and vigorously challenges old-established patterns of defensiveness, is crucial to the Malan approach. In his hands, BDP is always pushing towards a present moment, *in vivo* experience, as opposed to an intellectual detached discussion, the latter construed as a tactical defence.

Another standard psychoanalytic concept that animates much of the BDP therapist's activity is working with, or rather against, the 'sadistic superego'. This too can be traced back to Strachey (1934) and his idea that people's problems flow from the prohibitions located in an internalised parent figure – thou shalt not love, hate, cry, assert yourself, protest, etc. In the Strachey model, the patient assumes transferentially that the therapist will similarly be cruelly critical, but there is a discrepancy between that expectation and the therapist's benign and validating, albeit challenging, presence; that then leads to psychic reorganisation and the internalisation of a portion of a more loving superego.

The idea of the superego's 'sadism' derives in part from the Kleinian tradition, where the child's own death-instinct-derived hostile impulses are postulated as projected into the parents and then reintrojected in the form of the superego. In my view, the sadistic superego concept is questionable (Holmes, 2011) and, to some extent, incompatible with the idea of affect phobia. From this perspective, the reason why people try to stop unwanted feelings surfacing into consciousness is primarily because a) they are by definition painful and b) because to feel them threatens security. Expressing protest and manifestations of fear in situations of insecure attachment reduces further the sub-optimal security offered by the caregiver: their suppression is not a manifestation of sadism but the need to achieve a modicum of safety. Indeed, conceptualising emotional inhibition as deriving from a harsh anti-hedonic internal parent may in itself be a defence against a sense of helplessness and vulnerability (Fairbairn's 'it is better to be a sinner in a world ruled by God than to live in a world ruled by the Devil').

The therapeutic consequence of that perspective is that the key provision of the therapist is not so much that of a benign superego figure ousting a sadistic one as someone who provides conditions of real security, which in turn releases the capacity for exploration of affect. In the latter situation it becomes safe to vent feelings, whether these be angry protest at poor care-giving, grief at loss and absence, or cries of unrecognised distress.

Implicit acknowledgement of the limitations of the 'sadistic superego' concept leads to the idea of therapy as *maieusis* in contrast to Davaloo-esque challenge. The midwifery metaphor derives originally from Socrates (Feldman, 1966; Rycroft, 1985; Padel, 1991) but tends to be downplayed, as psychoanalysts like to emphasise the mutative impact of intelligent and apposite interpretation as opposed to the holding, soothing function they provide as the patient pushes to give birth to a new self – or, rather, a new version of the old self. Meanwhile, Malan remains a largely unacknowledged, good old self, or should it be 'good-old Self', undaunted, and much in need of celebration.

CHAPTER 19

ANTHONY STORR

Anthony Storr was one of that very select band of psychiatrists who have crossed the mysterious barrier between professional eminence and public recognition. He is one of only three who have appeared on the radio programme *Desert Island Discs* – an accolade coveted far more than a knighthood. Most educated people have heard of him, mainly through his best-selling books that throw psychological light on subjects of general interest, including aggression (1968b), gurus and their followers (1997), creativity (1972), solitude (1988), sex and sexual deviation (1968a) and music (1992), as well as accessible introductions to the work of Freud (1989) and Jung (1973). All illustrate his enviable capacity to communicate complex ideas without oversimplification.

The son of a distinguished cleric, Storr's parents were cousins; he was the youngest of four children by ten years, and thus virtually an only child. His childhood was unhappy, plagued by illness and loneliness. Educated at Winchester, he was bullied, but acquired there his life-long passion for music – he was a gifted pianist and viola player – and reading. A turning point in his life was his friendship with the novelist and scientist C. P. Snow, his tutor at Cambridge. Snow encouraged and valued him, and endorsed his wish to become a psychiatrist. Snow is best known for his phrase 'the two cultures' – science and the arts – and the deep divide in intellectual life between them (Snow, 1973). Storr was comfortably able to reconcile these two aspects in both his work and his writings. Having finally found his vocation and voice – and his first wife – Storr excelled at medical school and, after qualification as a physician, trained in psychiatry at the Maudsley Hospital, then dominated by its intimidating director and guru (see Storr, 1997), Sir Aubrey Lewis. Storr (Stevens, 2001) commented:

> I owed Lewis one thing, at least. Once you had suffered the experience of presenting a case at one of his Monday morning conferences, no other public appearance, whether on radio, TV or the lecture platform, could hold any terrors for you.

Storr's career can be divided into three main phases. On completing his psychotherapy training, and leaving the Maudsley, he set up in private practice in Harley Street as a Jungian psychoanalyst. Through his personal charisma and writings, especially the best-selling *The integrity of the personality* (Storr, 1960), he soon became a very successful and fashionable analyst, through whose consulting rooms passed many eminent men and women, academics, artists, writers, musicians and politicians.

Phase three started in 1974, when Storr gave up his private practice, left London, remarried, and moved to Oxford to take up a post as consultant psychotherapist at the Warneford Hospital, under the encouragement of his friend Professor Michael Gelder. He found the academic atmosphere of Oxford extremely congenial and became friends with leading local figures, such as the pianist Alfred Brendel and the philosopher Isaiah Berlin. Following retirement from the National Health Service, he remained highly productive in this third phase, continuing to write, and was an active member of Green College, where he was a fellow. He was made an honorary fellow of the Royal College of Psychiatrists in 1993, again one of the very few psychotherapists to be so chosen.

Storr's life illustrates many of the principles he sets out in *The art of psychotherapy*. The origins of a person's character and conflicts are to be found in childhood. Genetic inheritance sets the scene, both physically (Storr attributed his asthma to his parents' consanguinity) and mentally. Developmental pathways, both traumatic (sent to boarding school at an early age; bullying; physical illness) and resilience-enhancing (musical abilities; self-sufficiency), set up life-long dispositions. Solitude can be painful but productive. Creativity helps overcome unhappiness. Sex matters. Resentment and anger (Storr's response to bullying; parents who failed to recognise his unhappiness at school) need to be acknowledged and given vent; appropriate assertiveness has a necessary aggressive edge. Finding a sympathetic, older, wiser friend or parent figure (Snow) can make all the difference to a troubled adolescent. Stress can be strengthening as well as destructive. 'Success' carries narcissistic dangers as well as rewards. Mid-life is a moment for re-evaluation and reviving adolescent aspirations and abilities. Friendship is important to mental health, as is being part of a community. Life post-retirement can be productive and enjoyable.

CHAPTER 20

JONATHAN PEDDER

Psychoanalysis has no lack of eponymous heroes – the founder himself and his daughter, Jung, Klein, Winnicott, Lacan, Kohut – each of whom represents a rallying point for a faction of our fractious discipline. But unhappy the age that has need of heroes, and three cheers for the unsung, of whom Jonathan Pedder is an outstanding example.

Pedder's unique contribution, intrinsic to this modesty, is his capacity to remain loyal to the contradictory British blend of empiricism, romanticism and democracy while fully embracing the startling originality of the psychoanalytic *Weltanschaung*. Almost all his contributions are imbued with this spirit, whether arguing the case for psychoanalysis as an integral part of psychiatry; the need for simple human contact as well as interpretation in the consulting room; for a developmental account of depression that takes account of real trauma; or for parallels between catharsis in therapy and theatre.

Psychotherapeutic politics

I first met Jonathan when he was chair of the Psychotherapy Faculty of the Royal College of Psychiatrists. He was by far the best chair among the many under whom I served. One was immediately struck by his uprightness, both physical and moral – a man of total integrity, a good listener yet able to stick to his principles, combining an enviable overview of strategy with attention to minute detail of phraseology, spelling and punctuation. (It was from him that I learned that invaluable committee technique – in his case, an aspect of his conscientiousness – of homing in on typos imbedded in dense documents, thereby impressing the majority of committee members who habitually give papers little more than a cursory glance.) An enthusiastic sailor in his spare time, with him at the helm one knew one would be in utterly safe hands.

Jonathan's reticence, together with what I perceive as his instinctive aversion to the narcissistic lure of leadership, meant that he was more monarch-maker than king, the power behind the throne rather than the incumbent. But, although by nature cautious, he knew when to press home his point without deflection. At a coffee-fuelled cabal where the plot was hatched to establish the first psychotherapist president of the Royal College, the turning point came with Jonathan's quoting from *Julius Caesar*, 'There is a tide in the affairs of men, which, taken at the flood ...'. He insisted that the time was ripe and that we should *carpe diem* – perhaps also revealing himself, Brutus-like, as the noblest therapist of them all.

The capacity to grasp the essential point, simplify it, and then look at its ramifications and implications is to be found throughout Pedder's writings. Often he starts from an idea thrown out by one of his illustrious forbears – especially Balint and Winnicott – and develops it, clarifying, and adding his own original twist. I imagine he was an excellent therapist. His capacity to listen intently to the 'minute particulars' (Hobson, 1985), to get to the intellectual and emotional heart of the matter, to stick to his guns ('there is no such thing as peacetime', one of his memorable aphorisms, applicable both to psychoanalytic politics and perhaps no less to the unremitting ambivalence of the analytic relationship) while remaining open and receptive, is the essence of good therapy.

His Whiggish aliveness to historical forces and the importance of enlightened leadership enabled him to transcend the sometime narrow confines of psychoanalytic thinking in the social and political arena. A passionate and eloquent advocate for psychoanalysis as a necessary component of all the helping professions, he was always ready to endorse eclectic approaches in which psychoanalytic ideas are adapted to clinical and political realities without losing their essential nature.

Language

Pedder's theoretical contributions can be traced to his ability both to pay intense attention to the minutiae of language and, adopting Freud's railway metaphor, to follow wherever the words – as 'switches' or junction points – take one, often in new and unexpected directions. Depending on context, he could stay reassuringly on track or become enjoyably playful. Drawing on his natural balance and poise, he steered an even course through the ever present analytic pitfalls of wildness and dogmatism. It was hard to imagine his vessel capsizing or getting stuck in the doldrums.

I shall pick out three of these linguistic pirouettes that I have found particularly illuminating, and then delineate some of the ways in which Pedder epitomises the independent voice in British psychoanalysis.

As far as I know, Pedder was the first to point out the etymological link between the words *metaphor* and *transference*, the former derived from the Greek, the latter from Latin, but both meaning 'to carry over' or 'bring across'. Influenced by Winnicott, Pedder emphasises the essential playfulness of the analytic relationship and the importance of 'learning to play' as a positive aspect of both process and outcome in therapy.

To enter metaphorical mode is to find deeper likenesses between apparently dissimilar things. The 'work' of therapy (which in reality is more akin to 'play') relies greatly on metaphor/simile (some of which are 'dead' or conventional metaphors, some arising anew in the minds of the participants): 'What does your depression feel *like*?'; 'It sounds as though you sometimes are utterly *trapped* by your current role'; 'Listening to you made me think of someone *groping in the dark* with no reassuring hand to hold.'

Pedder's original insight was that transference itself is, via Matte-Blancoian symmetrisation, a species of metaphor – finding parallels between the superficially very different situations of being a patient seeking help and a child faced with parents towards whom he or she has a mixture of contradictory emotions. Thus the 'play' of therapy becomes utterly real as its links with the past reveal themselves, and 'reality' playfully mutable as the ways in which the assumptions and phantasies which colour and distort it are disclosed.

Staying with another linguistic association to the word 'play', Pedder likens therapy to the experience of theatre – the capacity of great works of the imagination, while bracketed off from reality, nevertheless to deepen our understanding of emotional and social life. Freud famously compared the analyst to a surgeon – cool, detached, self-effacing, able skilfully to wield the knife of interpretation in order to reveal and excise the offending pathology. Pedder switches – carries us across – from the operating theatre into the world of drama. He shows how the frame, analytic and theatrical, marks the boundary between the external and the internal world; the similarity of cathartic immersion in emotional reality; the trajectory from uncertain beginnings, through development of themes, to tension and its resolution; finally, at the end of the performance/session, the necessary return to 'real life', with all its rewards and uncertainties.

My third example of the acuteness of Pedder's ear is his critique of Strachey's translation of Freud's famous 1937 paper as 'Analysis terminable and interminable'. He points out that the title could more accurately have been translated into English as 'Psychoanalysis finite or infinite'. The very different linguistic harmonics of that road not taken might have steered therapists away from the abortive or guillotine-like implications of termination and irritable ones of interminability – suggesting instead themes of separation, death, a timeless unconscious, and the infinity of irreversible loss. As always, Pedder thinks through the practical implications of ideas, in this case suggesting, as compared with classical technique, a more titrated, attenuated approach to ending, and one that acknowledges the role of continuing 'mature dependency' of patients on their analysts.

Independent thinking in psychoanalysis

A paradox of the independent stream in psychoanalysis is that its very core values – suspicion of grand totalising theories and valuation of the tentative, dialogic and provisional – mean that it can appear to lack a clearly identified position or viewpoint. At its worst, the middle group appears to be more a muddle group. Close reading of Pedder's oeuvre counteracts this prejudice and reveals the key features of independent thought in an exemplary way.

I have already focused on Pedder's *sensitivity to language* and his valuation of *play* as a crucial mutative element in the analytic relationship. To these I would add five other aspects which I see as central to the independent tradition. First, the capacity *not to be hidebound* by tradition and a scholastic, quasi-Talmudic adherence to the psychoanalytic canon. Pedder draws on Bowlby, Fairbairn and Balint to argue that attachment and non-sexual love (*agape*) are of equal importance to *eros* and *thanatos* as motivators in human affairs.

From this flows the capacity – indeed, necessity – of *openness to relevant non-psychoanalytic findings and ideas*, leading to cross-fertilisation and hybrid vigour rather than sterility and repetitiousness. A good example here is the use of Brown and Harris's (1978) studies of depression in women and the finding that the early loss of a parent predisposes to depression in later life, and that the age at which this occurs influences whether the subsequent depression is neurotic or psychotic in character.

A third element, then, is Pedder's ability to remain *in touch with 'common sense'* while still drawing on analytic ideas. Indeed, it is this very capacity that makes him such a powerful ambassador for psychoanalysis among non-psychoanalytic colleagues such as psychiatrists and the non-psychoanalytic psychotherapists. Another example is 'Pedder's rule', that the period of notice which a patient should be given of an impending ending of therapy should be the square root of the number of months the patient has been in treatment.

Pedder drew on Balint's picture of 'pruning' as a metaphor for the role of the analyst in helping with patients' emotional growth. This Anglo-Saxon, 'Protestant' model can be contrasted with the more 'Catholic' approaches to found in some other psychoanalytic traditions. For Pedder, the role of the analyst is *'maieutic'* – that of a midwife – who does not interpose herself between the patient and his unconscious but helps shape, encourage and facilitate. Like Luther's God, in the independent tradition the unconscious speaks directly to the subject, never via an omniscient analyst.

Finally, the independent tradition is unequivocally interpersonal/relational, seeing *the therapeutic relationship as one between two human beings*, the contribution of the analyst never fully reducible to technique. Important though transference and counter-transference, projective identification, drives and defence are, there remains, *au fond*, two human beings in relationship, trying to understand each other and to find the support and succour that the suffering calls forth. Paradoxically, Pedder's medical and psychiatric background means that he is able to see the simple humanity that lies behind roles and titles, the inescapability of human suffering, and the requirement, never fully realisable, to alleviate it.

CHAPTER 21

CHARLES RYCROFT

To write about one's analyst, even after an interval of more than 30 years, is far from straightforward. The pitfalls of idealisation, denigration, sibling rivalry with fellow analysands, collusion and narcissistic identification all militate against objectivity. On the other hand, to have been in a position to test a particular analytic approach *in vivo* must count for something, and being a patient can stimulate curiosity and a fascination with the analyst's ideas which, with the passage of time, may reflect mature internalisation that goes beyond acting out or Oedipal intrusion. But, if this piece strays outside the bounds of balanced exposition, perhaps due allowances will be made.

My account falls into three parts. First, I summarise Rycroft's critique of psychoanalysis as he encountered it in the period 1940–1960 while training and working within the British Psychoanalytical Society. Second, I try to elaborate the theoretical perspective and psychotherapeutic methods which he developed in opposition to the conventional psychoanalysis of his day. Third, I link these with themes in contemporary psychoanalytic psychotherapy in an attempt to show how, without forming a distinct school or movement or acquiring overt followers, many of his ideas have passed into common currency.

First, I must say something about Rycroft's style. To say that *le style c'est l'homme* would certainly be true of him, in both his literary and his therapeutic persona. Clarity of thought, preciseness of phrase, freshness, wit, avoidance of cliché and jargon, a fondness for parenthesis, an ability to stack one clause neatly upon another as each sentence wends its way to a satisfying conclusion – to read Rycroft is to be taken on a journey through intellectual territory with which he is so utterly at home that he can point out interesting anomalies and curiosities without straying beyond the modest limits which he usually sets himself. There was something quintessentially *dapper* in Rycroft's whole approach – a lightness of touch, an ironic seriousness – that permeated his dress, his gait, his writing, his tentative yet authoritative interpretive stance, and his well-modulated tenor of voice and manner. He was, in short, a gentleman – in the Confucian sense of someone who is both true to himself and utterly respectful of others, polite but not conformist, caring but never controlling.

Peter Fuller, in his introduction to *Psychoanalysis and beyond* (Rycroft,1985), emphasises the *Englishness* of Rycroft in his response to a psychoanalysis, which had sprung up on European soil, had transplanted to America with apparent ease, but had never quite caught on in the mainstream of intellectual life in Britain. For someone of Rycroft's intelligence and breadth of vision, the oeuvre is modest, consisting mainly of essays and short pieces. Many of his best insights come as asides or throw-away lines. He displays all the virtues, and some of the limitations, of this English intellectual tradition: he is no system-builder; he is suspicious of grand theories and catch-all explanations and sensitive to illogicalities and paradox; and he both espouses common sense and abhors grandiosity and pretension.

To repeat, Rycroft's 'Englishness' is both a strength and a weakness. In sporting terms, now obsolete, one was either a gentleman or a player. Although after qualification in 1948 Rycroft rapidly established himself as a significant figure on the psychoanalytic scene, it was not long before he became increasingly reluctant to play psychoanalytic politics. He beat a 'strategic retreat' (his phrase), which meant that he never, in my view, fully developed his central ideas within an atmosphere in which they could be challenged and extended. Although for a while an insider – he was scientific secretary of the Institute of Psychoanalysis in the 1950s, and his admirable *Critical dictionary of psychoanalysis*, which has never been out of print since its publication in 1968, would be on the bookshelves of most practising psychoanalysts – he always felt somewhat excluded from the psychoanalytic inner circle, and he eventually ploughed a rather lonely furrow as psychoanalysis' psychoanalyst. As he put it, he took up 'a stance external to both psychoanalysis as a theoretical system and the psychoanalytical movement as a socio-historical phenomenon; one which would, hopefully, enable me to be objective about both' (Rycroft, 1985, p. 121).

This section could be seen in terms of the author's legacy – which at its most general can be understood as that which is handed down from one generation to the next. So it is perhaps legitimate to speculate how Rycroft's own legacy was cruelly interrupted by the death of his father when he was around 11 years old. This had a significant material effect – he was never particularly well off – and it made him highly sensitive to the impact of loss and bereavement (one of several connections with his fellow psychoanalytic renegade John Bowlby). To continue with this unwarranted psychobiographical speculation, when the process of identification with the father is interrupted, boys may veer between slavish imitation, in the guise of 'parentification', or 'negative identification' that is unmodulated rebellion. Perhaps the *Critical dictionary of psychoanalysis* and Rycroft's mature stance vis-à-vis psychoanalysis could be seen in part as a healthy transcendence of these two tendencies, born out of his response to his father's untimely death and an attempt to breathe fresh life into a psychoanalytic tradition which he felt had become ossified and infertile.

Rycroft's critique of psychoanalysis

Rycroft's central critique of classical psychoanalysis is that it presents itself as a *causal* theory of human behaviour rather than, as he chose to view it, as a theory of *meaning*. Psychoanalysis purports to find the causal or etiological origin of neurotic behaviour, and, armed with this knowledge, the patient is then supposedly liberated from its thrall. With his highly developed critical and sceptical sensitivity, Rycroft understood that *causes* in the strictly scientific sense are highly unlikely to be unravelled in the consulting room. His creative self saw the psychotherapeutic enterprise as an attempt to understand the patient's communications, direct and indirect. In this view, psychoanalytic expertise consists in unravelling confused, disguised or unwitting communication and in transmitting that understanding to patients, so that they may be better able to communicate with themselves. Most of Rycroft's major criticisms of psychoanalysis flow from this basic position.

He did not claim originality in this shift to a meaning-based meta-psychology, merely associating himself with a number of authors such as Home, Schafer and Erikson who had come to similar conclusions. Jaspers, not as far as I know cited by Rycroft, similarly distinguished between understanding (i.e. an empathic and ultimately semantic account of human experience) and explanation (a causal theory about the origins of mental states), albeit from a psychiatric rather than a psychoanalytic tradition.

Rycroft's history-of-ideas angle on this is that Freud and subsequent psychoanalysts were keen to claim intellectual respectability for their new discipline. They therefore dressed up their theories in pseudo-scientific garb, presenting psychoanalytic concepts such as ego or the unconscious or libido as though they had similar philosophical status to gravity or valency or genes. He questions the existence of these reified hypothesised psychological entities. For him there is no such thing as 'an unconscious' – a ghost in the machine which manipulates our waking consciousness – but, rather, unconscious *processes* which need to be taken into account when trying to understand the complexities of human behaviour. 'The unconscious is only a metaphor and ... mental processes do not really take place inside anything and do not have spatial relations to one another' (Rycroft, 1985, p. 115).

From a Rycroftian perspective, a dream or slip of the tongue is not 'caused' by the workings of the unconscious or repressed drives seeking discharge, but can be unravelled (or interpreted – Rycroft points out that Freud's most famous work was not called *The causes of dreams*) in terms of its personal meaning for the dreamer or malapropist.

Whether this radical espousal of hermeneutics and narrative really solves the problem of psychoanalysis' epistemological status is a question beyond the scope of this chapter. Psychoanalytic concepts can undoubtedly be subjected to scientific enquiry, although the consulting room is perhaps not the best arena for such investigation. Nevertheless, Rycroft's perspective has the huge advantage of liberating dreams and slips of the tongue, and psychoanalysis generally, from the tyranny of psychic determinism. Perhaps dreams sometimes have a personal meaning, sometimes not; perhaps the meanings we attribute to dreams are post hoc, imposed on them, as Wittgenstein suggested, by a meaning-making part of the mind that is distinct from the dream-forming process. This position is also compatible with Timpanaro's (1976) (Rycroft, 1985) famous critique of the Freudian theory of verbal slips of the tongue. Like Rycroft, Timpanaro is impressed by, but sceptical of, the virtuosity of Freud's explanations. As a Marxist social commentator who made his living as a proof-reader, he prefers to see most slips as resulting from compression and 'banalisation' – that is, the automatic elision of words and intrusion of standard phrases into complex text. Here too one can argue that a slip is sometimes of psychic significance, sometimes not, providing a more balanced and tentative perspective than the classical standard psychoanalytic approach.

This constructive tentativeness, coupled with rigorous logical criticism, coloured Rycroft's approach to therapy as well as theory. Although capable of being extremely tough, he would offer his interpretations in a questioning, provisional-seeming way, allowing the patient to disagree, elaborate and correct minor details on his own behalf. Thus, the whole process became open-ended and dialogic (to use an Americanism Rycroft would probably have disliked), rather than dogmatic or persecutory.

Although Rycroft saw psychoanalysis as a theory of meaning rather than causation, he sensed the danger of divorcing the discipline from its roots in medicine and evolutionary theory. Hence his description of psychoanalysis as a *'biological theory of meaning'* (his emphasis) – that is grounded in the body and its destiny, with sex, birth, illness and death as central themes. He saw the pseudo-scientific position of psychoanalysis as a trap which cut it off both from semantics and the emerging new sciences of cybernetics and ethology. He was impressed with Bateson's ideas about communication deviance and double binds and with Bowlby's introduction of attachment theory as an evidence-based ethological angle on psychoanalysis. This espousal of the biological became at one point an *ad hominem* (or rather *ad feminam*) assault – he viewed many psychoanalysts as essentially cerebral urban creatures who combined in a paradoxical way intense personal fastidiousness with a theoretical espousal of such primitive emotions as envy and hatred and greed:

> Most analysts ... had quite uncanny ideas about nature and animals. They had just no idea how animals or bodies work. They would be aghast if a cat brought in a bird it had killed in the garden. Absolutely appalled! ... Lots of analysts seemed to be determined to perform the sexual act by the use of intellect rather than instinct.
>
> (Rycroft, 1985, p. 28)

(I don't entirely agree with this – it seems rather that some highly cerebral people are attracted to psychoanalysis because it provides an entrée for the body into their intellect-dominated world, while at the same time providing a theoretical framework for this disturbing process of embodiment.)

A third consequence of the shift of psychoanalytic emphasis from causes to meaning, from the expression of drives to communication, was that it enabled Rycroft to dispense with the presumed conflict between the 'reality principle' and the 'pleasure principle', and the consequent muddle into which psychoanalysis tended to get itself in relation to creativity and the imagination.

In classical Freudian meta-psychology, maturation and psychic health is seen as a shift from domination by the pleasure principle towards that of the reality principle, whereas in neurosis, so the argument goes, the opposite is true. Since much imaginative activity and artistic creation is clearly pleasurable and not based in reality, and yet is only tendentiously 'neurotic', this creates serious theoretical difficulties. Here Rycroft, drawing heavily on Winnicott, but also on Coleridge and the romantic poets, argues that effective communication is both pleasurable *and* informative, and that there is a third zone, neither pure pleasure, nor pure reality, where interpersonal exchange, playfulness, humour and imagination hold sway. For him psychic health is associated with a species of *poise*: being able to hold a balance between primary and secondary processes, being in touch with both reality and imagination. Neurosis, from this perspective, arises when there is an imbalance, or an excess of one or the other. Here again we see the return of the notion of the Confucian gentleman, able to render (to change the religious metaphor) unto Caesar and unto God in equal measure.

Rycroft's critique of the pseudo-scientific stance of psychoanalysis extended to the politics of psychoanalysis and to clinical practice itself. Real science is open to refutation; pseudo-science retreats into a closed self-referential system. Real science tests its ideas against reality; pseudo-science depends on unsubstantiated opinion and special pleading. Psychoanalysis at its worst is guilty of all such sins and more. Rycroft was critical of what he saw as psychoanalytic over-valuation of interpretations, and especially transference interpretations, as the curative factor in therapy. Like Winnicott, he thought that 'being there', holding, humanity, attention and interest were as important as any special insights into the human psyche which psychoanalysis might claim. This position was not likely to endear him to those psychoanalysts who wanted to see their unique skills as the essential curative factors in neurosis and to devalue features which psychoanalysis might have in common with other psychotherapies.

> Transference interpretations do indeed indicate that the therapist possesses some theoretical ideas that enable him to elucidate matters that would otherwise be obscure; but ... they also indicate that the therapist has been listening attentively, has remembered what the patient said during previous sessions and has been sufficiently interested to listen .... Therefore [they] are not merely ideas generated by a conceptual framework possessed by the therapist and fed by him to the patient's psychic apparatus, but also sentences uttered by a real live person who is devoting time and attention to another real live person.
>
> (Rycroft, 1985, p. 63)

'Rycroftian' theory ?

Given his fairly comprehensive, albeit piecemeal, critique of psychoanalysis, what did Rycroft, as a thinker and therapist who would not have been content with a purely atheoretical stance, find to put in place of the psychoanalytic ideas he rejected?

Here I think three influences can be detected. First, as already implied, there is the tradition of British empiricism and sceptical enquiry, which in a late essay Rycroft himself put under the heading of 'Cambridge' (Rycroft, 1991). An offshoot of this was his capacity to locate both individual patients and psychoanalysis in a social and historical context, and thus to go beyond purely intrapsychic explanations and interpretations: 'We are creatures of biological and *historical* destiny' (Rycroft, 1985, p. 84, my emphasis).

This notion of historical determinism, with its flavour of the Marxism Rycroft imbibed at Cambridge in the 1930s, is balanced by a second major influence – the existential tradition – which can be summarised in the early Marxist idea that *man makes himself on the basis of prior conditions*. I am not sure how intellectually enamoured Rycroft was with the sometimes obscure and rambling writings of 'continental' philosophy, but he refers frequently to existentialism, and Rollo May and, of course, his analysand Laing get major entries in the *Critical dictionary of psychoanalysis*. He also cites John Macmurray, who could be described as a Scottish Christian existentialist. Macmurray was in turn one of Fairbairn's mentors, with whom Rycroft also clearly felt an intellectual affinity. The existentialist tenet that the essential humanness of man cannot be reduced to objective descriptors is consistent with Rycroft's critique of what he saw as psychoanalysis' reification and pseudo-objectification of the mind.

The notions of freedom, agency and authenticity crop up frequently in Rycroft's writings, all of which can be linked to the existentialist tradition. Therapy's job, as he saw it, was to help patients liberate themselves from the constraints of upbringing, social expectation and self-deception. He became a psychoanalyst at a time when to do so was slightly socially disreputable and, although he claimed not to be able to understand one word of Lacan (personal communication), I think he would have been sympathetic to the radical edge to psychoanalysis which contemporary Lacanians have tried to revive. He was impressed by Schafer's (1976) 'action language' for psychoanalysis, which views individuals as making and 'choosing' their own lives. I place 'choosing' in quotation marks because, clearly, the idea of unconscious choice is problematic, and we certainly do not choose our biological and historical destiny. Nevertheless the idea of a person, or a Self, ultimately responsible for his or her own life, able to live with and overcome 'angst' (another favourite existential concept), is implicit in much of Rycroft's writing. Paul Tillich's (1952) famous title *The courage to be* was a phrase of which Rycroft would have approved.

Similarly, Rycroft's emphasis on self-deception, false self-existence or defendedness generally centres on the existentialist notion of *authenticity*. This can perhaps be linked with the idea of the 'gentleman' as someone free from pretension and self-deception, who knows himself, who accepts himself and others as they are, who retains his independence of mind without trying to impose it on others, who cannot be crushed, and who avoids all unnecessary violence. To live authentically is to be true to oneself, to have integrity in the literal sense, to be all of a piece, to be the 'real thing', not some fake or simulacrum of a person, not conforming to expectations, inflating or adapting oneself for the sake of survival or self-aggrandisement or advancement.

Indeed Rycroft is not above accusing Freud of moments of inauthenticity:

> I ... have often felt that there was something less than straightforward, something disingenuous, about his selection of which details about himself or his patients he should disclose or withhold on grounds of discretion, about his capacity to pass over obvious weaknesses in his arguments as though he himself had not noticed them, and about his tendency to have it both ways by offering incompatible interpretations simultaneously.
>
> (Rycroft, 1985, p. 90)

Perhaps there is an element of an English gentleman's revenge here, from someone who had been accused of being an 'upper-class dilettante' (Fuller, in Rycroft, 1985) when he first applied for training at the Institute of Psychoanalysis and, once he did join, felt that non-Jews were treated as outsiders.

Authentic living is coherent living and is the antithesis of the 'splitting of the ego' (Freud, 1938), which came into prominence with Kleinian authors such as Rosenfeld and Segal. Like Klein, Rycroft saw Freud's late discovery of splitting as a defence mechanism (to use language he disliked) more profound than repression. It linked with such cultural notions as Eliot's 'dissociation of sensibility', and the existentialist idea of alienation and was clinically relevant to the kind of patient he describes in 'The analysis of a paranoid personality' (Rycroft, 1985), who today would more likely be seen as borderline. While focusing on splitting as the primary source of inauthenticity, Rycroft also saw the need for benign dissociation, in the sense of fostering through therapy a reflective self that is simultaneously actor and observer.

The third strand in Rycroft's non-analytic influences is, as I have mentioned, the Romantic tradition, and especially the writings of Keats and Coleridge. Without ever being quite explicit about it, I believe he saw psychotherapy at its best as an imaginative activity, akin to poetic responsiveness, and would have seen the contemporary notion of counter-transference, in which the analyst uses the feelings engendered in her by the patient to gain access to the patient's inner world, as a far more subtle and less automatic process than is often implied in psychoanalytic discourse. He was acutely aware of the implicit paradox in trying to legislate for spontaneity and creativity.

His paper 'Psychoanalysis and the literary imagination', published both in *Psychoanalysis and beyond* (Rycroft, 1985) and in *The innocence of dreams* (Rycroft, 1979), of which he was justly proud, tries to spell out the conditions under which imaginative activity is likely to flourish. These include 'negative capability', the capacity to tolerate uncertainty without 'irritably reaching after fact and reason'; the capacity to 'play' with ideas and feelings without knowing in advance what their outcome might be; being able to encompass both 'feminine' receptivity and 'masculine' penetrativeness without too much anxiety; and having permeable ego-boundaries, thus being able to bring a wide variety of emotional and intellectual responses together without worrying about their sanity, respectability or credentials. This benign splitting is the end result of a developmental process which includes both the therapist's parental handling in childhood and the training therapy. For the therapeutic imagination to flourish, the therapist has the capacity to be receptive to herself, to be able to 'hold' herself, to allow herself to be playful, and to tolerate awkward, embarrassing or unacceptable aspects of herself. Here Rycroft's 'biological theory of meaning' begins to come alive. Discovering meaning in therapy is no longer a scholastic exercise akin to code-breaking or dry lexicography, but an interpersonal activity that arises out of the sensitivities and subtleties of emotional communication, the prototype of which is, of course, mother–baby interaction. In their observational work with parents and infants, Trevarthen (1984) and others have shown these processes can be subjected to rigorous scientific enquiry without violating their essence.

Clearly there are links here with Bion's notion of 'maternal reverie' (1970), Winnicott's idea of transitional space as the 'place where we live' (1971), Bollas's advocacy of freedom and spontaneity in the analyst's responses to the patient (1987), and Ogden's 'analytic third' (1979). Rycroft's unique contribution comes not so much from the ideas he puts forward as, once again, from a particular *style* of thought and expression that illustrates the very stance he advocates. He is less subjective than, say, Bollas and Ogden, less idiosyncratic that Winnicott, less theory-driven and obscure than Bion. For example:

> If the self tries to observe itself while creating it inevitably fails, since the self-as-agent must, willy nilly, become located in the observing, introspecting self and not in the part of itself it is trying to observe .... The self that dreams, imagines, and creates is intrinsically nominative and can only be the subject of verbs, can only be 'I' and never 'me', and ... it does a disappearing trick if one tries to push it into the objective, accusative position.
>
> (Rycroft, 1985, p. 266)

This 'subjective-objective', experiential-philosophical narrative style typifies Rycroft's analytic stance. It is highly sensitive to logical inconsistencies; is concerned with the fundamentals of language and how people communicate not just with one another but also with themselves; mixes clarity of thought with colloquialism and metaphor – 'willy nilly', 'disappearing trick' – in a way that is illuminating and memorable; is driven by ethical conviction and commitment – in this case to the fragility and importance of the imagination; and contains an implicit 'accusation' that psychoanalysis has got it wrong if it tries to objectify creativity.

To conclude, how might Rycroft have viewed the contemporary psychotherapeutic and psychoanalytic scene? First, I think he would have welcomed the pluralistic world in which psychoanalysis, even if still in its own eyes *primus inter pares*, is but one among many psychotherapies, all of which are needed if the variety of human needs is to be met. (I once tried to explain to him the workings of psychodrama which I had been pursuing in tandem with my psychoanalytic therapy. 'Oh', he said, 'you mean it's a bit like playing charades at Christmas.') It is interesting, in thinking about Rycroft, to consider one of these new therapies, Hobson's conversational model, or Psychodynamic-Interpersonal Therapy as it is now called (Hobson, 1985; Margison, 2001). Hobson worked in public- sector psychotherapy in Manchester rather than in the somewhat rarefied atmosphere of Wimpole Street. Like Rycroft, Hobson combined an interest in psychoanalysis, existentialism and the romantic poetic tradition, was critical of persecutory tendencies within therapy, advocated a tentative negotiating style, and valued metaphor and meaning. Had Rycroft chosen to work in the National Health Service, or had there been a university tradition of psychoanalysis in Britain, one could imagine the development of a similar Rycroftian therapy, called perhaps Psychodynamic Existential Therapy, or even, given his interest in dreams, the Rycroftian-Existential Method (REM).

Second, Rycroft would have been reassured to find that psychotherapy research has confirmed the importance of 'common factors' in therapy (i.e. the non-specific conditions such as reliability, regularity, concerned interest, etc., are as important in producing change as specific interventions such as transference interpretations) and the significance of the therapeutic alliance as the most reliable predictor of favourable outcome in the psychotherapy of whatever persuasion.

Third, Rycroft would have been interested to see how psychoanalysis is once more gradually opening itself up to 'real' science – via attachment theory, child development studies and neurobiology (Schore, 1994). For example, the distinction between 'episodic' (*what* happened) and 'semantic' (*how* it happened) memory in cognitive science is akin to Freud's distinction between secondary and primary processes as explicated by Rycroft, and this in turn can be linked with neural network theory, which has come from computing science to neuroscience and now into psychoanalysis. Always an evolutionist, Rycroft would also have been interested in the applications of neo-Darwinism to psychotherapy (Holmes, 2010).

A final point concerns Rycroft's attitude towards 'support' in psychotherapy. Some authors (e.g. Caper, 1998), including Freud, have tried to define the difference between psychoanalysis and other psychotherapies in terms of its neutrality and militant avoidance of persuasion or support. Caper argues that patients are continually trying to manoeuvre therapists into superegoish condemnation or praise, and that therapists unconsciously collude with this and have continually, via scrutiny of their counter-transference, to bring themselves back to neutrality. I think Rycroft would have demurred here, arguing that Caper's project is inherently impossible and that, for two reasons, there can never be a neutral Archimedean point from which to observe human nature; there is an inherent paradox at the heart of psychoanalysis which simply has to be lived with. First, however well analysed and in touch with his counter-transference, the therapist is always affected by the phenomena he is trying to observe – there are always two unconsciousness in the consulting room communicating with each other, however 'well analysed' one of them purports to be. Second, at a theoretical level, psychoanalysis cannot escape from the conundrum that,

> since psychoanalysis aims at being a scientific psychology, psychoanalytic observations and theorising is involved in the paradoxical activity of using secondary process thinking to observe, analyse, and conceptualise precisely that form of mental activity, the primary processes, which scientific thinking has always been at pains to exclude.
>
> (Rycroft, 1962, p. 390)

I think Rycroft would argue that it is inevitable that the therapist will be to a degree supportive, simply by virtue of his commitment to the therapeutic process, and that therapy is unlikely to be helpful if it is not supportive. What is necessary, I think he might have said (more elegantly than this of course), is simultaneously to be supportive and to be able to reflect on the meaning and nature of that support and its impact on the patient. For instance, he would often allow sessions to proceed in quite a light, chatty way (in contrast to the uncompromising rigour of a Kleinian approach – at least, as it tends to be carica-tured), but then use seemingly light or irrelevant conversation to open up deeper themes, rather as one might a dream or a Rorschach test.

This is actually a more psychologically holistic approach than classical psy-chic determinism, as it assumes that whatever interaction is set up between therapist and patient – describing a dream, a slip of the tongue, an apparently irrelevant conversation, or a supportive stance of the therapist – will in one way or another reveal the key meanings and preoccupations of the patient. The therapist's skill lies in maintaining his benign split between support and under-standing meaning, and at the same time being able to communicate this to the patient – rather than being too preoccupied with staying on his or her high analytic horse.

Conclusion

Rycroft had a keen sense of history. When asked to describe 'the god I want', he chose *continuity* – the capacity simultaneously to look both forwards and back-wards. He saw how some people who are attracted to psychoanalysis wish to become, literally, self-made men and women and to deny, destroy or 'ablate' their past and their parents in favour of their new psychoanalytic family. He is implic-itly critical of this project, which denies the reality of the historical forces of which we are a product. At the same time he acknowledged, possibly with a touch of philosophical exasperation, that psychoanalysis is '*sui generis*', innova-tive, unclassifiable: 'A psychological theory ... which conforms to the canons of neither the natural sciences, the humanities nor the arts' (Rycroft, 1985, p. 230).

Kohon makes a similar point in his account of hysteria when he says that 'psy-choanalysis is like a nomadic tribe, never settling in one place ... it makes sense to talk about the double vision that the analyst needs to have' (Kohon, 1986, pp. 374–5). Rycroft possessed this double vision to the highest degree and used it with extreme tact. He was something of an intellectual nomad, but in this perhaps he was being more true to the paradox at the heart of psychoanalysis than his critics would like to think. He himself was certainly *sui generis*: highly individuated, deeply authentic, his own man, doing his own thing. He also embodied the spirit of continuity, both personally in his combination of conventionality and subversiveness and professionally in his ability to mine the intellectual tradition of psychoanalysis while embracing new ideas from cybernetics and attachment theory. In sum, he was both an actor and an agent and, to end with a Rycroftian pun, in an uniquely English way, a 'gent'.

PART VI

EPHEMERA

To paraphrase Keynes, in the end we are all ephemera, but I end this book with a heterogeneous selection of shorter, more journalistic pieces. Some were aimed at medical colleagues – 'Untied' (I am glad to record that in the UK doctors are now banned from wearing ties in on hygienic grounds) and 'The "good-enough" doctor', which is an attempt to challenge the NHS's persecutory managerial culture. The next two pieces are directed more at the analytic community and explore two controversial topics: frequency of sessions and fees. The book ends with 'What exactly do you *do*?', a confessional about my unresolved ambivalence about my role as a psychiatrist.

CHAPTER 22

UNTIED

Dress code in medicine has always been important, perhaps dating from the 1856 Medical Act, when barber surgeons needed to establish their respectability and equal standing with their Harley Street colleagues. For me, as an unreconstructed scruff, it has been a problem since medical school days. As London clinical students in the 1960s, we heard dark tales of students being sent home from St Elsewhere's down the road for not wearing suits with matching shoes. At liberal University College Hospital we were not exactly flower power, but we prided ourselves on a relaxed attitude towards jackets and woolly jumpers. For the men, though, ties were still *de rigueur* on the wards.

Evidence-based medicine reveals that patients like their doctors to look respectable. It would have been unthinkable for a male doctor progressing through the hospital grades in the 1970s to appear without a tie, although medical students were increasingly idiosyncratic in their dress. When I was doing a Saturday GP locum in casual clothes, but still wearing a tie, a patient, the daughter of a famous novelist, commented archly, 'This is the first time I have ever been treated by a doctor in jeans.' Luckily, she seemed to find it more amusing than disreputable.

Different medical specialties subtly proclaim themselves via dress code. A surgical colleague told me that he could always pick out the psychiatrists in the canteen by their corduroy suits – especially if bottle green. This from someone who had just come back from a year's sabbatical in Australia, who also told me that Hawaiian shirts and Bermuda shorts are commonly to be found there on professorial ward rounds. I reminded him that he and his anaesthetist colleagues often appeared at lunch in their operating pyjamas.

Clothing is eloquent: sometimes our sartorial vernacular says, 'Ignore my clothes, I am saving lives'; sometimes, 'Trust me, I am a pillar of the establishment'; occasionally, perhaps, 'I am making lots of money, so I must be good.' Recently, I encountered a distinguished cardiothoracic surgeon doing his Sunday rounds in the intensive care unit in track shoes and muddy jogging bottoms, which, it seemed to me, proclaimed modestly, 'I too am human; all that matters is skill and compassion and vigilance.'

Now to my continuing struggle with the tie: I hate the things, constricting and functionless in our overheated hospitals. For most of my working life I have dutifully worn one, ripping it off the moment I left for home at the end of the day (a spell in East Africa being the exception where not to be open necked was to risk heat exhaustion). Then, a few years ago, the rot began to set in. I started to allow myself a tieless, shirtsleeve drill in August. When speaking at conferences I began to carry my tie in my pocket, donning it just before mounting the podium. Finally, I suddenly decided that it was time to 'come out' completely and wear my elderly and wrinkled neck with pride.

Near enough to retirement to get away with it, I am almost always untied, except, naturally, when due to be questioned by the Mental Health Act Commission. Colleagues vary in their reactions. Some come up to me and whisper their support. Others say they enjoy their ties –one, recently remarried, now sports a different strip of sleek and colourful silk for each day of the week. I remain unrepentant, fondly hoping that the 'tie-de' is turning. Hence, I hereby announce a national 'tie off' campaign for male doctors. Members will be issued with a suitable neck garment, to be worn only at annual conventions, over a bare chest.

CHAPTER 23

THE 'GOOD-ENOUGH' DOCTOR

Let's face it – we doctors aren't saints. Have we not all sometimes felt bored and irritated by certain patients, longing for the consultation to end? Can any doctor honestly say that he or she has never felt a flicker of sexual interest in a patient? Have we never – and, post-Shipman, it is very difficult to say this – imagined the death of certain patients and the relief that would bring, not just to them but to us, their impotent carers? Do we not at times resent the demands of people for whom illness seems to have become a way of life? Whose thoughts have not sometimes drifted off towards their own concerns – to the need for sleep, food or distraction, or to some family, career or future plans?

Rather than being motivated by altruism and scientific integrity, are we merely using our patients to bolster our own fragile sense of competence and health? Most of us look reasonably healthy, physically and mentally, as we stride about 'our' hospitals and surgeries, strong and powerful in contrast to the vulnerability and distress with which we are surrounded. Are we not treating ourselves, our vulnerability and fear, as much as our patients?

So is none of us really fit to practise? In confessing to these failings, am I writing a professional suicide note? What are we to do with these normal human reactions? Are we to ignore them, repress them, speak out about them – or can we use them in the service of our work?

The crucial distinction is between thought and action. We aim, as far as possible, to be pure in word and deed, but we can allow ourselves to be as ugly as we like in thought. The more aware we are of our reactions to a patient – however bizarre, irrelevant or unprofessional these may seem – the less likely we are to use the power imbalance between us to act in untoward ways. When bad things happen between doctors and patients it is usually due to a confluence of the unconscious needs of both. If the lonely doctor had been aware of and been able to articulate the extent of his sexual fantasies, he would have been far less likely to end up in bed with his sexually abused and depressed patient. I often find that a few minutes' irreverent moaning about patients with colleagues before a ward round leads to better and more compassionate consultations.

The feelings a doctor has, or actions he or she carries out in relation to patients, are often a manifestation of the patient's inner world, via a mental mechanism known as 'projective identification'. If a doctor is bored with a patient, this may be because the patient is feeling dull or uninteresting or is angry about something but cannot express the anger. Excessive worry about a patient may be the result of being infected by the patient's anxiety – but out of proportion to the objective situation.

The GMC prescribes do's and don'ts for doctors. Although these are undoubt-edly useful, most doctors consciously subscribe to them anyway, and the question of why bad or harmful practice continues remains unanswered. This is because, like all human beings, we are less coherent than we like to think and are motivated by forces of which we are unaware as much as by the conscious wish to heal and do a good job. Ultimately the key to good doctoring is not regulation but the abil-ity to put ourselves in our patients' shoes – to imagine what it might be like to be on the receiving end of our treatment. There are many ways to acquire this capac-ity for reflexive practice: role play, listening to users' perspectives, being a patient (through illness or through therapy or counselling). 'Balint' groups, widely used in general practice, attempt to explore doctors' feelings about their patients through facilitated case discussion.

The search for the perfectly 'good' doctor is an illusion – our unconscious minds will make sure of that. The psychoanalyst Donald Winnicott reassured mothers that to be 'good enough' was preferable to striving to be ideal. Mothers who are good enough provide children with the opportunity to learn to cope effec-tively with disappointment and failure in the context of love. Similarly, if we can without complacency bring our good and bad parts together to become a 'good-enough doctor', we should be content. More importantly, so will our patients, despite sometimes feeling let down by us.

CHAPTER 24

IN PRAISE OF 'LOW INTENSITY' PSYCHOTHERAPY

Most social institutions have dominance hierarchies. Armies have their generals, universities their vice-chancellors, companies their CEOs; psychoanalysis is no exception. But, in the contemporary world of democratic, evidence-based transparency, such hierarchies are normally subject to checks and balances which ensure, in principle at least, that position bears at least some relationship to merit and performance. For psychoanalysis, however, therein lies a paradox. First, our work takes place within a bounded, private space whose very essence is its inviolable confidentiality; reports of what goes on within are unavoidably subject to distortion. Second, unlike most institutions, where generals and foot soldiers have very different roles, psychotherapists, whether training analysts or beginner counsellors, all do more or less the same thing – namely, sit in a room with a client, listening and talking.

One consequence of this is that, in the psychoanalytic world, rank and position tend to be determined by somewhat arbitrary criteria. These include:

- Where did she train? (old school tie criterion)
- How often does she see clients? (frequency criterion)
- Does she make transference interpretations? (content criterion, but reported not observed, so liable to self-serving distortion)
- How long are her therapies? (duration criterion)

Frequency of sessions

When it comes to frequency, the standard classification, and with it professional psychoanalytic status, runs as follows:

- 4+ sessions a week: psychoanalysis (gold standard)
- 3 sessions a week: psychoanalytic psychotherapy ('good enough')
- 1–2 sessions per week: psychodynamic psychotherapy ('low intensity')

Classifications ideally should, as Plato put it, 'cut nature at the joints'. Those that don't have their uses but are essentially arbitrary, and they may reflect vested interests rather than fundamental differences. The key features of psychoanalysis remain contested, but most would agree that they include working with transference and making interpretations rather than suggestions and encouragement. In psychoanalysis, frequency of sessions is therefore an arbitrary criterion, in that there is nothing intrinsic to frequency that makes it quintessentially 'psychoanalytic'. Five times a week therapies may function mainly in a supportive fashion, while once-weekly therapy can be transferential, interpretive and 'mutative'. In complex cases, duration of therapy correlates with better outcomes than briefer therapies, but this reflects length of therapy over time, not session frequency (Leichsenring & Raybung, 2011).

An argument and its resolution

During the course of a heated discussion with a group of metropolitan-based psychoanalysts about session frequency, the author vigorously defended the above views, arguing that what counted as 'high' or 'low' intensity depended on how frequency is calibrated and that, in psychoanalytically deprived areas, money shortage and distance mean that twice weekly can seem like a great deal. One interlocutor then felicitously moved the debate on from fractious rivalry with the suggestion that a differentiating feature of low-intensity therapy is the greater salience of *loss*, and that this may present special difficulties for both client and analyst. A theoretical rather than an arbitrary aspect of session frequency had come to the fore, making the conversation immediately more focused and collaborative.

I was reminded of this in the following semi-fictionalised clinical example.

Fortnightly

Adam, suffering from bipolar disorder, could afford no more than fortnightly sessions, negotiating time-limited therapy of 50 sessions spread over two years. After a year things were going well: he had married his partner, who was pregnant with their first child. He remained, however, also wedded to his cannabis, but had moved from oscillating between abstinence and binges of smoking to seeing that low-level regular use was probably his most realistic hope. During one session, in which he spoke of how he, his brothers and other sons of servicemen fathers were all cannabis-smokers, and how he gained comfort from knowing there was resin in his pocket if he needed it, I found myself unaccountably thinking about what it would be like to work five times week with Adam.

I then saw how this thought linked with Adam's 'absent' parents in childhood (the eldest of five children, at 15 months he had 'lost' his mother when the next baby arrived; his father was away in the army for long stretches and preoccupied on his return); a recent break (which had meant a month between sessions); and the impending birth, which meant that Adam was about to 'lose' exclusive closeness with his wife.

Trying to pull this together, and following the principle that any free associative thoughts that arise in therapists' minds should be put to interpretative use, I said something like: 'So cannabis is a "pocket parent", tiding you over the long gaps that have been present at every stage of your life, including now: you know that if you were in "proper" psychoanalysis you would be coming five times a week.' Adam's riposte was that when his wife had the baby she would have a new focus, which might free him to pursue his work as a musician; and that he liked the gaps between sessions as they gave him a sense of independence and resilience.

The trauma of his mother's too-frequent pregnancies was clear in this glass-half-full account, as was his yearning for intimacy but terror at its possibility. Nevertheless, this vignette served to remind me that it is not so much the concrete arrangements of therapy (session frequency, etc.) that matters as their psychic meaning; that resilience is something to be valued as well as regression; and that the absences may be as important to the therapeutic process as the sessions themselves.

The double session

This leads to a practice I have recently developed: the double session. In my semi-retired, semi-rural state, I see clients only one day per week. Many come from far away and public transport is non-existent. Four hours' driving for a 50-minute session is a big investment of time and fuel for a limited return. I have therefore experimented with offering these distant clients two consecutive sessions, weekly or fortnightly, with a 10-minute interval between each. At first I was worried that we would run out of things to talk about, and that client and/ or I would become fatigued. In fact it seems to works well, and I have discovered from informal conversations that colleagues experiment with similar flexible arrangements. The break enables client and therapist to retreat into themselves for a moment and fosters a reflexive, mentalising perspective in which, in session two, we can think about what was talked about in the previous hour, just as one might about the previous session in daily analysis. We can 'dream the session' while (half!) awake. There is less feeling of rush. A psychoanalytic culture is created out of an unconventional arrangement.

Conclusion

Innovative approaches to delivering psychoanalytically informed therapy are important. Skype supervision and therapy, or intensive weekends of several sessions at monthly intervals, are practised in less urbanised and compressed territories than the UK. I have suggested a) that there can be therapeutic congruence between 'low intensity' therapy and client need, and, if appropriately conceptualized, this can be mutative, not necessarily collusive or second best; b) that two consecutive sessions at weekly or fortnightly intervals can efficiently replicate some features of more intense psychoanalytic therapy.

CHAPTER 25

HOW MUCH DO YOU CHARGE?

When two or three psychotherapists are gathered together the conversation invariably drifts at some point to 'how many people are you seeing', prompting open, if sometimes exaggerated, responses. By contrast, when asked how much they charge, therapists tend to be evasive. Most are familiar with Freud's famous aspiration:

> It is possible to foresee that at some time or other the conscience of society will awake and remind it that the poor man should have just as much right to assistance for his mind as he now has to the life-saving help offered by surgery. ... Such treatments will be free. It may be a long time before the State comes to see these duties as urgent. Present conditions may delay its arrival even longer.
>
> (Freud, 1919: 166–8)

But not everyone is aware that there are places, one no further from Hampstead than is Manchester, where Freud's dream, even in these 'present [economic] conditions', is already realised. In Germany, 300 to 360 sessions of thrice-weekly psychoanalytic therapy is available, free at the point of need, to suitable patients, funded out of compulsory insurance or taxation. The only circumstance in which patients are obliged to pay is when they fail to turn up for a session unannounced (this is a private payment to the therapist, since the state understandably does not pay for sessions which do not occur). Similar, if less generous, provisions are to be found in Austria, Canada and Australia.

How is it that, while being almost unthinkable in Britain, countries not economically so different from the UK manage to provide psychoanalysis in this way? In the case of Germany there are several relevant factors. Perhaps the most important is that it was realised as early as the 1950s that systematic outcomes studies of psychoanalytic therapies would be necessary if the authorities were to be convinced of its efficacy. Germany today remains in the vanguard of psychoanalytic outcome research. By contrast, until recently, psychoanalysis in the UK adopted a cavalier resistance to exposure to any sort of academic rigour, including systematic research. A related issue – given the political clout of the medical profession – is the groundswell of pro-psychoanalytic medical doctors in Germany, both psychiatrists and psychosomatic physicians, whereas in the UK psychoanalytically minded psychiatrists are in a small minority and their physician counterparts almost nonexistent. A third aspect is the wish in Germany to make amends for the disgraceful treatment of the 'Jewish science' under the Nazis; by contrast, British xenophobia manifests itself in tacit resistance to 'new' and 'foreign' ideas, even those that have been around for over 100 years!

All this came to mind in a recent discussion with a colleague about the virtues and drawbacks of paying for psychoanalytic sessions. My friend argued cogently that the commitment entailed in paying, even a small amount, has an important existential effect. 'Free' psychoanalysis encourages a passive, helpless attitude, inimical to the facing up to one's privations, and the part one has played and continues to play in them, that is central to psychic change. He counter-quoted Freud:

> he [the analyst] should refrain from giving treatment free ... one may regret that analytic therapy is almost inaccessible to poor people ... [but] little can be done to remedy this ... The absence of the regulating effect offered by the payment of a fee makes ... the whole relationship removed from the real world.
>
> (Freud, 1913)

My riposte was that a) insisting on payment for analysis inevitably excludes a large swathe of people who would otherwise benefit from such treatment; b) the notion of 'commitment' extends beyond money – time, travel, space in one's life. etc. Searching for a 'fusion of horizons' led us to enumerate the various possible financial arrangements used in psychoanalytic therapy and to list their pros and cons:

1 *State-funded psychoanalysis*, along German lines, greatly widens the pool of potential patients and endorses the idea of psychoanalysis as a social good. It possibly encourages dependency rather than mutativity.
2 *A flat-rate fee* is non-negotiable; introduces realism into a patient's life; mobilises activity and a sense of self-worth in raising the funds through work, borrowing, etc. But it excludes the poor.
3 *Low-cost arrangements in training institutions* widen the potential pool of people who can afford therapy while ensuring some financial commitment. They reinforce the 'inverse care law' in which the most ill patients are seen by the least experienced therapists (albeit supervised), while senior therapists confine themselves mostly to training other analysts.
4 *A 'tithe' system in which therapists include a number of 'free' cases in their caseload, usually around 10 per cent*, widens the pool a fraction but makes an artificial and arbitrary division between payers and non-payers. It impacts on the transference and counter-transference and is a sop to therapists' conscience.
5 *A therapist-determined sliding scale where the therapist operates a 'progressive' fee system, in which the fee is determined by the patient's declared means, e.g. £1 for every £1000 income*, widens the pool of potential patients. Patients may not be entirely honest about their resources (e.g. failing to 'mention' unearned income) – which can undermine therapeutic honesty but also provide useful transferential material. This potentially reduces therapists' earnings but, given supply and demand, does not necessarily do so.
6 *A patient-determined sliding scale in which therapists declare their range (e.g. between £10 and £100 per session), and patients say what they can/will pay*, widens the pool and provides useful transferential information. The fee can change as therapy progresses. Potentially limits therapists' earnings.

As an NHS psychiatrist I remain eternally grateful that the taxpayer relieved me of having to charge my patients for my work. Nevertheless, by German standards NHS psychoanalytic therapy provision is pitiful. My friend might argue that those patients I did see would have got a better service, and been more motivated to change, had they had to pay something commensurate with their income.

Given that the German system is unlikely to be instituted in the UK in any foreseeable future, if therapists want to extend psychoanalytic therapy to the less well-off, genuinely sliding-scale practice will need to become much more widespread than I suspect is currently the case. Perhaps there should be an Association of Sliding Scale Psychoanalytic Psychotherapists (ASSPAP), whose members can be designated on the roster so that poorer patients can identify which therapists are likely to be within their means. They might also by the end of therapy be able to de-code the cryptic Kleinian message embedded in the acronym, or even come to the conclusion that, in its rightful place, money is 'good shit'.

CHAPTER 26

WHAT EXACTLY DO YOU *DO*?

Like many people in our profession, I have learned, rather painfully, to be wary in social situations when asked what it is that I 'do'. I usually begin by saying I work in a hospital or university, move on, but only if encouraged to do so, to explain that I am a 'medic'/doctor, and then await further expressions of interest before confessing that I am a psychiatrist. This can induce a variety of responses, including embarrassed laughter, a nonplussed conversational lacuna, an instant change of conversational direction, an extended enquiry about how to deal with an eating-disordered daughter or an alcoholic husband, or a probe about what species of psychiatrist I might be – the pill-pushing or psychoanalytic variety. If I am incautious enough to confess to being psychoanalytically minded (but not, as it happens, a 'proper' psychoanalyst, of which more later) the conversation will then turn to the mysterious conflation in the lay mind between psychotherapist, psychoanalyst, psychologist and psychiatrist. Finally, my interlocutor (if not by now beating a hasty retreat) will ask such questions as: 'Does that mean you are especially perceptive and can see things about us which normal people don't notice?'; 'Don't you find it depressing listening to people's problems all day long?'; 'Do you ever actually cure anybody?'; 'Aren't your patients just bored housewives with nothing better to do than come and talk to weird types like you?'

Faced with such an onslaught, it is hard not to be defensive. Once, in answer to the perceptiveness question, I found myself responding with mock portentousness: 'Yes, although we have only just met, I can see into the innermost recesses of your soul, instantly knowing everything about you, your sexual hangups laid bare before me without you having to utter a word ...'

What's going on here? Do psycho-babblers in Paris, New York or Tel Aviv have the same difficulties, or is it just we repressed Brits who cannot deal with our inner world and the sexual innuendo that surrounds the unconscious? Or is it my own ambivalence about our subject which prevents me from being more unabashed about promoting the vital importance of a psychological perspective?

This ambivalence runs not just through medicine but through psychiatry itself. Explaining to psychiatric colleagues that I am primarily a psychotherapist often elicits the response, 'Oh, so you're a *believer*...' Working, as I did, in a district general hospital, in which all medical specialties are represented, prejudice can be even more naked. When the hospital's chief surgeon first came to my quiet, comfortably furnished, yet essentially modest office, he was visibly envious that such a lowly specialty as psychiatry should be better endowed than his cramped space shared with a secretary. I tried to explain to him that my consulting room was the equivalent of his operating theatre, and that exploring the psyche can in its own way be as delicate a task as his most tricky operations. He remained unconvinced, but a grudging respect and friendship grew up between us, based mainly on a shared loathing for management-ese and devaluation of professionalism in the NHS. But the idea that psychiatry is a medical interloper, suitable only for doctors who are dim or disturbed, or both, and that psychiatric work doesn't really equate to the life-and-death theatre of 'real' medicine, dies hard.

How then to respond? Here I tend to adopt two main strategies. The first is to try to outplay my opponents at their own game. I emphasise the scientific basis of psychological therapies, citing evidence that psychotherapy is as effective in treating depression as anti-depressants, without concomitant side-effects. I quote effect sizes and the mechanisms of action of therapy: remoralisation, creating a secure base from which to explore, the activation of mastery and agency that psychotherapy alone can induce, and the importance of fostering mentalising in the intimate world of our intensely social species. At the same time I suggest that so-called evidence-based medicine can be a lot *less* scientific than it purports to be, that many physical problems are psychological in origin, and that good doctoring in all its guises contains a large psychotherapeutic component.

My second tack is reserved for the particular kind of sceptic whose objection to psychotherapy is more political than scientific – those who suggest it is an opiate which diverts people from facing the problems of material deprivation and the social causes of distress such as income inequality. Here I try to join with them in the idea that psychotherapy, at its best, is a form of humanism that celebrates the essential value of the individual and helps people to realise their true potential. I see psychotherapy as embodying an existential ethic that enables its subjects to take responsibility for themselves and their lives, facing up to the destructive and life-diminishing as well as the creative possibilities of the human condition.

It would be good to end on this upbeat note. But, as may be apparent throughout this volume, there is a part of me that identifies with psychotherapy's critics. Perhaps it is linked with my father's proud claim that, unlike his Jewish wife and son, *he* had no unconscious and, what's more, had no intention of ever developing one! When, some 40 years ago, I considered applying for training as a 'full' kosher psychoanalyst at the UK Institute of Psychoanalysis, in the end I did not go ahead, consciously at least because I did not wish to become part of what I perceived to be an esoteric cult. I have ever since been stuck with the consequences of that rather ill-informed and arrogant decision. But at least as a psychiatrist I was reasonably clear what my skills consisted of – being unfazed by madness or unprovoked violence, and knowing roughly what to do when someone is psychologically disturbed. Alongside that unglamorous but socially necessary work lies the elusive, fascinating, quasi-priestly role of the psychotherapist, a professional who can legitimately claim expertise in the field of the inner world and interpersonal relationships, and who is able to channel his or her own wounded-healer 'illness' in the service of others. If my original perception that analysts are people who tend to dine exclusively with other analysts has within it a grain of truth, that is perhaps because no such revelations are necessary. But I would still love someone to tell me, even at this late stage – as my professional identity begins slowly to dissolve – how to slip one's job description as a psycho-professional into dinner party talk without its becoming a conversation-stopper.

SOURCES

Chapter 1   Interview with Dianna Kenny. In D. Kenny (2013), *From id to inter-subjectivity: talking about the talking cure with master clinicians.* London: Karnac Books.

Chapter 2   Ten books. *British Journal of Psychiatry* (2001) 179: 468–71.

Chapter 3   Varicose veins: an optional illness. *Practitioner* (1970) 204: 549–54; J. Herman (1997) A paper that changed my practice. *British Medical Journal*, 315: 0.8.

Chapter 4   The sibling and psychotherapy: a review with clinical examples. *British Journal of Medical Psychology* (1980) 53: 297–305.

Chapter 5   The psychology of nuclear disarmament. *Psychiatric Bulletin* (1982) 6: 136–8.

Chapter 6   Psychoanalytic psychotherapy. In J. Holmes, ed. (1991), *A textbook of psychotherapy in psychiatric practice*, pp. 3–29. Edinburgh: Churchill.

Chapter 7   An attachment model of depression: integrating findings from the mood disorder laboratory. *Psychiatry: Interpersonal and Biological Processes* (2013) 76: 68–86; A doctor's perspective, postscript to Through the wasteland: chronic depression. *British Medical Journal* (2011) 342: d93.

Chapter 8   Bentall's black-and-white blast. *Cognitive Neuropsychiatry* (2011) 16: 562–6.

Chapter 9   Narrative in psychiatry and psychotherapy: the evidence? *Medical Humanities* (2000) 26: 92–6.

Chapter 10   Psychodynamic psychiatry: rise, decline and revival. In S. Bloch, S. A. Green & J. Holmes, eds (2014), *Psychiatry: Past, Present, and Prospect.* Oxford: Oxford University Press.

Chapter 11   Family and individual therapy: comparisons and contrasts. *British Journal of Psychiatry* (1985) 147: 668–76.

Chapter 12   Psychoanalysis and CBT: confluence of theory, watershed in practice? In D. Loewenthal & R. House, eds (2010), *Critically Engaging CBT.* New York: McGraw-Hill.

Chapter 13   Integration in psychoanalytic psychotherapy: an attachment meta-perspective. *Psychoanalytic Psychotherapy* (2010) 24: 183–201.

Chapter 14   Superego: an attachment perspective. *International Journal of Psychoanalysis* (2011) 92: 1221–40.

Chapter 15   Donnel Stern and relational psychoanalysis. *British Journal of Psychotherapy* (2011) 27: 305–15.

Chapter 16   On Bowlby's 'trilogy'. *British Journal of Psychiatry* (2013) 202: 371.

Chapter 17   Are we all Balintians now? *British Medical Journal* (2008) 337: a1549.

Chapter 18   David Malan. In F. Osimo & M. J. Stein, eds (2012), *Theory and practice of experiential dynamic therapy*. London: Karnac Books.

Chapter 19   Anthony Storr. In J. Holmes (2012), *Storr's The art of psychotherapy*. 3rd rev. ed., London: Hodder Arnold.

Chapter 20   Dr Jonathan Pedder. *The Psychiatrist* (2010) 34: 358.

Chapter 21   Charles Rycroft's contribution to contemporary psychoanalytic psychotherapy. *American Journal of Psychoanalysis* (2010) 70: 180–92.

Chapter 22   Untied. *British Medical Journal* (2000) 321: 999.

Chapter 23   Good doctor, bad doctor: a psychodynamic approach. *British Medical Journal* (2002) 325: 722.1.

Chapter 24   How often do you do it? *New Associations* (2011) 6.

Chapter 25   How much do you charge? *New Associations* (2012) 8.

Chapter 26   What exactly do you *do*? In J. Raphael-Leff, ed. (2002), *Between sessions and beyond the couch*, pp. 208–10. Colchester: University of Essex Press.

REFERENCES

Abbass, A. (2006) Intensive short-term dynamic psychotherapy of treatment-resistant depression: a pilot study. *Depression and Anxiety* 23: 449–52.

Abbass, A., Sheldon, A., Gyra, J., & Kalpin, A. (2008) Intensive short-term dynamic psychotherapy for DSM-IV personality disorders: a randomized controlled trial. *Journal of Nervous & Mental Disease* 196: 211–16.

Abraham, K. (1924) *Selected papers*, ed. E. Jones. London: Hogarth Press.

Ahktar, S. (2012) *Good stuff: generosity, resilience, humility, gratitude, forgiveness & sacrifice.* New York: Jason Aronson.

Ainsworth, M., Blehar, M., Waters, E., & Wall, S. (1978) *Patterns of attachment: a psychological study of the Strange Situation.* Hillsdale, NJ: Lawrence Erlbaum.

Allen, J. G. (2013a) *Restoring mentalizing in attachment relationships.* Arlington, VA: American Psychiatric Association.

Allen, J. (2013b) *Mentalising in the development and treatment of attachment trauma.* London: Karnac Books.

Altus, W. D. (1966) Birth order and its sequelae. *Science* 151: 44–9.

Andrews, G., Pollock, C., & Stewart, G (1989) The determination of defense style by questionnaire. *Archives of General Psychiatry* 46: 455–60.

Ansbacher, H. L., & Ansbacher, R. R. (1958) *The individual psychology of Alfred Adler.* New York: Harper & Row.

Aron, L. (1996) *A meeting of minds: mutuality in psychoanalysis.* Hillsdale, NJ: Analytic Press.

Artero, S., Touchon, J., Dupuy, Malafosse, A., & Richie, K. (2011) War exposure, 50-HTTLPR genotype and lifetime risk of depression. *British Journal of Psychiatry* 199: 43–8.

Avdi, E. (2008) Analysing talk in the talking cure: conversation, discourse, and narrative analysis of psychoanalytic psychotherapy. *European Psychotherapy* 8(1): 69–88.

Avdi, E., & Georgaca, E. (2007) Narrative research in psychotherapy: a critical review. *Psychology and Psychotherapy: Research and Practice* 78: 1–14.

Balint, M. (1957) *The doctor, his patient and the illness.* London: Pitman.

Barker, C. (1983) The psychotherapist. In N. T. Singleton (ed.), *The analysis of real skills: social skills.* London: Oxford University Press.

Barnett, B. (2007) *You ought to! A psychoanalytic study of the superego and conscience.* London: Karnac Books.

Bateman, A., & Fonagy, P. (2004) *Psychotherapy for borderline personality disorder: mentalization-based treatment.* Oxford: Oxford University Press.

Bateman, A., & Fonagy, P. (2008) 8-year follow-up of patients treated for borderline personality disorder: mentalization-based treatment versus treatment as usual. *American Journal of Psychiatry* 165: 631–8.

Bateman, A., Brown, D., & Pedder, J. (2010) *Introduction to psychotherapy: an outline of psychodynamic principles and practice.* 4th ed., London: Routledge.

Bateson, G. (1972) *Steps to an ecology of mind.* New York: Paladin.

Beebe, B., Lachmann, F., Markese, S., & Bahrick, L. (2012) On the origins of disorganized attachment and internal working models. *Psychoanalytic Dialogues* 22: 352–74.

Beiber, I., Dain, H. J., Dince, P. R., *et al.* (1962) *Homosexuality: a psychoanalytic study.* New York: Basic Books.

Belsky, J., Houts, R. M., & Fearon, R. M. (2010) Infant attachment security and the timing of puberty: testing an evolutionary hypothesis. *Psychological Science* 21: 1195–201.

Benjamin, J. (2004) Beyond doer and done to: an intersubjective view of thirdness. *Psychoanalytic Quarterly* 73: 5–46.

Bentall, R. (2010) *Doctoring the mind: why psychiatric treatments fail.* London: Penguin.

Bergin, A., & Garfield, S. (1994) *Handbook of psychotherapy and behaviour change.* Chichester: Wiley.

Berlin, I. (1953) *The hedgehog and the fox: an essay on Tolstoy's view of history.* London: Weidenfeld & Nicolson.

Bersani, L., & Phillips, A. (2008) *Intimacies.* Chicago: University of Chicago Press.

Bettelheim, B. (1969) *The children of the dream.* London: Thames & Hudson.

Bettelheim, B. (1982) *Freud and man's soul.* New York: Knopf.

Bion, W. R. (1967) *Second thoughts.* New York: Jason Aronson.

Bion, W. R. (1970) *Attention and interpretation.* London: Tavistock.

Bion, W. R. (1978) *Sao Paulo clinical seminars.* In *Clinical seminars and four papers.* Oxford: Fleetwood Press, 1987, pp. 131–222.

Blass, R. B. (2010) Affirming 'That's not psychoanalysis!': on the value of the politically incorrect act of attempting to define the limits of our field. *International Journal of Psychoanalysis* 91: 81–9.

Blatt, S. (2008) *Polarities of experience: relatedness and self-definition in personality development, psychopathology and the therapeutic process.* Washington, DC: American Psychological Association.

Bleiberg, E. (2006) Treating professionals in crisis: a mentalization-based specialized inpatient program. In J. Allen & P. Fonagy (eds), *Handbook of mentalization-based treatment,* pp. 233–48. Chichester: Wiley.

Bloch, S., & Crouch, E. (1985) *Therapeutic factors in group psychotherapy.* Oxford: Oxford University Press.

Bollas, C. (1987) *The shadow of the object: psychoanalysis of the unthought known.* London: Free Association Books.

Bollas, C. (2007) *The Freudian moment.* London: Karnac Books.

Bollas, C. (2011) *The Christopher Bollas reader.* London: Routledge.

Bolton, D., & Hill, J. (1996) *Mind, meaning and mental disorder.* Cambridge, MA: MIT Press.

Boston Change Process Study Group (2008) Forms of relational meaning: issues in the relation between the implicit and reflective verbal domains. *Psychoanalytic Dialogues* 18: 125–48.

Bowlby, J. (1971) *Attachment.* London: Penguin.

Bowlby, J. (1980) *Loss: sadness and depression.* London: Hogarth Press.

Bowlby, J. (1988) *A secure base.* London: Routledge.

Brearley, M. (2007) What do psychoanalysts do? In L. Braddock & M. Lacewing (eds), *The academic face of psychoanalysis,* pp. 20–32. London: Routledge.

Brenner, C. (1955) *An elementary textbook of psychoanalysis.* New York: Doubleday.

Brim, O. G. (1958) Family structure and sex role learning by children. *Sociometry* 21: 1–16.

Britton, R. (2006) Emancipation from the super-ego: a clinical study of the Book of Job. In D. Black (ed.), *Psychoanalysis and religion in the 21st century,* pp. 83–96. London: Routledge.

Brody, A.L., *et al.* (2001) Brain metabolic changes associated with symptom factor improvement in major depressive disorder. *Biological Psychiatry* 50: 171–8.

Bromberg, P. (2010) *Awakening the dreamer.* London: Routledge.

Brown, G. W., & Harris, T. O. (1978) *The social origins of depression.* London: Tavistock.

Brown, G. W., Bhrolchain, M. N., & Harris, T. (1975) Social class and psychiatric disturbance among women in an urban population. *Sociology* 9: 225–54.

Butler, A., Chapman, J., Forman, E., & Beck, A. (2006) The empirical status of CBT: a review of meta-analyses. *Clinical Psychology Review* 26: 17–31.

Byng-Hall, J. (1980) Symptom-bearer as marital distance-regulator: clinical implications. *Family Process* 19: 335–65.

Caper, R. (1998) *A mind of one's own*. London: Routledge.

Carhart-Harris, R., Mayberg, H., Malizia, A., & Nutt, R. (2008) Mourning and melancholia revisited: correspondences between principles of Freudian metapsychology and empirical findings of neuropsychiatry. *Annals of General Psychiatry* 7: 9–42.

Carmeli, Z., & Blass, R. (2010) The relational turn in psychoanalysis: revolution or regression. *European Journal of Psychotherapy and Counselling* 12: 217–24.

Casement, P. (1985) *On learning from the patient*. London: Tavistock.

Caspi, A., Moffitt, T., Taylor, A., Craig, I., Harrison, H., *et al.* (2003) Influence of life stress on depression polymorphism in the 5-HTT gene. *Science* 301: 386–9.

Castonguay, L. G., & Beutler, L. E. (2006) *Principles of therapeutic change that work*. Oxford: Oxford University Press.

Castonguay, L. G., Goldfried, M. R., Wiser, S. L., Raue, P. J., & Hayes, A. M. (1996) Predicting the effect of cognitive therapy for depression: a study of unique and common factors. *Journal of Consulting and Clinical Psychology* 64: 497–504.

Cavell, M. (2006) *Becoming a subject*. Oxford: Oxford University Press.

Champagne, F. (2010) Early adversity and developmental outcomes: interactions between genetics, epigenetics and social experiences across the lifespan. *Perspectives on Psychological Science* 5: 564–74.

Christie, G. (2009) Humour. In S. Akhtar (ed.), *Good feelings: psychoanalytic reflections on positive emotions and attitudes*. London: Karnac Books.

Clare, A. (1976) *Psychiatry in dissent*. London: Tavistock.

Clarkin, J. F., Frances, A., & Moodie, J. (1979) Selection criteria for family therapy. *Family Therapy* 18: 391–403.

Clarkin, J. F., Levy, K. N., Lenzenweger, M. F., & Kernberg, O. F. (2007) A multiwave RCT evaluating three treatments for borderline personality disorder. *American Journal of Psychiatry* 164: 922–8.

Coles, P. (2003) *The importance of sibling relationships in psychoanalysis*. London. Karnac Books.

Crandell, L. E., Patrick, M. P., & Hobson, R. P. (2003) 'Still-face' interactions between mothers with borderline personality disorder and their 2-month-old infants. *British Journal of Psychiatry* 183: 239–47.

Damacio, A. (1994) *Descartes' error*. New York: Jason Aronson.

Dare, C., Eisler, I., Russell, G., Treasure, J., & Dodge, L. (2001) Psychological therapies for adults with anorexia nervosa: randomised controlled trial of out-patient treatments. *British Journal of Psychiatry* 178: 216–21.

Deutsch, F. (1957) A footnote to Freud's 'Fragment of an analysis of a case hysteria'. *Psychoanalytic Quarterly* 26: 159–67.

Diamond, D., Stovall-McClough, C., Clarkin, J., & Levy, K. (2003) Patient–therapist attachment in the treatment of borderline personality disorder. *Bulletin of the Menninger Clinic* 67: 227–59.

Doi, T. (1989) The concept of *amae* and its psychoanalytic implications. *International Review of Psycho-Analysis* 16: 349–54.

Eagle, M. (2007) Attachment and sexuality. In D. Diamond, S. Blatt, & J. Litchenburg (eds), *Attachment and sexuality*. Hillsdale, NJ: Academic Press.

Eagleton, T. (2007) *How to read a poem*. Oxford: Blackwell.

Eliot, G. (1876) *Daniel Deronda*. New York: Harper.

Eliot, T. S. (1986) *Collected poems*. London: Faber & Faber.

Elkin, I., *et al.* (1989) National Institute of Mental Health Treatment of Depression Collaborative Research Program. *Archives of General Psychiatry* 46: 971–82.

Erikson, E. (1950) *Childhood and society*. New York: Basic Books.

Erikson, E. (1959) *Young man Luther*. London: Faber & Faber.

Erikson, E. (1965) *Childhood and society*. 2nd ed., London: Penguin.

Etchegoyen, H. (2005) *The fundamentals of psychoanalytic technique*. London: Karnac Books.

Fairbairn, W. (1954) *An object-relations theory of the personality*. London: Hogarth Press.

Farber, B. (2006) *Self-disclosure in psychotherapy*. New York: Guilford Press.

Farber, B., & Metzger, J. (2008) The therapist as secure base. In J. Obegi & E. Berant (eds), *Clinical applications of adult psychotherapy and research*, pp. 46–70. New York: Guilford Press.

Feldman, A. (1966) Psychoanalysis and Shakespeare by Norman Holland: review. *Psychoanalytic Review* 53: 148–53.

Fingarette, H. (1963) *The self in transformation*. New York: Basic Books.

Fink, B. (1997) *A clinical introduction to Lacanian psychoanalysis*. Cambridge, MA: Harvard University Press.

Fleugel, J. C. (1921) *The psychoanalytic study of the family*. London: Hogarth Press.

Fonagy, P. (1998) Moments of change in psychoanalytic theory: discussion of a new theory of psychic change. *Infant Mental Health Journal* 19: 346–53.

Fonagy, P. (2006) The failure of practice to inform theory and the role of implicit theory in bridging the transmission gap. In J. Canestri (ed.), *Psychoanalysis from practice to theory*. Chichester: Wiley.

Fonagy, P. (2009) Postscript. *Psychoanalytic Psychotherapy* 23: 276–80.

Fonagy, P., & Bateman, A. (2006) Progress in the treatment of borderline personality disorder. *British Journal of Psychiatry* 188: 1–3.

Fonagy, P., & Target, M. (2007) The rooting of the mind in the body: new links between attachment theory and psychoanalytic thought. *Journal of the American Psychoanalytic Association* 55: 412–56.

Fonagy, P., Gergely, G., Jurist, E., & Target, M. (2002) *Affect regulation, mentalization, and the development of the self*. New York: Other Press.

Fonagy, P., Gergely, G., & Target, M. (2008) Psychoanalytic constructs and attachment theory and research. In J. Cassidy & P. Shaver (eds), *Handbook of attachment*, pp. 783–810. 2nd ed., New York: Guilford Press.

Frank, J. (1986) Psychotherapy: the transformation of meanings. *Journal of the Royal Society of Medicine* 79: 341–6.

Freud, A. (1936) *The ego and the mechanisms of defence*. London: Hogarth Press.

Freud, A. (1969) *Indications for child analysis*. London: Hogarth Press.

Freud, A. (1998) *Selected writings*. London: Penguin.

Freud, S. (1905) Fragment of an analysis of a case of hysteria. *SE*, 7: 1–122.

Freud, S. (1911–15) Papers on technique. *SE*, 12.

Freud, S. (1913) On beginning the treatment (further recommendations on the technique of psycho-analysis, I). *SE*, 12.

Freud, S. (1914) On narcissism: an introduction. *SE*, 14: 67–102.

Freud, S. (1916) Introductory lectures on psychoanalysis. *SE*, 16, 17.

Freud, S. (1917) Mourning and melancholia. *SE*, 14: 243–58.

Freud, S. (1919) Lines of advance in psychoanalytic therapy. *SE*, 17: 157–68.

Freud, S. (1921) Group psychology and the analysis of the ego. *SE*, 18.

Freud, S. (1923) The ego and the id. *SE*, 19.

Freud, S. (1926) The question of lay analysis. *SE*, 20.

Freud, S. (1927) Humour. *SE*, 21: 159–66.

Freud, S. (1930) Civilisation and its discontents. *SE*, 19: 57–145.

Freud, S. (1933) New introductory lectures in psychoanalysis. *SE*, 22: 1–182.

Freud, S. (1938) Splitting of the ego in the process of defence. *SE*, 23.

Fromm-Reichman, F. (1959) *Psychoanalysis and psychotherapy: collected papers*. Chicago: University of Chicago Press.

Fulford, W. (1988) *Moral theory and medical practice*. Cambridge: Cambridge University Press.

Gabbard, G. (1989) *Sexual exploitation of professional relations*. Washington, DC: American Psychiatric Press.

Gabbard, G. (1994) *Psychodynamic psychiatry in clinical practice: the DSM-IV edition*. Washington, DC: American Psychiatric Press.

Gabbard, G. (2004) *Long-term psychoanalytic psychotherapy: a basic text*. Arlington, VA: American Psychiatric Press.

Gabbard, G. (2005) Major modalities of psychotherapy: psychodynamic. In G. Gabbard, J. Beck, & J. Holmes (eds), *Oxford textbook of psychotherapy*. Oxford: Oxford University Press.

Gabbard, G., Lazar, S., Horngerger, J., & Spiegel, D. (1997) The economic impact of psychotherapy: a review. *American Journal of Psychiatry* 154: 147–55.

Gabbard, G., & Westen, D. (2003) Rethinking therapeutic action. *International Journal of Psycho-analysis* 84: 823–41.

Gadamer, H.-G. (2004 [1965]) *Truth and method*, trans. J. Weisheimer & D. Marshall. London: Continuum.

Garland, C. (1982) Taking the non-problem seriously. *Group Analysis* 12: 4–14.

Garland, C. (1998) *Understanding trauma: a psychoanalytic perspective*. London: Butterworth.

Gelder, M. G., López-Ibor, J. J., & Andreasen, N. C. (2000) *New Oxford textbook of psychiatry*. Oxford: Oxford University Press.

Gergely, G. (2007) The social construction of the subjective self. In L. Mayes, P. Fonagy, & M. Target (eds), *Developmental science and psychoanalysis*, pp. 39–63. London: Karnac Books.

Gibson, R. F. (ed.) (2004) *The Cambridge companion to Quine*. Cambridge: Cambridge University Press.

Gilbert, P. (2006). Evolution and depression: issues and implications. *Psychological Medicine* 36: 287–97.

Gladwell, M. (2008) *Outliers*. New York: Little, Brown.

Goffman, I. (1961) *Asylums*. London: Penguin.

Goldberg, D. (2009) The interplay between biological and psychological factors in determining vulnerability to mental disorders. *Psychoanalytic Psychotherapy* 24: 236–47.

Grant, S., Margison, F., & Powell, A. (1991) The future of psychotherapy services. *Psychiatric Bulletin* 15: 174–9.

Gray, P. (1994) *The ego and analysis of defense*. Northville, NJ: Jason Aronson.

Greenberg, H., Mayer, D., Guerena, R., et al. (1963) Order of birth as a determinant of personality and attitudinal characteristics. *Journal of Social Psychology* 60: 221–30.

Greenberg, J., & Mitchell, S. (1983) *Object relations in psychoanalysis*. Cambridge, MA: Harvard University Press.

Grossmann, K., Grossmann, K. & Waters, E. (2005) *Attachment from infancy to adulthood: the major longitudinal studies*. New York: Guilford Press.

Grotstein, J. (2007) *A beam of intense darkness*. London: Karnac Books.

Gustafson, J. (1986) *The complex secret of brief psychotherapy*. New York: Norton.

Guthrie, E., Creed, F., Dawson, D., & Tomenson, B. (1991) A randomized control trial of psychotherapy in patients with refractory irritable bowel syndrome. *Gastroenterology* 100: 450–57.

Haley, J. (1977) *Problem-solving therapy*. San Francisco, CA: Jossey-Bass.

Hall, A., & Fagan, R. (1956) Definition of system. *Yearbook for the Advancement of General Systems Theory* 1: 18–28.

Hamilton, V. (1982) *Narcissus and Oedipus*. London: Routledge.

Hare, E. H., & Price, J. S. (1969) Birth order and family size: bias caused by changes in birth rate. *British Journal of Psychiatry* 15: 647–57.

Hart, J. T. (1971) The inverse care law. *The Lancet* 297: 405–12.

Hayes, A. M., Castonguay, L. G., & Goldfried, M. R. (1996) Effectiveness of targeting the vulnerability factors of depression in cognitive therapy. *Journal of Consulting and Clinical Psychology* 64: 623–7.

Heard, D., & Lake, B. (1997) *The challenge of attachment for care-giving*. London: Routledge.

Hill, D. (1954) Psychotherapy and the physical methods of treatment in psychiatry. *Journal of Medical Science* 100: 360–74.

Hobson, J. (1985) *Forms of feeling*. London: Routledge.

Hobson, P. (2002) *The cradle of thought.* London: Macmillan.

Hobson, R. (1985) *The heart of psychotherapy.* London: Routledge.

Hoffman, L. (1981) *Foundations of family therapy.* New York: Basic Books.

Hoglend, P., Kjell-Petter, B., Svein, A., *et al.* (2008) Transference interpretations in psycho-analytic psychotherapy: do they yield sustained effects? *American Journal of Psychiatry* 165: 763–84.

Holmes, J. (1983) Psychoanalysis and family therapy: Freud's Dora case reconsidered. *Journal of Family Therapy* 5: 235–51.

Holmes, J. (1985) The language of psychotherapy. *British Journal of Psychotherapy* 1: 240–54.

Holmes, J. (1993/2013) *John Bowlby and attachment theory.* 2nd ed., London: Routledge.

Holmes, J. (1997) *Attachment, autonomy, intimacy.* New York: Jason Aronson.

Holmes, J. (2001) All you need is CBT. *British Medical Journal* 324: 288–94.

Holmes, J. (2010) *Exploring in security: towards an attachment-informed psychoanalytic psychotherapy.* London: Routledge.

Holmes, J. (2011) Superego: an attachment perspective. *International Journal of Psychoanalysis* 92: 1221–40.

Holmes, J. (2012) *Storr's The art of psychotherapy.* London: Hodder Arnold.

Holmes, J. (2013) *The therapeutic imagination: using literature to deepen psychodynamic understanding and enhance empathy.* London: Routledge.

Holmes, J., & Bateman, A. (2002) (eds) *Integration in psychotherapy.* Oxford: Oxford University Press.

Holmes, J., & Lindley, R. (1997) *The values of psychotherapy.* London: Karnac Books.

Hopkins, G. M. (1953) *Poems and prose.* Harmondsworth: Penguin.

Hrdy, S. (1999) *Mother Nature.* London: Penguin.

Humphrey, N. (1983) *Consciousness regained.* Oxford: Oxford University Press.

Imber, S., Pilkonis, P., Sotsky, S., *et al.* (1990) Mode-specific effects among three treatments for depression. *Journal of Consulting and Clinical Psychology* 58: 352–9.

Ito, T. (1998) Negative information weighs more heavily on the brain: the negativity bias in evaluative categorizations. *Journal of Personality and Social Psychology* 75: 887–900.

Jackson, D., & Haley, J. (1963) Transference revisited. *Journal of Nervous and Mental Disease* 137: 363–71.

James, O. (2007) *Affluenza.* London: Vermillion.

Kächele, H., Schachter, J., & Thomä, H. (2009) *From psychoanalytic narrative to empirical single case research: implications for psychoanalytic practice.* London: Routledge.

Kandel, E. R. (1999) Biology and the future of psychoanalysis: a new intellectual framework for psychiatry revisited. *American Journal of Psychiatry* 156: 505–24.

Karasu, T. (1986) The psychotherapies: benefits and limitations. *American Journal of Psychotherapy* 40: 324–42.

Kelly, G. A. (1955) *The psychology of personal constructs.* New York: Norton.

Kenny, D. (2011) *The psychology of music performance anxiety.* Oxford: Oxford University Press.

Kernberg, O. (1984) *Object relations and clinical psychoanalysis.* Northville, NJ: Jason Aronson.

Kernberg, O. (2009) The concept of the death-drive: a clinical perspective. *International Journal of Psychoanalysis* 90: 1009–23.

Khan, M. (1983) *Hidden selves: between theory and practice in psychoanalysis.* London: Hogarth Press.

King, P. (2003) *No ordinary psychoanalyst: the exceptional contribution of John Rickman.* London: Karnac Books.

Klein, M. (1948) *Contributions to psychoanalysis.* London: Hogarth Press.

Klein, M. (1957) *Envy and gratitude.* London: Hogarth Press.

Klein, M. (1969) *Collected writings,* vol. 3, ed. R. Money-Kyrie. London: Hogarth Press.

Koch, H. L. (1955) Some personality correlates of sex, sibling position and sex of sibling among five- and six-year-old children. *Genetic Psychology Monographs* 52: 3–50.

Koch, H. L. (1956) Some emotional attitudes of the young child in relation to characteristics of his sibling. *Child Development* 27: 393–426.

Kohon, G. (1986) *The British school of psychoanalysis: the independent tradition*. London: Free Association Books.

Kohut, H. (1977) *The restoration of the self*. New York: International University Press.

Kuhn, T. (1977) *The essential tension: selected studies in scientific tradition and change*. Chicago: University of Chicago Press.

Kuyken, W., Watkins, E., & Beck, A. (2005) CBT for mood disorders. In G. Gabbard, J. Beck, & J. Holmes (eds), *Oxford textbook of psychotherapy*, pp. 111–26. Oxford: Oxford University Press.

Kuyken, W., et al. (2010) How does mindfulness-based cognitive behavioural therapy work? *Behaviour Research and Therapy* 48: 1105–12.

Laing, R. (1960) *The divided self*. London: Penguin.

Lambert, M. (2003) *Bergin & Garfield's Handbook of psychotherapy and behaviour change*. 5th ed., New York: Wiley.

Larkin, P. (1955). *The less deceived*. London: Marvell Press.

Lasko, J. K. (1954) Parent behaviour towards first and second children. *Genetic Psychology Monographs* 49: 96–137.

Lear, J. (1993) An interpretation of transference. *International Journal of Psycho-analysis* 74: 739–55.

Lear, J. (2003) *Therapeutic action: an earnest plea for irony*. London: Karnac Books.

Lear, J. (2009) Technique and final cause in psychoanalysis: four ways of looking at one moment. *International Journal of Psycho-analysis* 90: 1299–317.

Lederer, J. (2009) *Family Action Newham: perinatal support project*. London: Family Action.

LeDoux, J. (1994) Emotion, memory and the brain. *Scientific American* 270: 32–9.

Leichsenring, F., & Rabung, S. (2008) Effectiveness of long-term psychodynamic psychotherapy: a meta-analysis. *Journal of the American Medical Association* 300: 1551–65.

Leichsenring, F., & Rabung, S. (2011) Long-term psychodynamic psychotherapy in complex mental disorders: update of a meta-analysis. *British Journal of Psychiatry* 199: 15–22.

Leichsenring, F., Rabung, S., & Leibing, E. (2004) The efficacy of short-term psychodynamic psychotherapy in specific psychiatric disorders: a meta-analysis. *Archives of General Psychiatry* 61: 1208–16.

Leiman, M. (1995) Early development. In A. Ryle (ed.), *Cognitive analytic therapy: developments in theory and practice*. Chichester: Wiley.

Lemma, A. (2009) Commentary on Christie. In S. Akhtar (ed.), *Good feelings: psychoanalytic reflections on positive emotions and attitudes*. London: Karnac Books.

Lemma, A., Fonagy, P., & Target, M. (2012) *Dynamic interpersonal therapy*. London: Routledge.

Lemma, A., Roth, A., & Pilling, S. (2008) *The competences required to deliver effective psychoanalytic/psychodynamic psychotherapy*. London: Research Department of Clinical, Educational and Health Psychology, UCL; www.ucl.ac.uk/clinical-psychology/CORE/Psychodynamic_ Competences/Background_Paper.pdf.

Lemma, A., Target, M., & Fonagy, P. (2010) The development of a brief psychodynamic protocol for depression: dynamic interpersonal therapy. *Psychoanalytic Psychotherapy* 24: 329–46.

Lesser, M., & Lesser, B. Z. (1983) Alexithymia. *American Journal of Psychiatry* 140: 1305–8.

Levy, D. M. (1935) Maternal over-protection and rejection. *Archives of Neurology and Psychiatry* 25: 886–9.

Levy, D. M. (1939) Sibling rivalry studies in children of primitive groups. *American Journal of Orthopsychiatry* 9: 205–15.

Levy, K. (2008) Psychotherapies and lasting change. *American Journal of Psychiatry* 165: 556–9.

Lewin, B. D. (1951) *The psychoanalysis of elation*. London: Hogarth Press.

Linehan, M., Comtois, K., Murray, A., Brown, M. Z., Gallop, R. J., Heard, H. L., et al. (2006) Two-year randomized controlled trial and follow-up of dialectical behavior therapy vs. therapy by experts for suicidal behaviors and borderline personality disorder. *Archives of General Psychiatry* 63: 757–66.

Lorenz, K. (1959) *King Solomon's ring*. London: Butterworth.

Luborsky, L., Crits-Cristoph, P., Mintz, J., & Auerbach, A. (1989) *Who will benefit from psychotherapy?* New York: Basic Books.

Luborsky, L., & Singer, B. (1975) Comparative studies of psychotherapies: is it true that 'Everyone has won and all must have prizes'? *Archives of General Psychiatry* 32: 995–1008.

Luyten, P., & Blatt, S. (2011) Psychodynamic approaches to depression: whither shall we go? *Psychiatry* 74: 1–3.

Lynch, D., Laws, K., & McKenna, P. (2009) CBT for major psychiatric disorder: does it really work? A meta-analytical review of well-conducted trials. *Psychological Medicine* 57: 1–16.

Lyons-Ruth, K. (1999) The two-person unconscious: intersubjective dialogue, enactive relational representation, and the emergence of new forms of relational organisation. *Psychoanalytic Enquiry* 19: 576–617.

Lyons-Ruth, K., & Boston Change Process Study Group (2001) The emergence of new experiences: relational improvisation, recognition process and non-linear change in psychoanalytic psychotherapy. *Psychologist/Psychoanalyst* 21: 13–17.

Lyons-Ruth, K., & Jacobvitz, D. (2008) Attachment disorganization. In J. Cassidy & P. Shaver (eds), *Handbook of attachment*, pp. 666–97. 2nd ed., New York: Guilford Press.

McArthur, C. (1956) Personalities of first and second children. *Psychiatry* 19: 47–54.

McCluskey, U. (2005) *To be met as a person*. London: Karnac Books.

McCullough, L., Kuhn, N., Andrews, S., Kaplan, A., Wolf, J., & Hurley, C. L. (2003) *Treating affect phobia: a manual for short-term dynamic psychotherapy*. New York: Guilford Press.

McGlashan, T. (1988) A selective review of North American long-term follow-up studies of schizophrenia. *Schizophrenia Bulletin* 14: 515–42.

McGowan, P. O., Sasaki, A., D'Alessio, A. C., Dymov, S., Labonte, B., Szyf, M., *et al.* (2009) Epigenetic regulation of the glucocorticoid receptor in human brain associates with childhood abuse. *Nature Neuroscience* 12: 342–8.

MacIntyre, A. (2013) *After virtue*. London: Bloomsbury.

Madanes, C., & Haley, J. (1977) Dimensions of family therapy (1956). *Journal of Nervous and Mental Diseases* 165: 88–98.

Main, M. (1991) Metacognitive knowledge, metacognitive monitoring and singular (coherent) vs multiple (incoherent) models of attachment: findings and directions for future research. In C. Parkes, J. Stevenson-Hinde, & P. Marris (eds), *Attachment across the lifecycle*, pp. 127–59. London: Routledge.

Main, M. (1995) Recent studies in attachment: overview with selected implications for clinical work. In S. Goldberg, R. Muir, & J. Kerr (eds), *Attachment theory: social, developmental and clinical perspectives*, pp. 276–89. Hillsdale, NJ: Analytic Press.

Main, T. (1989) *The ailment and other psychoanalytic essays*. London: Free Association Books.

Malan, D. (1979) *Individual psychotherapy and the science of psychodynamics*. London: Butterworth.

Malan, D., & Della Selva, P. (2006) *Lives transformed: a revolutionary method of dynamic psychotherapy*. London: Karnac Books.

Mallinckrodt, B., Porter, M. J., & Kivlighan, D. M., Jr (2005) Client attachment to therapist, depth of in-session exploration, and object relations in brief psychotherapy. *Psychotherapy: Theory, Research, Practice, Training* 42: 85–100.

Margison, F. (2001) Psychodynamic interpersonal therapy. In J. Holmes & A. Bateman (eds), *Integration in psychotherapy: models and metaphors*. Oxford: Oxford University Press.

Martin, F. (1977) Some implications from the theory and practice of family therapy for individual therapy (and vice versa). *British Journal of Medical Psychology* 50: 53–64.

Matte-Blanco, I. (1975) *The unconscious as infinite sets*. London: Routledge.

Mayberg, H. S. (2009) Targeted electrode-based modulation of neural circuits in depression. *Journal of Clinical Investigation* 119: 717–25.

Mayberg, H. S., *et al.* (2000) Regional metabolic effects of fluoxetine in major depression: serial changes and relationship to clinical response. *Biological Psychiatry* 48: 830–43.

Mayer-Gross, W., Slater, E., & Roth, M. (1969) *Clinical psychiatry*. 3rd ed., London: Baillière-Tindall & Cassell.

Meares, R. A., & Hobson, R. F. (1978) The persecutory therapist. *British Journal of Medical Psychology* 50: 349–59.

Medawar, P. (1984) *Pluto's republic*. Oxford: Oxford University Press.

Meins, E. (1999) Sensitivity, security and internal working models: bridging the transmission gap. *Attachment and Human Development* 3: 325–42.

Mikulincer, M., & Shaver, P. (2008) Adult attachment and affect regulation. In J. Cassidy & P. Shaver (eds), *Handbook of attachment*, pp. 503–31. 2nd ed., New York: Guilford Press.

Mikulincer, M., Shaver, P., Cassidy, J., & Berant, E. (2008) Attachment-related defensive processes. In J. Obegi & E. Berant (eds), *Attachment theory and research in clinical work with adults*, pp. 293–327. New York: Guilford Press.

Milner, M. (1971) *On not being able to paint*. London: Heinemann.

Milrod, B. (2009) Psychodynamic psychotherapy outcome for generalized anxiety disorder. *American Journal of Psychiatry* 166: 841–4.

Milrod, B., Leon, A. C., Busch, F., Rudden, M., Schwalberg, M., Clarkin, J., *et al.* (2007) A randomized controlled clinical trial of psychoanalytic psychotherapy for panic disorder. *American Journal of Psychiatry* 164: 265–72.

Milton, J. (2001) Psychoanalysis and CBT – rival paradigms or common ground? *International Journal of Psychoanalysis* 82: 431–47.

Minuchin, S. (1974) *Families and family therapy*. Cambridge, MA: Harvard University Press.

Mitchell, S. (2000) *Relationality*. Hillsdale, NJ: Analytic Press.

Mollon, P. (2009) The NICE guidelines are misleading, unscientific, and potentially impeded good psychological care and help. *Psychodynamic Practice* 15: 9–24.

Murray, L. (2009) The development of children of post-natally depressed mothers: evidence from the Cambridge longitudinal study. *Psychoanalytic Psychotherapy* 23: 185–99.

Music, G. (2009) What has psychoanalysis got to do with happiness? Reclaiming the positive in psychoanalytic psychotherapy. *British Journal of Psychotherapy* 25: 435–55.

Nagel, T. (1986) *The view from nowhere*. Oxford: Oxford University Press.

Nemiroff, R., & Colarusso, C. (eds) (1985) *The race against time*. New York: Plenum Press.

Nesse, R. (2005) Is depression an adaptation? *Archives of General Psychology* 57: 14–20.

NICE (2005) *Depression: management of depression in primary and secondary care*. National Clinical Practice Guideline no. 23, http://guidance.nice.org.uk/CG23 (accessed 18 March 2011).

NICE (2009) *Depression in adults (update): draft NICE guideline for consultation*, www.nice.org.uk.

Oberlander, T. F., Weinberg, J., Papsdorf, M., Grunau, R., Misri, S., & Devlin, A. M. (2008) Prenatal exposure to maternal depression, neonatal methylation of human glucocorticoid receptor gene (NR3C1) and infant cortisol stress responses. *Epigenetics* 3: 97–106.

Ogden, T. (1979) On projective identification. *International Journal of Psycho-analysis* 60: 357–73.

Ogden, T. (1987) *The matrix of the mind*. Northvale, NJ: Jason Aronson.

Ogden, T. (1989) *The primitive edge of experience*. London: Karnac Books.

Osuch, E. A., *et al.* (2000) Regional cerebral metabolism associated with anxiety symptoms in affective disorder patients. *Biological Psychiatry* 48: 1020–23.

Padel J. (1991) Fairbairn's thought on the relationship of inner and outer worlds. *Free Associations* 2: 589–615.

Palazolli, M., *et al.* (1978) *Paradox and counter-paradox*. New York: Jason Thomson.

Panksepp, J., & Watt, D. (2011) Why does depression hurt? *Psychiatry* 74: 5–13.

Papp, P. J. (1976) Family choreography. In P. J. Guerin (ed.), *Family therapy*. New York: Gauden Press.

Parker, G. (1979) Parental characteristics in relation to depressive disorders. *British Journal of Psychiatry* 134: 138–47.

Parkes, C. M. (1975) *Bereavement*. London: Penguin.

Parkes, C. M. (1996) *Bereavement: Studies of Grief in Adult Life*. 3rd ed., London: Penguin.

Parkes, C. M. (2006) *Love and loss: the roots of grief and its complications*. 2nd ed., London: Routledge.

Parry, G., Roth, A., & Kerr, I. (2005) Brief and time-limited therapy. In G. Gabbard, J. Beck, & J. Holmes (eds), *Oxford textbook of psychotherapy*, pp. 507–22. Oxford: Oxford University Press.

Parsons, T., & Bales, R. F. (1955) *Family, socialization and interaction process*. Glencoe, IL: Free Press.

Paul, G. (1986) Strategy of outcome research in psychotherapy. *Journal of Consulting Psychology* 31: 109–18.

Paykel, E., & Herbert, K. (1989) *Depression: an integrated approach*. London: Butterworth.

Pedder, J. (1979) Transitional space in psychotherapy and theatre. *British Journal of Medical Psychology* 52: 377–84.

Pedder, J. (1989) How can psychotherapists influence psychiatry? *Psychoanalytic Psychotherapy* 4: 43–54.

Pedder, J. (2010) *Attachment and new beginnings*, ed. G. Winship. London: Karnac Books.

Piaget, J. (1954) *The child's construction of reality*. London: Routledge & Kegan Paul.

Pickett, K., & Wilkinson, R. (2010) Inequality: an underacknowledged source of mental illness and distress. *British Journal of Psychiatry* 197: 426–9.

Piper, W. E., Ogrodniczuk, J. S., Joyce, A. S., McCallum, M., Rosie, J. S., O'Kelly, J. G., et al. (1999) Prediction of dropping out in time-limited, interpretive individual psychotherapy. *Psychotherapy* 36: 114–22.

Polan, H., & Hofer, M. (2008) Psychological origins of infant attachment and its role in development. In J. Cassidy & P. Shaver (eds), *Handbook of attachment*, pp. 158–72. 2nd ed., New York: Guilford Press.

Power, M. (2002) Integrative therapy from a cognitive-behavioural perspective. In J. Holmes & A. Bateman (eds), *Integration in psychotherapy*, pp. 27–48. Oxford: Oxford University Press.

Racker, H. (1968) *Transference and counter-transference*. London: Hogarth Press; repr. London: Karnac Books, 1982.

Renn, P. (2012) *The silent past and the invisible present*. London: Routledge.

Risch, N., Herrell, R., Lehner, T., Liang, K. Y., Eaves, L., Hoh, J., et al. (2009) Interaction between the serotonin transporter gene (5-HTTLPR), stressful life events, and risk of depression: a meta-analysis. *Journal of the American Medical Association* 301: 2462–71.

Rogers, C. (1951) *Client-centered therapy*. London: Constable.

Rollman-Branch, H. (1966) The first-born child, male. *International Journal of Psycho-analysis* 47: 404.

Rorty, R. (1989) *Contingency, irony, and solidarity*. Cambridge: Cambridge University Press.

Roth, A., & Fonagy, P. (2006) *What works for whom?* New York: Guilford Press.

Roth, P. (2001) *The superego*. Cambridge: Icon Books.

Rycroft, C. (1962) Beyond the reality principle. *International Journal of Psycho-analysis* 43: 388–94.

Rycroft, C. (1968) *Imagination and reality*. London: Hogarth Press.

Rycroft, C. (1972) *A critical dictionary of psychoanalysis*. London: Penguin.

Rycroft, C. (1979) *The innocence of dreams*. London: Tavistock.

Rycroft, C. (1985) *Psychoanalysis and beyond*. London: Chatto.

Rycroft, C. (1991) *Viewpoints*. London: Hogarth Press.

Ryle, A. (1990) *Cognitive analytic therapy*. Chichester: Wiley.

Safran, J., & Muran, J. (2000) *Negotiating the therapeutic alliance: a relational treatment guide*. New York: Guilford Press.

Sagan, C., Mack, J., Hehir, J., & Gould, S. (1986) *The long darkness: psychological and moral perspectives on nuclear winter*. New Haven, CT: Yale University Press.

Samuels, A., & Veale, D. (2009) Improving access to psychological therapies: for and against. *Psychodynamic Practice* 15: 41–56.

Sandell, R., Blomberg, J., Lazar, A., Carlsson, J., Broberg, J., & Rand, H. (2000) Varieties of long-term outcome among patients in psychoanalysis and long-term psychotherapy: a review of findings in the STOPP. *International Journal of Psycho-analysis* 81: 921–42.

Sandler, J. (1976) Countertransference and role responsiveness. *International Journal of Psycho-analysis* 3: 43–7.

Sandler, J., Dare, C., & Holder, A. (1973) *The patient and the analyst*. London: Allen & Unwin.

Sandler, J., & Rosenblatt, B. (1962) The concept of the representational world. *Psychoanalytic Study of the Child* 17: 128–45.

Schafer, R. (1976) *A new language for psychoanalysis*. New Haven, CT: Yale University Press.

Schore, A. (1994) *Affect regulation and the origin of the self: the neurobiology of emotional development*. Hove: Erlbaum.

Schore, A. (2003) *Affect regulation and the repair of the self*. New York: Norton.

Searles, H. (1965) *Collected papers on schizophrenia*. London: Hogarth Press.

Segal, H. (1987) Silence is the real crime. *International Review of Psycho-analysis* 14: 3–12.

Segraves, R. T. (1982) *Marital therapy*. New York: Plenum Press.

Shafer, R. (1960) The loving and beloved superego. *Psychoanalytic Study of the Child* 15: 163–88.

Shakespeare, W. (1974) Sonnet 111. In *Sonnets*. London: Nonesuch.

Shapiro, D. A. (1981) Comparative credibility of treatment rationales: three tests of expectancy theory. *British Journal of Clinical Psychology* 21: 111–22.

Shapiro, D. A., Barkham, M., Rees, A., Hardy, G. E., Reynolds, S., & Startup, M. (1994) Effects of treatment duration and severity of depression on the effectiveness of cognitive/behavioral and psychodynamic-interpersonal psychotherapy. *Journal of Consulting & Clinical Psychology* 62: 522–34.

Shapiro, D. A., & Firth-Cozens, J. (1987) Prescriptive v. exploratory psychotherapy: outcomes of the Sheffield Psychotherapy Project. *British Journal of Psychiatry* 151: 790–98.

Sharpe, E. (1937) *Dream analysis*. London: Hogarth Press.

Shaver, P., & Hazan, C. (eds) (2008) *Handbook of attachment*. 2nd ed., New York: Guilford Press.

Shaver, P., & Mikulincer, M. (2008) An overview of attachment theory. In J. Obegi & E. Berant (eds), *Clinical applications of adult psychotherapy and research*, pp. 17–45. New York: Guilford Press.

Shedler, J. (2010) The efficacy of psychodynamic psychotherapy. *American Psychologist* 65: 98–109.

Shepherd, M. (1984) What price psychotherapy? *British Medical Journal* 288: 809–10.

Simpson, J., & Belsky, J. (2008) Attachment theory within a modern evolutionary framework. In J. Cassidy & P. Shaver (eds), *Handbook of attachment*, pp. 131–57. 2nd ed., New York: Guilford Press.

Skynner, A. C. R. (1976) *One flesh: separate persons*. London: Constable.

Slade, A. (2005) Parental reflective functioning: an introduction. *Attachment and Human Development* 7: 269–82.

Slade, A. (2008) The implications of attachment theory and research for adult psychotherapy: research and clinical perspectives. In J. Cassidy & P. Shaver (eds), *Handbook of attachment*, pp. 762–82. 2nd ed., New York: Guilford Press.

Slade, A., & Holmes, J. (2013) *Attachment: collected papers* (6 vols). London: Sage.

Slater, P. (1961) Towards a dualistic theory of identification. *Merrill–Palmer Quarterly* 7: 113–21.

Snow, C. (1973) *The two cultures*. Cambridge: Cambridge University Press.

Steele, H. (2002) State of the art: attachment. *The Psychologist* 15: 518–28.

Steele, H., & Siefer, L. (2010) An attachment perspective on borderline personality disorder: advances in gene–environment considerations. *Current Psychiatry Reports* 12: 61–7.

Steiner, J. (2002) *Psychic retreats*. London: Routledge.

Stepansky, P. (2009) *Psychoanalysis at the margins*. New York: Other Press.

Stern, D. B. (1997) *Unformulated experience: from dissociation to imagination in psychoanalysis*. Hillsdale, NJ: Analytic Press.

Stern, D. B. (2010) *Partners in thought: working with unformulated experience, dissociation and enactment*. London: Routledge.

Stern, D. N. (1985) *The interpersonal world of the infant*. New York: Basic Books.

Stern, D. N. (2004) *The present moment in psychotherapy and everyday life.* New York: Norton.

Stern, D. N. (2010) *Forms of vitality: exploring dynamic experience in psychology, the arts, psychotherapy, and development.* New York: Oxford University Press.

Stern, D. N., Sander, L. W., Nahum, J. P., Harrison, A. M., Lyons-Ruth, K., Morgan, A. C., Bruschweiler-Stern, N., & Tronick, E. Z. (1998) Non-interpretive mechanisms in psychoanalytic therapy: the 'something more' than interpretation. *International Journal of Psycho-analysis* 79: 903–21.

Stevens, A. (2001) Anthony Storr obituary, *The Guardian*, 21 March.

Stiles, W., & Shapiro, D. (1989) Abuse of the drug metaphor in psychotherapy process-outcome research. *Clinical Psychology Review* 9: 521–43.

Stiles, W., Shapiro, D., & Firth-Cozens, J. (1988) Verbal response mode in contrasting psychotherapies. *Journal of Consulting and Clinical Psychology* 56: 727–33.

Stoller, R. (1984) Psychiatry's mind–brain dialectic, or the Mona Lisa has no eyebrows. *American Journal of Psychiatry* 141: 554–8.

Storr, A. (1960) *The integrity of the personality.* London: Heinemann.

Storr, A. (1968a) *Sexual deviation.* London: Penguin.

Storr, A. (1968b) *Human aggression.* London: Penguin.

Storr, A. (1972) *The dynamics of creation.* London: Secker & Warburg.

Storr, A. (1973) *Jung.* London: Fontana.

Storr, A. (1988) *Solitude.* New York: Free Press.

Storr, A. (1989) *Freud.* Oxford: Oxford University Press.

Storr, A. (1992) *Music and the mind.* New York: Ballantine.

Storr, A. (1997) *Feet of clay.* London: HarperCollins.

Strachey, J. (1934) The nature of the therapeutic action of psychoanalysis. *International Journal of Psycho-analysis* 18: 139–45.

Strenger, C. (2013) Why psychoanalysis must not discard science and human nature. *Psychoaanlytic Dialogues* 23: 197–210.

Sturge, C. (1977) Personal communication.

Sullivan, H. S. (1954) *The interpersonal theory of psychiatry.* New York: Norton.

Sutton-Smith, B., & Rosenberg, B. G. (1971) *The sibling.* New York: Holt, Rinehart & Winston.

Symington, N. (1983) The analyst's act of freedom as an agent of therapeutic change. *International Journal of Psycho-analysis* 64: 283–91.

Taylor, D. (2009) Consenting to be robbed so as not to be murdered. *Psychoanalytic Psychotherapy* 23: 263–75.

Thomä, H., & Kächele, H. (1986) *Psychoanalytic practice.* London: Springer.

Tillich, P. (1952) *The courage to be.* London: Nisbet.

Timpanaro, S. (1976) *The Freudian slip: psychoanalysis and textual criticism.* London: Verso.

Trevarthen, C. (1984) Emotions in infancy. In K. Scherer & P. Ekman (eds.), *Approaches to emotion*, pp. 293–310. Hove: Erlbaum.

Tronick, E. (1998) Dyadically expanded states of consciousness and the process of therapeutic change. *Infant Mental Health Journal* 19: 290–99.

Tuckett, D., Basile, R., Birkstead-Breen, D., et al. (2008) *Psychoanalysis comparable and incomparable.* London: Routledge.

Vaillant, G. (1977) *Adaptation to life.* Boston: Little, Brown.

Waldrop, M. F. (1965) Effects of family size and density on newborn characteristics. *American Journal of Orthopsychiatry* 35: 342–3.

Wallace, E. (1989) The philosophy of psychiatry. *Current Science* 2: 667–75.

Wallerstein, R. (1989) Psychoanalysis and psychotherapy: an historical perspective. *International Journal of Psycho-analysis* 70: 563–91.

Wampold, B. (2001) *The great psychotherapy debate.* New York: Erlbaum.

Wang, L., et al. (2008) Prefrontal mechanisms for executive control over emotional distraction are altered in major depression. *Psychiatry Research* 163: 143–55.

Warren, J. R. (1966) Birth order and social behaviour. *Psychological Bulletin* 65: 38–49.

Watson, P., & Andrews, P. (2002) Towards a revised evolutionary adaptionist analysis of depression: the social navigation hypothesis. *Journal of Affective Disorders* 72: 1–14.

Watts, A. (1961) *Psychotherapy East and West*. New York: Random House.

Watzlawick, P., Beavin, J., & Jackson, D. (1967) *Pragmatics of human communication*. New York: Norton.

Weaver, I. C., Champagne, F. A., Brown, S. E., Dymov, S., Sharma, S., Meaney, M. J., *et al.* (2005) Reversal of maternal programming of stress responses in adult offspring through methyl supplementation: altering epigenetic marking later in life. *Journal of Neuroscience* 25: 11045–54.

Westen, D. (2005) Implications of research in cognitive neuroscience for psychodynamic psychotherapy. In G. Gabbard, J. Beck, & J. Holmes (eds), *Oxford textbook of psychotherapy*, pp. 443–8. Oxford: Oxford University Press.

Wilkinson R. (2006) *Unhealthy societies: the afflictions of inequality*. London: Routledge.

Will, D. (1984) The progeny of positivism: the Maudsley school and anti-psychiatry. *British Journal of Psychotherapy* 1: 50–67.

Wing, J., & Brown, G. (1970) *Institutionalism and schizophrenia*. Cambridge: Cambridge University Press.

Winnicott, D. W. (1971) *Playing and reality*. London: Penguin.

Winnicott, D. W. (1972) *The maturational processes and the facilitating environment*. London: Hogarth Press.

Wittgenstein, L. (1958) *Philosophical investigations*. Oxford: Oxford University Press.

Wolff, H. H. (1972) Psychotherapy: its place in psychosomatic management. *Psychotherapy Psychosomatics* 22: 223–39.

Wright, K. (1991) *Vision and separation*. London: Free Association Books.

Young, J. (1990) *Cognitive therapy for personality disorders: a schema-focused approach*. Sarasota, FL: Professional Resource Exchange.

Zeki, S. (2009) *The splendours and mysteries of the brain*. Chichester: Wiley-Blackwell.

Žižek, S. (2006) *How to read Lacan*. London: Granta.

Zobel, I., Kech, S., van Calker, D., Dykierek, P., Berger, M., Schneibel, R., & Schramm, E. (2011) Long-term effect of combined interpersonal therapy and pharmacotherapy in a randomized trial of depressed patients. *Acta Psychiatrica Scandinavica* 123: 276–82.

INDEX